Assessment Methodology in Orthopaedics

Assessment Methodology in Orthopaedics

Edited by:

PB Pynsent PhD
Director of Research, Research and Training Centre, Royal
Orthopaedic Hospital NHS Trust, Birmingham, UK

JCT Fairbank MD FRCS
Consultant Orthopaedic Surgeon, Nuffield Orthopaedic Centre,
Headington, Oxford, UK

AJ Carr ChM FRCS
Consultant Orthopaedic Surgeon, Nuffield Orthopaedic Centre,
Headington, Oxford, UK

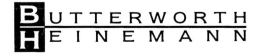

Butterworth-Heinemann
Linacre House, Jordan Hill, Oxford OX2 8DP
A division of Reed Educational and Professional Publishing Ltd

℞ A member of the Reed Elsevier plc group

OXFORD   BOSTON   JOHANNESBURG
MELBOURNE   NEW DELHI   SINGAPORE

First published 1997

British Library Cataloguing in Publication Data

A catalogue record for this book is available from the British Library

Library of Congress Cataloguing in Publication Data

A catalogue record for this book is available from the Library of Congress

ISBN 0 7506 2214 8

Typeset by E & M Graphics, Midsomer Norton, Bath
Printed and bound by Hartnolls Ltd, Bodmin, Cornwall

Contents

List of contributors

P Alderson BA PhD
Senior Research Officer, Social Science Research Unit, Institute of Education, University of London, London

EN Biden DPhil
Director, Institute of Biomedical Engineering, University of New Brunswick, Canada

R Brooks BA MSc
Senior Lecturer, Department of Economics, University of Strathclyde, Glasgow

M Burton BA(Hons.) MCSP
Lecturer in Physiotherapy, Royal Hallamshire Hospital, University of Sheffield, Sheffield

RG Burwell BSc MD FRCS
Emeritus Professor in Human Morphology and Experimental Orthopaedics, formerly Honorary Consulting Orthopaedic Surgeon, Department of Human Morphology, The Queen's Medical Centre, Nottingham

LA Cox BSc PhD CBiol MIBiol
Institute of Child Health, University College, London

JCT Fairbank MD FRCS
Consulting Orthopaedic Surgeon, Nuffield Orthopaedic Centre, Oxford

JA Finnegan MB FRCP
Consulting Clinical Neurophysiologist, Queen Elizabeth Hospital, Birmingham

R Fitzpatrick BA MSc PhD
Fellow, Nuffield College Oxford; Professor, Department of Public Health and Primary Care, University of Oxford, Oxford

HS Gill BEng DPhil
Oxford Orthopaedic Engineering Centre, University of Oxford, Nuffield Orthopaedic Centre, Oxford

AC Macey FRCS(Orth)
Consulting Orthopaedic Surgeon, Sligo General Hospital, Sligo, Ireland

PF McCombe FRACS
Consulting Orthopaedic Surgeon, Watkins Medical Centre, Brisbane, Australia

A Milne DCR DMS
Specialist in Trauma, Orthopaedic and Sports Injury Radiography, Northern General Hospital, Sheffield

RW Morris BSc MSc PhD
Senior Lecturer in Medical Statistics, Department of Primary Care and Population Sciences, The Royal Free Hospital School of Medicine, London

DW Murray MD FRCS
Consulting Orthopaedic Surgeon, Nuffield Orthopaedic Centre, Oxford

JJ O'Connor BE MA PhD
Research Director, Nuffield Orthopaedic Engineering Centre, Nuffield Orthopaedic Centre, Oxford

DP O'Doherty MD FRCS(Ed)
Consulting Orthopaedic Surgeon, Cardiff Royal Infirmary, Cardiff

JF Orr BSc PhD C.Eng MIMechE
Department of Mechanical and Manufacturing Engineering, The Queen's University of Belfast, Belfast

MA Preece
Professor of Child Health and Growth, University College, London

IC Revie
Department of Mechanical and Manufacturing Engineering, The Queen's University of Belfast, Belfast

M Saleh MB ChB MSc FRCS
Professor of Orthopaedic and Traumatic Surgery, Northern General Hospital, Sheffield

M Sims RGN
Clinical Nurse Specialist, Limb Reconstruction Service, Northern General Hospital, Sheffield

R Smith MD PhD FRCP
Consulting Physician in Metabolic Diseases, Nuffield Orthopaedic Centre, Oxford

R Tattersall
Northern General Hospital, Sheffield

TN Theologis MD MSc
Clinical Fellow in Orthopaedic Surgery, Nuffield Orthopaedic Centre, Oxford

Preface

Clinical research and clinical audit have been practised by orthopaedic surgeons for years. We found in our clinical practice that many of the available methods of assessment were unsatisfactory and that, although many measures had been proposed, it was not always easy to find them. When we did find them, they often lacked a proper validation and there was no guidance available to select the best for the task.

In the first two volumes in this series we have set out the methods and problems of measuring outcome both in orthopaedic surgery and trauma. As the writing of the latter volumes progressed, it became evident that the researcher into outcome must have an armamentarium of special skills. Hence the birth of this volume that seeks to set out some of the methods required and their associated errors. A knowledge of these is necessary not only to develop the instruments of outcome measurement but also to apply them with intelligence. Once again, we found this knowledge widely scattered. In contrast to the earlier books, which were largely written by authors at the end of their orthopaedic training, we have sought more senior authors for this book. This has meant that we have had to bully our contributors more vigorously to obtain our copy; in one or two cases we have had to forego including contributions which never appeared.

We are very grateful to all our contributors, some of whom have rewritten sections at our request. We apologise for the omission of chapters on measurement of images, clinical trials and medical history taking.[1]

We are very grateful to Ann Weaver for all the hard work she has put into this volume, which could not have appeared without her contribution.

---

[1] For readers with an interest in the methods and science of medical history, the subject is discussed at length in *The Medical Interview*, edited by M Lipkin, S M Putnam and A Lazare, Springer-Verlag, New York (1995). Although the volume does not deal with direct computer interviewing of the patient, this is an area in which we have a special interest.

Chapter 1

Assessing the reliability of clinical measurement

RW Morris

Introduction

Measurement in clinical practice and research must necessarily address the question of accuracy of the measure. An example is the comparison of leg alignment in two radiographs from a single patient taken before and after a knee replacement operation. Apparent changes may be due to (i) a real change in the patient's leg alignment, or (ii) an inaccurate measurement technique. The general problem was reviewed by Wright and Feinstein (1992), who named three sources of variability: the patient, the procedure and the clinician. They gave some practical hints on how to reduce these sources of variability in routine clinical measurement. Accepting, however, that such sources of variability will persist, studies should be undertaken to quantify this variability. In this way, from the example above, the surgeon will be better equipped to decide whether a patient's knee alignment has really changed since the operation. Similarly, the researcher seeking to compare the outcome between two groups of patients treated differently will need to know how reliably the outcome variable has been measured.

Confusion arises between a number of terms used in connection with the issue of measurement accuracy. Perhaps the two which are best known and agreed upon are *validity* and *reliability* (Fitzpatrick, 1993). Validity relates to whether the measurement procedure really measures what it purports to measure. Reliability concerns the ability of a measure 'to yield the same results on repeated trials under the same conditions' (Cox *et al.,* 1992). Thus a measurement which is not perfectly reliable cannot be perfectly valid. Other terms are sometimes used instead of reliability, but have arisen in particular contexts. *Reproducibility* tends to be concerned with the variation of a clinical measurement in the hands of different observers, or the same observer repeating the measurement (British Standards Institution, 1979). *Repeatability* often relates to comparing answers from patients on repeated administrations of a questionnaire (Chinn and Burney, 1987). *Agreement* was described by Bland and Altman (1986) when comparing two different methods for measuring the same variable. The term reliability seems to act as an umbrella term for all these applications.

When evaluating a new clinical measurement, it is in fact quite hard to find a gold standard. Some techniques may seem to be more precise than others, but perfect precision is an unattainable ideal. Some statistics such as sensitivity and specificity require the assumption of a gold standard diagnosis, so that we then evaluate the *validity* of a new diagnostic procedure; in general, we concentrate on assessing just how well two methods agree with one another. The majority of this chapter will be concerned with various facets of reliability rather than validity.

Handling different types of variable

The statistics required to quantify reliability depend on the type of variable being measured. The diagram below attempts to classify the data types for the purpose of this chapter, although different classifications could be offered. The diagram also points to the relevant sections of the chapter concerned with specific types of variable.

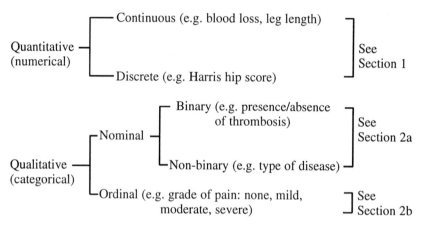

From the examples given above, it may be noted that *ordinal* and *discrete* variables differ only in the number of categories. A Harris hip score is, arguably, an ordinal variable with 101 categories (0,1,2,3,4,... 99,100). If the number of categories exceeds 10, such a variable may be safely regarded as discrete and thus amenable to statistical techniques described in Section 1 . If the number of categories is below five, the variable is ordinal and the techniques of Section 2b are required. Ordinal variables with five to 10 categories are harder to judge but are probably better regarded as discrete as far as quantifying their reliability is concerned.

1 Quantitative (numerical) variables

(a) Comparing methods of measurement

This section will summarise the approach of Bland and Altman (1986); readers requiring more detail would be well advised to consult their paper.

Application
Two methods of measuring the same variable may be compared when neither method can be regarded as perfect. The variable concerned will be quantitative,

either continuous or discrete. As an example, artificial data have been generated on two methods of measuring leg length inequality (a continuous quantitative variable); by ultrasound and by radiography. The data represent 20 subjects in whom leg length inequality ranges from 0 to 45 mm. Plausible differences between the two methods in measured leg length inequality have been based on the results of Terjesen *et al.* (1991).

Method

Figure 1.1 shows a scatter plot of leg length inequality for the 20 subjects according to the two measurement techniques. The graph appears to show good agreement. This apparent agreement would be spuriously enhanced if a regression line were fitted. A better approach would be to draw the line of identity; this is the line on to which all the points would have fallen had there been perfect agreement.

While Figure 1.1 is helpful, much of the graph consists of empty space. Bland and Altman (1986) recommend plotting the difference between the two variables against their average, for each of the subjects in the sample. In addition the mean of the differences and the 95% limits of agreement (i.e. Mean difference between methods $\pm$ 2 $\times$ standard deviation of differences)[1] are calculated. The values of the mean difference and the limits of agreement are then drawn as horizontal lines from the y axis so that variability and trends can easily be observed.

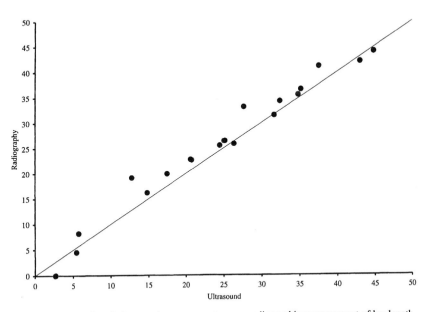

Figure 1.1 Scatterplot of ultrasound measurement versus radiographic measurement of leg length inequality (simulated data)

[1] The use of 2 as a multiplier for the standard deviation of the differences is a very adequate approximation, though 1.96 is recommended by Bland and Altman (1986) as technically more correct.

Worked example

This manoeuvre has been carried out for the data in Figure 1.1 and the result is shown in Figure 1.2. If the ultrasound and radiographic techniques had agreed perfectly in every case, the data points would lie along a horizontal line (parallel to the *x* axis) where the difference (shown on the *y* axis) equals 0. Points above this line represent cases when the ultrasound values are higher than the radiographic ones, and points below the line represent cases where ultrasound values are lower. Some differences are quite substantial; in one case ultrasound leads to values 6 mm lower than radiography. The mean difference is −1.387 mm, the standard deviation is 2.166 mm, so the 95% limits of agreement are −5.719 to +2.945 mm (shown in Figure 1.2).

The study of Terjesen *et al.,* which referred to 45 patients (as opposed to the artificial data generated here), quoted 95% limits of agreement of −9.1 to +5.3 mm. So in such a patient population, we predict that for 95% of subjects, the ultrasound measures will be anything between 9.1 mm lower and 5.3 mm higher than the radiographic measures. A difference of 9.1 mm may be large enough to be of concern. In most cases the differences between the two measurements will be smaller than this, but in 5% of cases the differences will lie outside even these limits.

Discussion

The above method is basically a simple graphical display and the limits of agreement formalise what the graph already shows. Investigators who produce a graph such as Figure 1.2 are often disconcerted when they realise how poor the agreement between two measuring techniques can be. Figure 1.1 is liable to produce a false sense of optimism concerning the degree of agreement. Such a

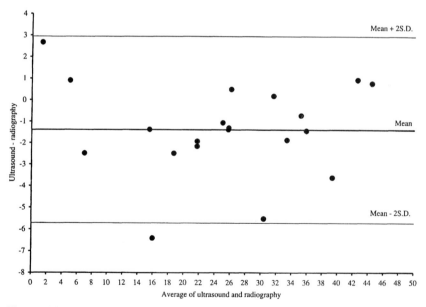

Figure 1.2 Scatterplot of difference in measurements (ultrasound - radiographic) versus average for data shown in Figure 1.1

false sense is reinforced by the spurious use of correlation, which is completely inappropriate in this context.

The data shown in Figure 1.1 have a correlation of 0.984. Many medical researchers have found r values exceeding 0.9 for this type of data and have incorrectly concluded that the methods agreed well with each other. There are several reasons why such a conclusion is misleading.

- We should really only declare perfect agreement if the points in Figure 1.1 lay on the line of identity. However, $r = 1$ could be obtained if the points lay on any other straight line.
- The higher the range of the variable being measured, the greater the correlation that will be obtained. The correlation for those values obtained for radiographic values less than 20 mm was 0.954, while for those obtained for radiographic values greater than 20 mm it was 0.974. Clearly it would be absurd to argue that agreement is poorer for both low *and* high radiographic values than it is over the whole spectrum of values.
- The worst possible error is to quote the P value for the correlation coefficient. This would be less than 0.001 for the data in Figure 1.1. Many computer programmes will provide a P value by default. This only tests the null hypothesis that the quantities produced by the two measuring techniques are completely unrelated. Obviously we would not evaluate the ultrasound against radiography if we seriously thought there may be no relationship between the two.

Another analysis which could be carried out is a paired t-test. This seems plausible, because each subject produces a value for each measurement technique. On average the ultrasound values in Figure 1.1 are 1.387 mm lower than the radiographic values. The standard deviation of the differences is 2.166 mm, and with a sample size of 20, the paired t-test gives a P value of 0.0099. This is a significant difference, showing that ultrasound values tend to be consistently lower than radiographic values. Again, this moderately useful information could have been guessed by noting that more of the data points in Figure 1.2 are below the zero line than are above it. However care must be taken if a paired t-test does not show a significant difference. A non-significant difference does *not* indicate that the methods agree. There may be a good deal of non-systematic variation which goes in no consistent direction. It is far more important to quantify this unsystematic variation, which will typically be larger and more important than any systematic variation.

If two methods of measurement do not agree with one another, it is quite possible that one or both of the methods are not sufficiently reliable. This brings us to a slightly different statistical issue.

(b) Observer variation

Application
Quantitative (either continuous or discrete) variables are again under consideration. The same value may not be obtained by two different observers, nor even by the same observer making the measurement twice or more. Information on how well two ultrasound measurements of leg length inequality under the same conditions agree with each other may have helped us understand why the ultrasound measures did not agree with the radiographic measures.

Terjesen *et al.* also compared the results from two observers using ultra-sonography.

The best studies will investigate both *inter* (between) and *intra* (within) observer variation. Conboy *et al.* (1996) studied 25 patients from a shoulder clinic, suffering dislocator syndrome ($n = 5$), impingement syndrome ($n = 15$) or arthritis ($n = 5$). These were assessed by three different observers using the Constant–Murley score which takes values from 0 to 100 and is based on pain, activity level, positioning, flexion, abduction, internal and external rotation, and power. In addition, three patients were selected to be assessed by each of the three observers on three separate occasions. The three subjects included one with dislocator syndrome, one with impingement syndrome and one with arthritis.

Quantifying the inter-observer variation will first be considered. Analysis shown here will be based on the total score rather than its components.

Method
Had only two observers taken part, the difference between them could have been plotted against the mean for the 25 subjects, in a similar way to the Bland and Altman (1986) plot shown for the previous data set. There would have been no purpose on this occasion in calculating the mean difference, or the 95% limits of agreement. While we may be interested to know whether one method of measurement tends to give consistently higher readings than the other, we are not interested in this for comparing two observers' readings. The two observers are of no particular interest in themselves; they are meant to represent the population of all possible orthopaedic surgeons who might attempt to assess the Constant–Murley score for shoulder patients. Instead we wish to calculate the inter-observer standard deviation.

The same principle applies in the present data set. Instead of plotting the difference against the mean, we calculate for each of the subjects, the mean and the standard deviation of the observers' readings. A plot of the standard deviation against the mean is carried out.

To be more formal, we could square all the standard deviations to obtain a set of variances. The average of these variances could be calculated, and the square root taken to give the inter-observer standard deviation. If s is this standard deviation, we may say with 95% confidence that the largest difference likely to occur between a single observation by a randomly chosen observer and the subject's true value is $2 \times s$.

The same technique could be applied to quantify the intra-observer variation, when each observer makes more than one reading per subject. Finally, when we have data on inter- and intra-observer variation, it is possible to disentangle the effects of the two.

Worked example
The mean and standard deviation of the three observers' readings for each of the 25 subjects may be plotted as shown in Figure 1.3. Some standard deviations are quite small (indicating good agreement for those particular subjects), whereas others are substantial. The largest standard deviation occurs for the individual with the lowest mean score (scores of 0, 30 and 0 for the three observers).

We will need to calculate an overall standard deviation for all the subjects. Squaring each of the 25 standard deviations, and averaging them gives an inter-observer variance of 78.5. The square root of this gives the inter-observer

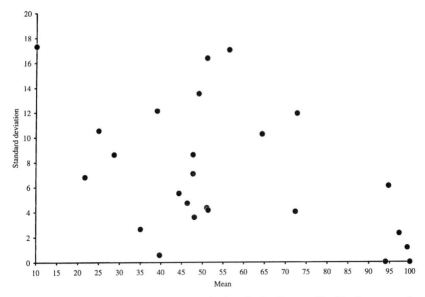

Figure 1.3 Standard deviation of three observers' values for the Constant Shoulder Score on each of 25 subjects, plotted against the mean for the subjects

standard deviation, 8.86. The largest difference likely to occur between a single observation by a randomly chosen observer and the subject's true value is thus $2 \times s_r = 17.7$ points on the Constant–Murley scale. This is rather large and thus a single observation may be unreliable.

The inter-observer variance may be obtained directly from a statistical package by carrying out a one-way analysis of variance, where subjects form the grouping factor. The 'within groups mean square', sometimes known as the 'residual mean square' is the quantity required. Brown and Swanson Beck (1994) provide details on the use of suitable packages.

As mentioned above, three subjects were measured by three observers on three occasions each. Taking each observer's trio of observations on the three subjects gives nine data trios on which intra-observer variability may be quantified. Once again, a graph analogous to Figure 1.3 can be produced (Figure 1.4). The standard deviation appears greater for lower average scores (i.e. for the arthritis subject). Little intra-observer variability is evident for those average scores close to 100 (i.e. for the subject with dislocator syndrome). An informal comparison of Figures 1.3 and 1.4 suggests that intra-observer variability is less than inter-observer variability but is still substantial. If the same manoeuvre is carried out on the data in Figure 1.4 as was done for Figure 1.3, we find that the intra-observer variance is 64.4 and thus the intra-observer standard deviation is 8.02. This is almost as large as the intra-subject standard deviation calculated above.

The first study, in which three observers took a single reading on each of 25 subjects, allowed us to estimate inter-observer variation. One subject obtained scores of 0, 30 and 0 for the three observers. However, part of the reason for the second, the observer's apparent deviation from the others, may have been the observer's own *intra*-observer variation. Had the assessment by the second

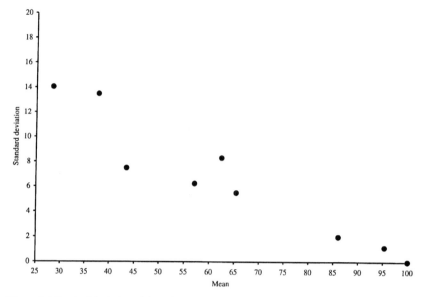

Figure 1.4 Standard deviation of three Constant Score readings taken by three different observers on three different subjects, plotted against the mean

observer been repeated on that particular subject, a score closer to 0 may have been obtained. In fact,

Apparent inter-observer variance = True inter-observer variance + Intra-observer variance.

From the second study, we have estimated intra-observer variance as 64.4. From the first study apparent inter-observer variance was 78.5. Thus the true inter-observer variance is estimated as only 14.1. Most of the apparent variation between observers may thus be attributed to variation of observers within themselves.

It is of clinical interest to know how important such variations are. We need to consider how much variation we could expect due to measurement error (whether inter-observer, intra-observer or a combination of the two) when a patient makes a return visit for a repeat assessment.

1. If a patient is seen on two visits by different observers, then the sum of inter-observer and intra-observer variance is required. This was 78.5, giving a standard deviation of 8.86. The maximum difference likely to occur according to the British Standards Institution (the *coefficient of reproducibility*) and recommended by Bland and Altman (1986), is $2.83 \times 8.86 = 25.1$. Thus unless a difference exceeds 25 points, we cannot be confident that the change is real.
2. If a patient is seen on two visits by the same observer, the intra-observer variance is required (64.4). Again, taking the square root to gain the standard deviation, and multiplying by 2.83, we get 22.7. So even in this situation, a patient will need to change his/her score by at least 23 points before we may attribute the change to anything beyond measurement error. There seems no

great point in insisting on the same observer assessing the patient on the two visits.

3. If it was practical for an observer to make two assessments of the patient at each visit, the average obtained on each visit may be more reliable. The expected variance would then be halved, from 64.4 to 32.2. Taking the square root and multiplying by 2.83 now gives a required change in the average score on the two visits of at least 16.1 points.

Discussion

Since observers vary within themselves as well as between themselves, studies should involve repeated measurements by the same observer as well as by different observers. Each observer should do the same number of repeated measurements and the same observers should assess each patient.

It may be felt that such studies should involve a small number of subjects assessed by a large number of observers on a large number of occasions, because the observers seem to be the whole focus. In fact this would be a misconception. It is important that a wide spectrum of subjects should be included for study, to increase the representatives from the true population. As was seen above, intra-observer variation seemed less for the dislocator syndrome patient than the arthritis patient.

The implications of observer variability carry over into method comparison. For data on leg-length inequality, if researchers were able to repeat each radiographic measurement made, and similarly each ultrasound measurement, they could calculate the average of these repeated measurements made with each technique. The agreement between the two techniques may then have been closer. Bland and Altman's (1986) example of repeating measurements for two different peak flow meters on each of 17 subjects provide a good example of disentangling measurement error from actual differences between the two techniques.

The limits of agreement calculated for comparing two measuring techniques and the coefficient of reproducibility for assessing observer variation, both give values in the same units in which the variables were measured. For the data in Figure 1.1, the ultrasound method varied from the radiographic method by up to 5.719 mm, the coefficient of reproducibility of the Constant Score by a single observer is 23 points. This may be meaningful for orthopaedic surgeons used to working with the Constant Score but others may not know whether 23 points would represent a clinically important shift. Lee (1992) has argued that a statistic which quantifies reproducibility relative to the normal variation between subjects is desirable. He proposes the *intra-class correlation,* which is to be distinguished from the ordinary correlation coefficient.

In the example where 25 subjects were measured by three different observers (once each), it is possible to break the variance down into apparent inter-observer variance (already calculated above as 78.5) and inter-subject variance. The latter may be derived from the 'Between subject sum of squares' in the one-way analysis of variance. However, subjects appear to vary between themselves partly because of measurement error, so an adjustment has to be made (details shown in Armitage and Berry, 1987, pp. 198–200). It turns out that inter-subject variance is 624.6. If we add these two sources of variance (78.5 and 624.6), we discover that the latter is 89% of the total. Thus the intra-class correlation is 0.89, and we can say that 89% of the total variance seen is 'explained' by the variability between subjects.

2 Qualitative (categorical) variables

(a) Nominal variables

(i) Validity

Application
Nominal variables often consist of only two categories (i.e. binary values). Examples in orthopaedics are the presence/ absence, of a fracture, of a cruciate ligament tear, of a congenital dislocation of the hip, of a postoperative complication such as a deep vein thrombosis and so on. Diagnoses of such conditions range from a quick test that may cost little either financially or in patient discomfort, to an invasive and expensive piece of sophisticated technology. From most points of view, it would be preferable to use the 'quick and dirty' test if it can be proved to be reasonably accurate. For each patient, the quick method will have the verdict 'positive' or 'negative', while the gold standard will establish whether the condition of interest is truly 'present' or 'absent'.

Statistics relating to the agreement between two diagnostic tests where neither is regarded as the gold standard, will be considered later.

Method
If we regard 'Yes' and 'No' as establishing the definite presence or absence of a diagnosis according to a gold standard test, and 'Positive' and 'Negative' as being the results of a quick test, data may be displayed as in Table 1.1.

There are $(a + c)$ patients who have the condition, but only a of these are positive on the quick test, while c are missed by the test: there are thus c false negatives. We define

> *Sensitivity* = Number of individuals with condition who are positive to the test divided by the total number with the condition
> $$= \frac{a}{a + c}$$

There are also $(b + d)$ patients without this condition, of whom d are negative on the test, but b are 'false positives'. We define

> *Specificity* = Number of individuals without condition who are negative to the test divided by the total number without the condition
> $$= \frac{d}{b + d}$$

Both sensitivity and specificity are then usually multiplied by 100 to give the result as a percentage. If the test were perfect, they would both be 100%.

The clinician who has applied the quick test might find the positive and negative predictive values of more direct use. If a positive result has been obtained, how likely is it that the condition is really present? Similarly, if a

Table 1.1 Standard layout of data showing relationship between test result and presence or absence of a specific characteristic

| According to quick test | According to gold standard | | |
	Yes	No	Total
Positive	a	b	$a + b$
Negative	c	d	$c + d$
Total	$a + c$	$b + d$	

negative result has been obtained, how likely is it that the condition is absent? We have

Positive predictive value = Number of individuals with condition who are positive to the test divided by the total number with a positive test

$$= \frac{a}{a + b}$$

Negative predictive value = Number of individuals without condition who are negative to the test divided by the total number negative to the test

$$= \frac{d}{c + d}$$

Worked example

Magnetic resonance imaging (MRI) and arthroscopy were evaluated on 1014 patients with new knee conditions who needed more than clinical examination for diagnostic purposes (Fischer *et al.,* 1991). Arthroscopy was seen as the 'gold standard'. Table 1.2 shows the results of diagnoses of a tear of the medial meniscus. Altogether 473 cases of meniscal tear were found by arthroscopy, but only 440 of these were detected by MRI. Thus the sensitivity of MRI is 440/473 = 93%. Arthroscopy demonstrated that 438 subjects did not have a meniscal tear but MRI only classed 367 of these as negative. Thus the specificity of MRI was 367/438 = 84%.

It may be more useful to a clinician to know the probability of a meniscal tear if the result of the MRI scan is positive. In the above data, 511 patients had a positive MRI result, but only 440 of these really had a meniscal tear according to arthroscopy. Thus the PPV is 440/511 = 86%. Similarly the negative predictive value is 367/400 = 92%.

Table 1.2 Relationship between diagnosis of medial meniscal tear on arthroscopy and MRI (Fischer *et al.,* 1991)

| According to MRI | According to arthroscopy | | |
	Yes	No	Total
Positive	440	71	511
Negative	33	367	400
Total	473	438	911

Discussion

It is important not to be confused between sensitivity and PPV. Sensitivity is expressed as a proportion of those who really have the condition, whereas PPV is expressed as a proportion of those with a positive test. The same sort of confusion is possible between specificity and NPV.

Although PPV is an intuitively appealing quantity, it can be misleading. The type of data shown in Table 1.2 refer to a patient group who were *a priori* at high risk of a medial meniscal tear. Had the MRI technology been applied to a wider spectrum of patients reporting new knee conditions, the sensitivity and specificity of the test would have been the same, since these quantities refer to fixed properties of the test. However, the PPV would have been much lower. In the data shown in Table 1.2, the true prevalence of a medial meniscal tear (according to arthroscopy) was 473/911 = 52%. If the test were applied in a population where the true prevalence was as low as 10%, the PPV would be only 39%.

In general, PPVs decrease with the true prevalence of the condition, however good the sensitivity and specificity happen to be. This fact has led to debate about the usefulness of screening neonates for congenital dislocation of the hip. However accurate ultrasound may be (in terms of a high sensitivity and specificity), the PPV would be very low if it was applied to every baby. In other words, the vast majority of those deemed positive by ultrasound would not have CDH requiring surgical treatment. The PPV would improve if we were to apply the screening only to a high risk group, in the manner reported by Clarke *et al.* (1989). However, the cost here is that some babies in a low risk group who actually have CDH will be missed and will present late.

The quantities' sensitivity and specificity, PPV and NPV, may be confusing, and a novel approach has been recommended by Sackett *et al.* (1991). They suggest that the diagnostic test should be defined in terms of its likelihood ratio (this equals sensitivity/(100 – specificity), if both are expressed as a percentage). Thus the likelihood ratio for the data in Table 1.2 is 93/(100 – 84) = 5.8. Thus the odds of a true medial meniscal tear, if diagnosed by MRI, would increase 5.8 fold. Sackett *et al.* have published a user friendly nomogram to show how the results of a diagnostic test modify a patient's disease probability. Their book is rich with clinical examples of diagnostic reasoning, based on knowledge of the accuracy of a diagnostic test.

(ii) Reliability

Application

The above quantities (in particular sensitivity and specificity) are dependent on the existence of a gold standard against which another test may be compared. Although the notion of a gold standard will often be illusory, it is perhaps more acceptable since we are dealing with categorical variables rather than exact quantities. The gold standard itself needs to be reliable in order to have any claim of validity. This requires the need for indices of reliability.

Other examples in the literature where the reliability of a nominal variable has been tested include the classification of ankle fractures (Thomsen *et al.*, 1991) and the presence or absence of scaphoid fractures according to radiographs (Dias *et al.*, 1990). In both these applications, inter-observer and intra-observer variation were considered. Perhaps a more frequent application concerns the repeated use of a patient questionnaire to elicit symptoms and disabilities.

Method
If a binary variable is observed separately on two occasions, the agreement may be shown by arranging the data into a table (Table 1.3). It can be seen that for *a* subjects, the binary variable was recorded as 'yes' on both occasions, and for *d* subjects, 'no' was recorded on both occasions. In all, therefore, the proportion of subjects where there was agreement on the two occasions was $(a+d)/N$, which we shall call p_o. However, a number of subjects would have agreed just on the basis of chance: we would have expected $(a + b)\cdot(a + c)/N$ to have been recorded as 'yes' on both occasions, and $(b + d)\cdot(c + d)/N$ as 'no' on both occasions. The principle here is that we multiply together the appropriate row total by the appropriate column total, and divide by the grand total. We can define the expected proportion in agreement as

$$p_e = \frac{\dfrac{(a + b)(a + c)}{N} + \dfrac{(b + d)(c + d)}{N}}{N}$$

Cohen (1960) devised the *Kappa* statistic to measure the amount of agreement over and above what would be expected by chance. The Kappa statistic contrasts p_o and p_e as follows

$$Kappa = \frac{p_o - p_e}{1 - p_e}$$

A Kappa statistic has a maximum value of 1 for perfect agreement. A value of 0 denotes no more agreement than could be expected by chance, while negative Kappa values imply agreement is even worse than could be expected by chance. It is not intuitive to know whether given Kappa values are acceptable. As it happens, Landis and Koch (1977) suggested a series of arbitrary cut-off points to demarcate varying amounts of agreement, and suggested that Kappa values exceeding 0.8 represented almost perfect agreement. In a later publication Fleiss (1981) suggests that values equal to or greater that 0.75 represent good agreement whereas values below 0.4 represent poor agreement. Fleiss (1981) also shows how to derive confidence intervals for Kappa statistics.

Worked example
As part of a study to assess outcome of knee replacements, a postal questionnaire was sent to patients of nine different surgeons. The questionnaire consisted of items on functional activities and visual analogue scales to rate perceived success

Table 1.3 Standard layout of data showing relationship between observed values of binary variable on two occasions

1st occasion	2nd occasion		
	Yes	No	Total
Yes	a	b	a + b
No	c	d	c + d
Total	a + c	b + d	N

Table 1.4 Relationship between responses by the same subjects to a question on ability to bend knee, on the same questionnaire sent a second time 1 month after the first occasion

Response on 1st occasion	Response on 2nd occasion		Total
	Yes	No	
Yes	18	4	22
No	2	37	39
Total	20	41	61

of the operation. Some of the patients were asked to fill in the questionnaire twice, at monthly intervals, to test the reliability of their answers. In particular, one item asked was 'Are you able to bend this knee as much as you would wish?', and the possible answers were 'Yes' or 'No'. The data on responses to this question for 61 knees in 47 patients are given in Table 1.4 (full details supplied by Morris, 1993). Of the total of 61 enquiries, the same response on the two occasions was obtained in 55 cases, giving an agreement of 90.2%. Although this sounds impressive, there are a certain number of subjects who would agree just by chance even if there was no relationship between what subjects answered on the two occasions.

Altogether 22 subjects said they could bend their knee as much as they liked on the first occasion and 20 said so on the second occasion. The 'expected' number who just by chance would agree on the two occasions that they could bend their knee as much as they liked is $22 \times 20/61 = 7.2$. We can similarly compute the expected number who would agree on the two occasions that they could not bend their knee as much as they liked, as $41 \times 39/61 = 26.2$. In all the expected number of agreements is 33.4, compared with 55 observed agreements. So the expected proportion in agreement is $33.4/61 = 54.8\%$. Kappa is then

$$\frac{0.902 - 0.548}{1 - 0.548} = 0.78$$

This represents good agreement for the two occasions. However, the 95% confidence interval for Kappa is 0.62–0.95, suggesting the true agreement may be anything from moderate to nearly perfect.

Discussion
The use of the kappa statistic has been well expounded by Fleiss (1981). It may be extended to the case where the nominal variable has more than two categories. Thomsen *et al.* (1991) reported the classification of 94 ankle fractures, both by the Weber system (four categories allowed) and the Lauge Hansen system (14 possible categories). Fleiss also shows how Kappa may be calculated when the categorical item is assessed more than twice. This is useful for studies of inter-observer agreement, as in Thomsen *et al.*'s study where four observers were involved.

The simplest and most common situation involves two observations of a binary variable, as illustrated above. It can be shown, however, that kappa will depend on the prevalence of the condition being tested. In the table above, it would have been more difficult to achieve high Kappa had the proportion of subjects who could bend their knee as much as they liked been nearer to 0% or

100%. High Kappa is easiest to achieve when the yes/no balance of the variable is 50/50.

It has been recognised (Grant, 1991) that Kappa measures the *relative* amount of agreement for categorical variables. Just as the intra-class correlation coefficient measures relative agreement between two observers for a quantitative measure such as the Constant Shoulder Score, so Kappa measures relative agreement for categorical variables. Chinn and Burney (1987) have argued that just as there should be absolute measures of agreement for quantitative variables (such as the coefficient of reproducibility), so there should be absolute measures for categorical variables. They have devised a statistic known as the *average correct classification rate*. This is intuitively simpler to interpret than Kappa. For the data on ease of knee bending shown in Table 1.4, the average correct classification was 94.8%.

(b) Ordinal variables — reliability

Application
In attempting to categorise the existence of such aspects of human experience as pain or disability, a yes/no dichotomy is clearly inadequate and classifications such as none/ mild/ moderate/ severe are more common. Such variables are called *ordinal*. The agreement in responses between repeated administrations of a questionnaire is of interest when such variables are being measured.

Method
In essence, the Kappa statistic may be applied in this situation also, just as for binary variables. The same principle of comparing observed and expected agreements would apply again. A slight modification is required, however, in terms of the disagreements. We should attribute more serious disagreement to a respondent who reported 'no pain' and 'severe pain' respectively on successive administrations of a questionnaire than we would if the responses were 'no pain' and 'mild pain' on the two occasions. The concept of partial agreement becomes relevant here, and Fleiss (1981) has shown how disagreements of varying seriousness may be taken into account using the *weighted Kappa* statistic. Weighted Kappa may also take a range of values, with 1 representing perfect agreement among the sample of subjects tested and 0 representing agreement no better than chance. The quadratically weighted Kappa described by Fleiss is used in this example.

Weighted Kappa is less easily calculated by hand than the ordinary Kappa and suitable computer programmes are probably necessary.

Worked example
Data from the study of knee replacement patients (Morris, 1993) are again used. Here we consider the questionnaire item 'Can you dress yourself?' with possible responses being 'Not without someone's help', 'By myself with difficulty' and 'By myself without difficulty'. The data are displayed in Table 1.5. Forty-three patients out of 47 (91%) gave the same response on the two occasions; 21.5 subjects (46%) would have agreed just by chance, giving an ordinary Kappa value of 0.84.

The quadratically weighted Kappa requires that the seriousness of disagreement be equal to the square of the difference between the categories.

Table 1.5 Relationship between responses by the same subjects to a question on ease of dressing, on the same questionnaire sent a second time 1 month after the first occasion

| Response on 1st occasion | Response on 2nd occasion | | | |
	Need help	Difficult	Not difficult	Total
Need help	3	0	0	3
Difficult	0	15	1	16
Not difficult	1	2	25	28
Total	4	17	26	47

Thus in Table 1.5, those 43 subjects who agreed on the two occasions had a disagreement weighting of 0, the three who disagreed by one grade had a disagreement weighting of 1, while the one subject who disagreed by two grades had a disagreement weighting of 4. The resulting weighted Kappa statistic was 0.81, a slight (though trivial) deterioration on the 'ordinary' Kappa value. This is because out of four subjects who disagreed in their responses on the two occasions, one disagreed to a serious extent.

Discussion

If an ordinal variable with a small number of categories were regarded as quantitative (so the categories in the data in Table 1.5 would be assigned numerical values of 1, 2, 3), then the intra-class correlation coefficient referred to in Section 1 for quantitative variables bears a very close relationship to the quadratically weighted Kappa. The idea of weighting various types of disagreement in the above example thus seems attractive in theory. However, it is unlikely to make a vast difference to the Kappa value. If it does do so, it is probably because a small sample size is involved.

Kappa has become very popular in recent years for qualitative variables. Like correlation coefficients, it is a dimensionless statistic which is both its strength and its weakness. Its strength is that its values may be compared between studies but a Kappa value standing on its own does not have an intuitive interpretation. The simple proportion in agreement or the average correct classification of Chinn and Burney (1987) are perhaps stronger in this regard.

In Section 1, inter- and intra-observer components of variation were separated out for quantitative variables. Methods to do this for categorical variables involve more sophisticated algorithms, and one approach has been described by Baker *et al.* (1991). The general lessons learned from quantitative variables will be relevant; apparent variation between observers may well be due to variation within observers. Thus repeat measures by single observers will be the first step towards understanding measurement error in categorical variables.

Statistics thus obtained may not be easily gleaned from raw data. As in all statistical analyses, tables of data which give the reader a proper feel for the raw data may be more valuable than sophisticated methods.

Conclusion

Inaccurately measured variables may mislead clinicians into wrongly imputing a disease state to a particular patient, or wrongly assuming an improvement (or deterioration) in condition. For researchers concerned with trials comparing different treatments, their outcome variables may be subject to measurement error. If so, they will lose power to demonstrate true relative benefits of one treatment over another.

Studies need to be carried out to compare results from two techniques for measuring the same variable (especially if it is a variable frequently used for diagnosis and management), and to quantify inter- and intra-observer variation. Some common methods used to analyse data arising from such studies may be misleading. A number of possible approaches have been outlined here. Data presentation in graphical or tabular form may well be more helpful than summary statistics. The latter should not be presented without the former.

References

Altman DG, Bland JM (1983) Measurement in medicine: the analysis of method comparison studies. *The Statistician*; **32**: 307–317

Armitage P, Berry G (1987) *Statistical Methods in Medical Research*, 2nd edition. Oxford: Blackwell

Bland JM, Altman DG (1986) Statistical methods for assessing agreement between two methods of clinical measurement. *Lancet*; **i**: 307–310

Baker SG, Freedman LS, Parmar MKB (1991) Using replicate observations in observer agreement studies with binary assessments. *Biometrics*; **47**: 1327–1338

British Standards Institution (1979) *Precision of test methods I: Guide for the determination and reproducibility for a standard test method.* (BS5497, part I). BSI, London

Brown RA, Swanson Beck J (1994) *Medical Statistics on Personal Computers,* 2nd edition. London: BMJ

Chinn S, Burney PGJ (1987) On measuring repeatability of data from self-administered questionnaires. *Int. J. Epidemiol.*; **16**: 121–127

Clarke NMP, Clegg J, Al-Chalabi AN (1989) Ultrasound screening of hips at risk for CDH. *J. Bone Jt Surg.*; **71B**: 9–12

Cohen J (1960) A coefficient of agreement for nominal scales. *Educ. Psychol. Measurement*; **20**: 37–46

Conboy VB, Morris RW, Kiss J, Carr AJ (1996) An evaluation of the Constant–Murley shoulder assessment. *J. Bone Jt Surg.*; **78B**: 229–232

Cox DR, Fitzpatrick R, Fletcher AE, Gore SM, Spiegelhalter DJ, Jones DR (1992) Quality-of-life assessment: can we keep it simple? (with discussion). *J. R. Statist. Soc. A*; **155**: 353–393

Dias JJ, Thompson J, Baston NJ, Gregg PJ (1990) Suspected scaphoid fractures. The value of radiographs. *J. Bone Jt Surg.*; **72B**: 98–101

Fischer SP, Fox JM, Del Pizzo W, Friedman MJ, Snyder SJ, Ferkel RD (1991) Accuracy of diagnoses from magnetic resonance imaging of the knee. *J. Bone Jt Surg.* [Am.]; **73-A**: 2–9

Fitzpatrick R (1993) Patient satisfaction and quality of life measures. In:Pynsent PB, Fairbank JCT, Carr A (eds) *Outcome measures in orthopaedics.* Oxford: Butterworth-Heinemann

Fleiss JL (1981) *Statistical Methods for Rates and Proportions,* 2nd edition. New York: Wiley

Grant JM (1991) The fetal heart rate trace is normal, isn't it? *Lancet*; **337**: 215–218

Lee J (1992) Evaluating agreement between two methods for measuring the same quantity: a response. *Comput. Biol. Med.*; **22**: 369–371

Landis JR, Koch GG (1977) The measurement of observer agreement for categorical data. *Biometrics*; **33**: 159–174

Morris RW (1993) *Comparative Evaluation of Outcome of Knee Replacement Operations Using Alternative Knee Prostheses.* PhD thesis. London: University of London

Sackett DL, Haynes RB, Guyatt GH, Tugwell P (1991) *Clinical Epidemiology: a Basic Science for Clinical Medicine*, 2nd edition. Boston: Little, Brown and Company

Terjesen T, Benum P, Rossvoll I, Svenningsen S, Floystad Isern AE, Nordbo T (1991) Leg-length discrepancy measured by ultrasonography. *Acta Orthop. Scand.*; **62**: 121–124

Thomsen NOB, Overgaard S, Olsen LH, Hansen H, Nielsen ST (1991) Observer variation in the radiographic classification of ankle fractures. *J. Bone Jt Surg.*; **73B**: 676–678

Wright JG, Feinstein AR (1992) Improving the reliability of orthopaedic measurements. *J. Bone Joint Surg.*; **74B**: 287–291

Chapter 2

Survival analysis

DW Murray

Introduction

This chapter describes how survival analysis can be used to assess the outcome of orthopaedic procedures. It also describes how survival rates for different procedures or different groups of patients can be compared. It is intended to enable orthopaedic surgeons without statistical training to use survival analysis, or when such analyses are presented, to appreciate them more critically.

The analysis

Survival analysis is a statistical technique that is used to determine the survival rate or failure rate of a particular procedure after a series of different time intervals. Although it is usually used for joint replacement, it can be used for many other procedures. It is particularly useful as patients can be followed up for different lengths of time, allowing patients to enter and be withdrawn from a trial at any stage and for whatever reason. For the analysis it is assumed that all patients received their operation simultaneously. The chance of the implant surviving for a particular length of time is then calculated. Any definition of failure can be used, although in joint replacement analysis, revision is usually considered to be the end point. A number of different end points can be analysed separately. Survival analysis does not assess pain or function unless they are included in the definition of failure.

Survival analysis can be undertaken with a life table or by the product limit method (Armitage and Berry, 1987). The life table was first used by the astronomer Edmund Halley (1656–1742) and is the most commonly used method in orthopaedics. It was first used in orthopaedics by Dobbs in 1980. With the life table method the survival rate is usually calculated at regular intervals. This is in contrast to the product limit method, described by Kaplan and Meier, where the survival rate is calculated every time a failure occurs (Kaplan and Meier, 1958). There are advantages and disadvantages of both methods. Both are suitable for graphical representation. With the product limit method, because of the frequent recalculations, a table cannot be constructed. A table is an advantage, as it can include details of the number of joints followed, the number of failures and the number lost to follow-up. Another advantage of the life table method is that confidence limits can be determined and displayed more readily.

The theoretical advantages of the product limit method are first that the arbitrary choice of time intervals is avoided and secondly, that it is more accurate as the survival rate may change during the intervals. However, in orthopaedics these are not real advantages as patients are usually reviewed annually. In the subsequent discussion only the life table method will be considered.

Before undertaking a survival analysis, the definition of failure, the starting date, the finishing date, the entry criteria and the assessment interval must be determined. For all patients in the trial the length of follow-up during the trial and the outcome is determined. The patients are sorted by length of follow-up, which is grouped into intervals. A life table is then constructed (Table 2.1). For each interval of follow-up, the number of patients still in the trial at the start of the interval, the number of failures occurring within the interval, and the number withdrawn during the interval are determined. (Once a failure has occurred the patient is no longer in the trial.) The number withdrawn includes those that died, those that reached the end of the trial, and those that were lost to follow-up. (Ideally the number lost to follow up should be included in a separate column.) The number at risk during the year is then calculated: it is the number of patients at the beginning of the year less half the number of withdrawals. The percentage failure rate for the year is determined by dividing the number of failures by the number at risk and multiplying by 100. The percentage success rate is determined by subtracting the failure rate from 100. The success rate for the interval being analysed and all previous intervals are then cumulated to give the survival rate for that interval. This is sometimes known as the cumulative survival rate (usually expressed as a percentage). A survival curve is then plotted with the cumulative survival rate on the vertical axis and the time after operation on the horizontal axis (Figure 2.1).

Confidence limits

In a survival analysis, data from patients with different lengths of follow-up are amalgamated. Therefore, although there may be large numbers of patients in the trial, only a small number will have been followed for a long period. The difference between different procedures is only likely to become apparent with long follow-ups. At this stage because of the small numbers involved, the survival rates may not be reliable. It is therefore essential that the number of patients at risk in each time interval is quoted. Some authors end their survival curves when the number of patients at risk drops below a predetermined level. For the larger studies this is often 50 (Malchau *et al.,* 1993). There is, however, some justification for presenting the whole data.

Confidence limits can be calculated in a number of different ways. For routine use, when the failure rates and the number of patients followed are relatively large, the method of Peto is recommended (Appendix) (Peto *et al.,* 1977). This method is simple to use but under some circumstances is not very accurate. When either the failure rate is low, or the number of patients followed is low it is preferable to use an 'exact' method. This should be based on the 'effective number at risk' described by Murray (Appendix) (Murray *et al.,* 1993). Various different 'exact' methods can be used. These include calculations, tables or use of the *F* distribution (Armitage and Berry, 1987). The method of Rothman is

Table 2.1 Life table for metal on metal THR, with confidence intervals (CI) determined by the method of Peto. (The raw data are from Dobbs, 1980)

Year	No. at start	Failures	Withdrawn	No. at risk	Failure rate	Success rate	Survival	95% CI
1	173	3	10	168	1.8%	98.2%	98.2%	2.0%
2	160	5	5	157.5	3.2%	96.8%	95.1%	3.3%
3	150	12	4	148	8.1%	91.9%	87.4%	5.0%
4	134	9	8	130	6.9%	93.1%	81.3%	6.0%
5	117	8	12	111	7.2%	92.8%	75.5%	7.0%
6	97	3	11	91.5	3.3%	96.7%	73.0%	7.8%
7	83	3	12	77	3.9%	96.1%	70.2%	8.6%
8	68	5	21	57.5	8.7%	91.3%	64.1%	9.9%
9	42	2	11	36.5	5.5%	94.5%	60.5%	12.3%
10	29	1	13	22.5	4.4%	95.6%	57.9%	15.5%
11	15	1	4	13	7.7%	92.3%	53.4%	19.8%
12	10	2	8	6	33.3%	66.7%	35.6%	22.9%

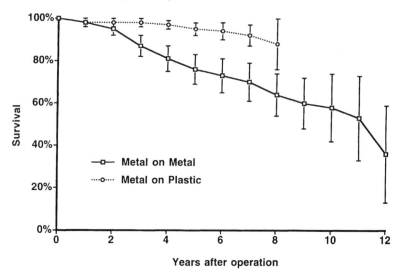

Figure 2.1 Survival curves comparing metal on metal and metal on plastic THR with 95% confidence limits determined by the method of Peto. The raw data were taken from Dobbs (1980)

described in the appendix as it can be used relatively easily with a personal computer (Rothman, 1978). The confidence limits should ideally be plotted with the survival curve and should always be quoted with survival rates (Figure 2.1).

Loss to follow-up

A fundamental assumption in survival analysis is that patients who are lost to follow-up and patients who die have the same failure rate as those that complete the trial. Although this may be valid for those that die, it is not valid for those that are lost to follow-up (Britton, 1995). If an operation fails, a patient may well go elsewhere to seek 'better' treatment. In studies, for example, of the best joint replacements, where the failure rate is very low, the possibility that even a single failure is hidden within the patients who are lost to follow-up will have a profound effect on the results. It is therefore essential that information about patients lost to follow-up is included, ideally in a column in the life table. Any patient not reviewed during the last time interval of the trial, or after the trial has finished, is a patient lost to follow-up, providing the patient has not died. This definition of loss to follow-up must be rigidly applied to all survival analyses so that patients lost to follow-up can be identified. One way of portraying the possible consequences of loss to follow-up is to plot a worst case survival curve derived by assuming that all patients lost to follow-up have failed (Murray *et al.,* 1993). The reader can then be certain that the true curve lies somewhere between this and the standard curve. If the loss to follow-up rate is high, the worst case curve degrades the results so dramatically that it would also serve as a powerful incentive to all authors to avoid losing patients to follow-up.

Definition of failure in joint replacement surgery

Any definition of failure may be used for a survival analysis. Many different definitions have been used and, not surprisingly, generate different survival rates (Nelissen *et al.,* 1992). Revision is the most widely used definition, as it is simple to identify and reproducible. However, revision may be delayed or even postponed indefinitely if the service lacks resources, if the patient is deemed too ill, or if the surgery is too complex. If this occurs, an early failure will be classified as a continuing success. There is no simple solution to this problem. One option is to analyse separately several outcomes. These should include an outcome which could be considered to be a total failure of the implant, an outcome which could be considered to be a partial failure, and an outcome which is an early predictor of failure. A total failure would be revision and/or development of severe pain or pain as bad as before the original operation. The primary indication for a joint replacement is pain. Therefore, for a joint replacement, development of moderate pain could be considered to be a partial failure (Britton, 1995). Currently roentgen stereophotogrammetric analysis is the only method that has been shown to predict joint replacement in the early stages. This, however, is complex and expensive. Until a simple method is available, the development of radiolucent lines, and/or subsidence seen on x-rays could be used as an end point. None of these outcomes in themselves is reliable, but each assess different facets and used together they may contribute useful information. Until a consensus is reached about what outcomes should be assessed it will remain difficult to compare survival analyses.

Pitfalls

Although survival analysis is a powerful tool, it does have major drawbacks when the failure rates are very low. With modern joint replacements which have very low failure rates (less than 1% per year) survival analysis can actually be abused to give a false impression. When reviewing a survival analysis it is important to consider a number of points (Murray *et al.,* 1993):

a) Were the start and finish date selected so as to exclude some failures?

b) Is failure clearly defined?

c) How many patients were there at risk in the year in which the survival rates are quoted? With numbers as low as 10, the possible error is of the order of 20% (Peto, 1984) and is therefore usually larger than the cumulative failure rate.

d) What proportion of patients were lost to follow-up? How does the number lost compare with the number of failures?

e) What method was used to determine confidence limits? During a period of time in which there were no failures, if the confidence interval does not widen then it can be deduced that the method of Greenwood was used (Greenwood, 1926). This method is inappropriate for low failure rates as it is too optimistic.

f) Are the conclusions drawn from the results valid when the confidence limits are considered?

g) If all the above questions cannot be answered, or if the conclusion is that a new joint replacement is better than traditional ones, the analysis needs to be treated with some caution.

Comparing results

The most important use of clinical trials is to compare different methods of treatment. Survival curves allow such comparisons to be made, although different numbers of patients may be at risk at different times. However, to make a formal comparison additional statistical techniques are necessary.

The log-rank test

The simplest statistical method that can be applied is the log-rank test (Mantel, 1966), which is described with examples by Peto *et al.* (1977) and used for comparing knee replacements by Curtis (Curtis *et al.,* 1992). Its underlying principle is simple: if, at some given time, two-thirds of the patients still at risk were treated by operation A and one-third by operation B then we should expect, if operations A and B are equally effective, that two-thirds of the failures in the next interval would be in group A and one-third in group B. The number of patients at risk at any time is calculated as for the survival table and the expected number of failures in each interval is calculated for each group. The log-rank test compares the observed failures with the expected failures in the two groups (Appendix). If differences are found, it is important to make certain that the 'lost to follow up' in both groups are not significantly different.

Stratification

The log-rank method can be used to investigate the effect of variables such as age, sex, weight or disease type on survival. Statisticians refer to these as explanatory variables and to the process of forming groups as stratification. Ideally, the groups should be formed at the outset of the trial. Analytical methods are designed to discover prognostic determinants so that they can be taken into consideration when two procedures are compared. It is important to know if an apparent difference is due to the presence of more 'good-prognosis' cases in one group than in the other. An advantage of dividing patients into groups is that one procedure may only be noticeably better than another in a subset of patients. The process of stratification, however, diminishes the numbers so that spuriously significant results may be produced.

Cox's proportional hazards model

Another method for taking into account the effect of prognostic variables is the proportional hazards model of Cox (1972). The method has been described with worked examples by Christensen and Kalbfleisch (Kalbfleisch and Prentice, 1980; Christensen, 1987). As in the case of the log-rank test, it makes the assumption that the ratio of failures to the number at risk is the same for group A and group B. The value of the model is that it can be used to assess the influence of several variables at once, including that of the use of either operation A or B. It is therefore possible to assess a difference in outcome between two operations while taking account of the effects of other influential variables.

Table 2.2 Observed and expected failures of metal on metal and metal on plastic total hip replacements. (The raw data are from Dobbs, 1980)

Year	Metal on metal No. at risk	Observed	Metal on plastic No. at risk	Observed	Total No. at risk	Observed	Metal expected	Plastic expected
1	168	3	236.5	4	404.5	7	2.9	4.1
2	157.5	5	218.5	0	376	5	2.1	2.9
3	148	12	214	1	362	13	5.3	7.7
4	130	9	208	2	338	11	4.2	6.8
5	111	8	190.5	4	301.5	12	4.4	7.6
6	91.5	3	152	2	243.5	5	1.9	3.1
7	77	3	86	1	163	4	1.9	2.1
8	57.5	5	22.5	1	80	6	4.3	1.7
9	36.5	2	0.5	0	37	2	2.0	0.0
Total		50		15		65	29.0	36.0

These methods of analysis are complex and require the co-operation of a statistician. There is a considerable risk of finding spurious associations, particularly if many variables are examined and if the failure rate is low.

Randomised trials

Orthopaedic surgeons should be aware that serious errors may occur when comparisons are made with published results of other investigators (Sacks *et al.*, 1982). When comparing survival rates it is preferable to use randomised rather than historical controls. There are a number of reasons why randomised trials have seldom been used in evaluating surgical procedures (Stirrat *et al.*, 1992). Neither blinding of the surgeon nor the use of a placebo is possible. In addition, when an established technique is compared with a new method, surgical experience tends to favour the accepted method. Despite these difficulties, randomised trials should be encouraged. In many fields of orthopaedics, and especially joint replacement surgery, the failure rates are low, so the detection of significant differences between operations requires large numbers of patients to be followed for long periods. Such numbers may not be attainable by one surgeon or even one centre, so multi-centre trials or meta-analysis may be necessary (Chalmers, 1990).

Conclusions

Any new surgical procedure or implant should be properly compared with currently accepted standards before it is accepted into general use. This should not be regarded as an optional requirement: failure to make such comparisons is unethical. Orthopaedic surgery is full of unresolved questions; well-constructed clinical trials offer the best hope of answering them. Such trials are onerous and time and money are needed to collect, record and analyse the data. The relatively few clinicians who undertake such trials must have an understanding of the statistical methods used and the problems that may be encountered. It is equally important that the much larger number of clinicians who read the reports of such trials should be able to criticise them in an informed way so that the practice of orthopaedics rests on a sound scientific basis.

Appendix

The Peto equation (Peto *et al.*, 1977)

If after a certain length of follow-up the cumulative survival is P and the number at risk is N then:

The confidence interval is $C = ZP \sqrt{\dfrac{1-P}{N}}$ and the confidence limits are $P* = P \pm C$

For 95% confidence limits $Z = 1.96$. It is recommended that this type of equation should not be used unless $N(1 - P)$ is greater than 10 (Armitage and

Berry, 1987). For example, for $N(1 - P)$ to be greater than 10, there should be at least 100 patients at risk if the survival rate is 90%.

The 'effective number at risk' and Rothman's (1978) method

If either the failure rate or the numbers followed up are small then the confidence limits should be determined by an 'exact method' and should be based on the 'effective number at risk'.

The 'effective number at risk' is the harmonic mean $M = t \div \sum \dfrac{1}{n_i}$ (Murray et al., 1993).

Where there are t intervals of equal length and in interval i there are n_i patients at risk.

The confidence limits are $P^* = \dfrac{MP}{(M + Z^2)} + \dfrac{Z^2}{2M} \pm Z \sqrt{\dfrac{P(1 - P)}{M} + \dfrac{Z^2}{4M^2}}$ (Rothman, 1978).

The log-rank test

Life tables are constructed for the treatments being compared (Table 2.1). For each treatment in each interval the number of patients at risk (N_i) and the observed number of failures is determined (Table 2.2). In each interval, by combining the different treatments, the total number at risk (T_i) and the total number of failures (F_i) is determined. Assuming the chance of failing is the same for both treatments, the expected number of failures (E_i) for each treatment is determined $(E_i = F_i N_i / T_i)$. For each treatment the total number of observed (O) and expected (E) failures is determined and $(O - E)^2/E$ is calculated. These are then summed for the different treatments. The P value is determined using chi-square tables, where the degree of freedom is one less than the number of different treatments. In the example (Table 2.2) the sum of $(O - E)^2/E$ is $(50-29)^2/29 + (15-36)^2/36 = 27.4$. Comparison of this value with the tabulated behaviour of chi-square with one degree of freedom (2 treatments – 1) shows that the observed difference between treatments is highly significant ($P < 0.001$).

References

Armitage P, Berry G (1987) *Statistical Methods in Medical Research*, 2nd edition. Oxford: Blackwell Scientific Publications

Britton AR, Murray DW, McPherson K, Bulstrode CJ, Dehan R (1995) Lost to follow up - Does it matter? *Lancet*; **345**: 1511–1512

Britton AR, Murray DW, Bulstrode CJ, McPherson K, Denham RA (1996) Long term comparison of Charnley and Stanmore design total hip replacement. *J. Bone Jt Surg.*; **78B**: 802–808

Chalmers I (1990) Evaluating the effects of care during pregnancy and childbirth. In: Chalmers I, Enkin M, Keirse MJNC (eds) *Effective Care During Pregnancy and Childbirth*. Oxford: Oxford University Press, pp. 3–38

Christensen E (1987) Multivariate survival analysis using Cox's regression model. *Hepatology*; **7**: 1346–1358

Cox DR (1972) Regression models and life tables. *J. R. Stat. Soc.*; **34**: 187–220

Curtis MJ, Bland JM, Ring PA (1992) The Ring total knee replacement: a comparison of survivorship. *J. R. Soc. Med.*; **85**: 208–210

Dobbs HS (1980) Survivorship of total hip replacement. *J. Bone Jt Surg.*; **62B**: 168–173

Greenwood M (1986) The error of sampling of the survivorship tables. In: *Reports on Public Health and Medical Subjects, No. 33, Appendix 1*. London: HM Stationary Office, pp. 23–25

Kalbfleisch JD, Prentice RL (1980) *The Statistical Analysis of Failure Time Data*. New York: John Wiley and Sons

Kaplan EL, Meier P (1958) Nonparametric estimation from incomplete observations. *J. Am. Stat. Assoc.*; **53**: 457–481

Malchau H, Herberts P, Ahnfelt L (1993) Prognosis of total hip replacement in Sweden. Follow-up of 92,675 operations performed 1978–1990. *Acta Orthop. Scand.*; **64**: 497–506

Mantel N (1966) Evaluation of survival data and two new rank order statistics arising in its consideration. *Cancer Chemother. Rep.*; **50**: 163–170

Murray DW, Bulstrode CJK, Carr A (1993) Survival analysis of joint replacements. *J. Bone Joint Surg.*; **75B**: 697–705

Nelissen RGHH, Brand R, Rozing PM (1992) Survivorship analysis in total condylar knee arthroplasty: a statistical review. *J. Bone Jt Surg.*; **74A**: 383–389

Peto J (1984) The calculation and interpretation of survival curves. In: Buyse ME, Staquet MJ, Sylvester RJ (eds) *Cancer Clinical Trials: Methods and Practice*. Oxford: Oxford University Press, pp. 361–380

Peto R, Pike MC, Armitage P, Breslow NE, Cox DR, Howard SV, Mantel N, McPherson K, Peto J, Smith PG (1977) Design and analysis of randomised clinical trials requiring prolonged observation of each patient. *Br. J. Cancer*; **35**: 1–39

Rothman KJ (1978) Estimation of confidence limits for the cumulative probability of survival in life table analysis. *J. Chron. Dis.*; **31**: 557–560

Sacks H, Chalmers TC, Smith H (1982) Randomised versus historical controls for clinical trials. *Am. J. Med.*; **72**: 233–240

Stirrat GM, Farndon J, Farrow SC, Dwyer N (1992) The challenge of evaluating surgical procedures. *Ann. R. Coll. Surg. Eng.*; **74**: 80–84

Chapter 3

Nomenclature, classification and coding

AC Macey

And to-day, to-day we shall have naming of parts

Henry Reed (1914–1986) *Lessons of War,* 1946

Orthopaedics defined

In 1952, the American Academy of Orthopaedic Surgeons (AAOS) defined orthopaedics as:

The medical specialty that includes the investigation, preservation, restoration, and development of the form and function of the extremities, spine, and associated structures by medical, surgical, and physical means.

Orthopaedics described

Orthopaedics is a highly technical and in many respects, an increasingly demanding discipline. It is perhaps one of the last specialties which covers all anatomical areas and is faced with a myriad of pathological problems and potential procedures from the cradle to the grave. Blauvelt and Nelson (1994) correctly state that a proper understanding of the morphology and function of the musculo–skeletal system in health or disease is based on a 'proper understanding of the language of the specialty' and that the imparting of accurate knowledge to others 'demands that precise language be used'.

An exponential change has occurred in all aspects of medicine, as basic science research has advanced and become absorbed into clinical practice. This is well illustrated by the changes in the latest edition of *A Manual of Orthopaedic Terminology* (Blauvelt and Nelson, 1994) which, in the past 17 years, has gone through five editions, with the surgery chapter alone having some 300 new procedures added.

As the Manual notes, research terminology is unique and, unlike that used in a clinical setting, it 'includes the language of biochemistry, biomechanics, immunology, physics, engineering, and prosthetics'. Disciplines as diverse as electrobiology, diagnostic imaging, oncology and immunology are also changing and are rapidly altering the language of clinical orthopaedics with a continuous requirement for new nomenclature and a reclassification of accepted terminology.

Rising costs have placed additional burdens on surgeons, these burdens are remote from clinical practice, whilst the challenge of naming, classifying and perhaps coding the wide variety of clinical work has still not been attained. In addition, a deluge of other concepts – manpower, training, clinical budgeting, management, purchasing, quality assurance, planning, personnel management, etc. – demand attention and distract from the surgeon's clinical work.

What clinical work do orthopaedic surgeons do?

The rising cost of health care and the perception of orthopaedic surgery as an expensive specialty has caused purchasers to look for justification or 'value for money' from the service. This in turn has provided the impetus for many overburdened orthopaedic surgeons to draw back from what is a busy coal face and make an assessment of their activities. These must now extend beyond the purely clinical to include training, teaching, education, audit, outcome and administration. Each area requires agreed terminology and accepted norms.

Clinical work

An American Academy of Orthopaedic Surgeons Technical Consulting Panel met in 1986 at the School of Public Health, Harvard to report on precisely what American orthopaedic surgeons do. Orthopaedic surgeons were classified as 3.1% of all doctors. 97% reported patient care as their major professional activity; 5% of all visits to physicians are to orthopaedic surgeons. On average 58 h per week were worked for 47 weeks a year. Twelve days were spent in continuing medical education. In all, 32% of time was spent seeing outpatients, 18% operating and 14% on rounds. The ten most common diagnoses made during the outpatient visits (January 1980–December 1981) are shown in Table 3.1. The distribution of cases treated by anatomical site and disease category is shown in Table 3.2. The nine most common disease categories are shown in Table 3.3. The surgical procedures that amount to 50% of orthopaedic operating are shown in Table 3.4.

Diagnosis

The first step in the clinical assessment of an orthopaedic patient is to make a diagnosis. Without this, treatment cannot be specific and becomes empirical.

Table 3.1 The ten most common diagnoses made during the above outpatient visits

	Diagnosis	% of visits
1	Knee symptoms	12.3
2	Back symptoms	7.4
3	Postoperative visit	5.5
4	Foot and toe symptoms	5.5
5	Low back symptoms	5.0
6	Progress visit, not elsewhere classified	4.8
7	Shoulder problems	4.8
8	Neck symptoms	3.7
9	Hand and finger symptoms	3.5
10	Ankle symptoms	2.9

Table 3.2 The distribution of cases treated by anatomical site

Anatomical site	Mean % of cases treated
Knee/leg	21.7
Thoracic/lumbar spine	18.1
Pelvis/hip/thigh	14.2
Foot/ankle	12.3
Hand/forearm	12.0
Shoulder/elbow	9.7
Neck (cervical spine)	7.5
Other (non-localised)	3.1

Table 3.3 The nine most common disease categories

Disease category	Mean % of cases treated
Trauma	42.3
Degenerative/rheumatoid	25.7
Congenital/developmental	8.2
Neurological	7.6
Infection	3.6
Other	3.4
Metabolic	2.6
Neoplastic	2.3
Vascular (circulatory)	2.3

Table 3.4 The surgical procedures that amount to 50% of orthopaedic operating

Procedure	%
Repair and plastic operations on bone	14.3
Reduction of fracture and fracture dislocation of hip	12.9
Other operations on joint structures	11.6
Incision and excision of joint structures	11.5
Operations on skin and subcutaneous tissue	11.0
Reduction of other fracture and fracture dislocation	10.5
Incision and excision of bones	8.2
Reduction of fracture and fracture dislocation of ankle and wrist	7.0
Operations – muscles, tendons, fascia, and bursa, not including hand	3.7
Operations on peripheral nerves	1.7

Engle (1964) defined diagnosis as 'the art, science or act of recognising disease from symptoms, signs and laboratory data'; this definition still remains appropriate (Engle, 1964). The debate on the difference between disease and diagnosis can be followed from Scadding's writings (Scadding, 1967; Campbell, 1979). Those requiring more *precision in diagnosis* may wish to peruse Patricia Fraser's thoughts, from her contribution to the book of the same name (Fraser, 1969).

Wenger and Rang (1993) observe that the Greek origin of the word *dia gnosis* means *through knowledge* but that the problem often facing the clinician is one of incomplete knowledge. 'Mostly we reach a diagnosis in the same way that Brigham Young reached Salt Lake City – we have come far enough and this looks right.' They propose four methods of reaching a diagnosis:

1. Gestalt or pattern recognition.
2. Algorithms.
3. Working through the differential diagnosis.
4. Guess and question, or the hypothetico–deductive method, i.e. make a guess about the most likely diagnosis and then test it by looking for positive features. (This is how most of us work!)

Most clinicians, if uncertain about diagnosis, will fall back on the surgical sieve approach to establish which of the broad categories is likely to be relevant (Pynsent and Fairbank, 1990). The more the emphasis from the patient is symptomatic and subjective, the greater the tendency to use this approach.

Normality

It is obvious that normality must be defined as a baseline before it is possible to recognise and name the abnormal. Limited data are available to help in this definition. Defining normal *structure* in the adult is helped by the long evolution that anatomy has undergone. At a microscopic level, histology has followed a similar course to a largely accepted terminology. Growth presents particular problems (see also Chapter 11), many of which have been addressed by Hensinger (1986) in his book *Standards in Pediatric Orthopaedics*. The criterion for inclusion of standards in the text was its relevance to the clinical assessment of patients or as a possible aid in future research.

Accepted norms may vary from case to case; this is a situation that makes comparisons between individuals or series difficult. There is a need for standardisation that has been addressed, for example, in hand surgery, when Swanson (1987) developed a system for the evaluation of physical impairment in the hand and upper extremity, that has been approved for use by the International Federation of Societies for Surgery of the Hand (IFSSH).

Nomenclature, classification and coding in clinical practice

In 1965 an expert group on Medical Terminology and Lexicography, convened by the World Health Organisation (WHO), produced the following definitions:

Nomenclature: a systematic list, of all or as many names as possible of members of a clearly defined conceptual or linguistic family, usually without accompanying definitions. Thus the names of all plants constitute a botanical nomenclature, and so with animals, tumours, diseases, etc., e.g. SNOMED the Systematised Nomenclature of Medicine.

Classification: a list of all the concepts belonging to a well defined group (e.g. of diagnoses etc.) compiled in accordance with criteria enabling them to be arranged systematically, and permitting the establishment of a hierarchy based on the natural or logical relationship between them.

Code: word or symbol or number used for secrecy or convenience instead of ordinary name.

The group emphasised the difference in philosophy between the two, a nomenclature being a list of names and a classification a list of concepts. In describing the origin of OPCS codes, Ashley and Aitken make the essential point that classifications are not designed to enable records to be retrieved for research purposes (Ashley and Aitken, 1988).

In the United Kingdom, all inpatients must have their diagnosis(es) and operation(s) recorded for Körner data collection (Windsor, 1986), when discharged from hospital. This text information is then converted into code, either by, often disinterested, clinicians or by coding clerks. Diagnoses are coded according to *The International Classification of Diseases* ICD-9 or 10 (World Health Organisation). Operations are coded according to *The Classification of Operations* OPCS IV (The Office of Population, Censuses and Surveys).

Deficiencies in the coding process

Coding is known to be at least 20% inaccurate (Scott-Samuel, 1978; Whates, 1982). It is also inadequate, inaccessible and frequently subject to long delays. As a result, clinicians (and management) are unable to extract useful information from the system and it falls into further decline.

The difficulties are caused by three distinct but related factors within the coding process:

i. Inconsistencies in the English (or natural language) description ascribed to each code. (Also referred to as the lexicon or rubric.)
ii. The codes themselves and their construction, i.e. whether they are multi-axial (modular) or uni-axial (integrated).
iii. The method by which the codes are arrived at – the user interface.

These problems are not new and were recognised over 20 years ago by a British Orthopaedic Association (BOA) sub-committee on disease indexing. They accepted that orthopaedic surgeons were 'too overworked with service needs to be involved with the ICD', yet needed 'a simple classification of diseases for the purpose of research'. However, as Ashley and Aitken note, long standing classifications, such as the International Classification of Diseases, have been designed explicitly for the compilation of statistics, especially those of a routine nature (Ashley and Aitken, 1988). They are not designed for, nor can they provide, an index to enable records to be retrieved for research purposes. Inevitably, they fail to answer the needs of the enquiring clinician and those enthusiastic enough to add additional digits to increase detail, will be disappointed by limited data retrieval capabilities.

Inconsistencies in the English (or natural language) description

'When I use a word,' Humpty Dumpty said in a rather scornful tone, 'it means just what I chose it to mean – neither more nor less'

Lewis Carroll. *Through the Looking Glass*, 1872, Ch 6

Wenger and Rang (1993) purposely elected to use the 'language of the orthopaedic workplace' when writing their textbook. All orthopaedic surgeons can relate to and understand workplace terminology instinctively. That this must also be a precise language is increasingly recognised. Unfortunately, this is not the language and terminology used in the statutory classification and coding systems that we are obliged to comply with, such as the International Classification of Diseases.

The essential first step in constructing a nomenclature, classification or coding system is the fall of Humpty Dumpty's assertion. The language of the workplace must be both precise and universally agreed. English (or other natural language) lends itself to ambiguity and uncertainty both in meaning and context. For example, there are a number of interpretations of the words 'the light red car'. Agreed terminology avoids this problem, but requires a long evolution. Nomina Anatomica, extant only since the 1960s, had a gestation dating back 500 years.

The *Manual of Orthopaedic Terminology* (Blauvelt and Nelson, 1994) succinctly states that a proper understanding of the morphology and function of the musculo–skeletal system in health or disease is based on a 'proper understanding of the language of the specialty' and that the imparting of accurate knowledge to others 'demands that precise language be used'.

Agreed terminology should follow from precise language and within most areas of orthopaedics and trauma this agreement is still evolving. Skeletal dysplasias are an example. Sir Thomas Fairbank was the first to synthesise the known dysplasias in one book (Fairbank, 1951). However, some of the terminology used was confusing until international agreement was achieved by the adoption of the Paris nomenclature of 1970. Continuing advances in understanding of the genetic basis for many dysplasias may soon prompt a review and revision of this work.

Terminology for hand surgery gained international acceptance as a result of the work of the IFSSH sub-committee for Standardisation of Nomenclature. Their document included both Nomina Anatomica and the 1956 American Academy of Orthopaedic Surgeons work on joint motion, with the aim of promoting communication by increasing precision and understanding. In 1983 a similar exercise was undertaken for the language of clinical hand surgery as required for the three areas of Symptoms, Signs and Investigations; Pathology and Disease; Treatment and Operations (Barton, 1986).

In 1986, McManus wrote that a standardised lexicon of orthopaedic surgery terms would be desirable (McManus, 1986). In 1990 the BOA Information Technology Committee undertook the task of committing to paper a lexicon that would adequately describe current trauma and orthopaedic practice. Unaware that Johnson had described the lexicographer as a 'harmless drudge', it took the unsuspecting committee some 4 years to publish two BOA 'blue books', one covering orthopaedics and the other trauma (British Orthopaedic Association, 1993a,b). These also formed the Association's contribution to the National

Clinical Terms Project (CTP) which concluded in 1994. The committee's effort has allowed some improvement and perhaps some standardisation in the language and terminology used. The resulting lexicon has been incorporated into the descriptive section (rubric) of the Read Clinical Classification (Read, 1986). However, the latter classification is simply a 'super set' of ICD and remains constrained by the limited and inflexible structure of ICD. Attempts have been made to circumvent this by the use of site codes as 'qualifying terms' but this has produced difficulties.

Problems with the codes and their construction

It should now be clear that the language of the workplace must be precise and comprise an agreed terminology or lexicon; however, the next difficulty lies in ensuring that the terminology is correctly used and appropriately structured into a coding system that will 'playback' the precise natural language description when the code is selected. Searching for phrases such as 'application of internal fixation' as one commercially available encoder requires, is a fruitless task. It is not the language of the workplace, so the use is incorrect and the context inappropriate, such that the search cannot succeed.

The 1974 BOA sub-committee on disease indexing suggested a basic system for orthopaedic diseases, based on the surgical sieve. Trauma was considered on an anatomical basis (Wainwright, 1974). The essential criteria for a coding system set out in the 1974 report remain valid and bear repetition:

Simplicity:

Brevity: it should be concise.

Acceptability: a classification system must be generally acceptable.

Utility: it should enable defined objectives to be more easily achieved with the coding system than without it.

Consistency: any disease or procedure should have the same identification from day to day.

Precision: any two or more items that can usually be distinguished should be allocated separate identifiers, provided always that this separation is required by sufficient users of the system.

Generality: it should be possible to aggregate separate codes with a minimum difficulty to achieve broader groupings. To this end, a hierarchical structure is helpful.

Economy: a coding system should be easy to use by a clerk rather than by a doctor, i.e. by as low a level of skills as possible.

Uniqueness: it should be possible to make comparisons over as wide an area and time interval as possible; this requires a degree of standardisation.

Adaptability: extensions of knowledge and new techniques should permit the system to be coded by the allocation of new identifiers. The sub-division should be made in such a way that the codes before and after this sub-division are easy to relate.

The report also commented on other contemporary efforts to include site with the ICD and OPCS codes. A pocket book similar to that in use at the Royal National Orthopaedic Hospital, London was recommended, noting that the rapid development of orthopaedic surgery required an annual authoritative issue of new conditions and procedures (RNOH, 1973). It was concluded that the BOA would be an appropriate body to undertake this annual exercise. Although laudable and sound in principle these efforts did not survive, probably due to the fact that funding has always been directed exclusively towards ICD and OPCS, as these are relevant to financial and management systems, this has been to the detriment of clinical systems. In 1990 the BOA formed an Information Technology committee – a phoenix of the 1974 committee, to address the issue of nomenclature, classification and coding once again.

The structure of systems

Systems of nomenclature, classification and coding can be constructed from a number of small discrete 'blocks' of information as a modular (multi-axial) approach or, from larger single 'blocks' containing longer strings of text, an integrated or uni-axial approach. The key distinction between the systems listed in Table 3.5 is based on whether they are uni-axial (integrated) or multi-axial (modular). The latter invariably have site as an axis and are ideally suited to trauma and orthopaedics.

Table 3.5 Nomenclature, classification and coding systems in use (the suffix U is appended to uni-axial systems and M to multi-axial systems)

ICD-9	U
ICD-9-CM	U
ICD-9-CM vol. 3 – procedures	U
Orthopaedic ICD-9-CM Expanded	U
ASSH ICD-9-CM	U
ICD-10	U
Read codes	U
BOA Trauma Lexicon	U
BOA Elective Lexicon	U
OPCS IV	U
Diagnosis Related Groups (DRGs)	U
Healthcare Resource Groups (HRGs)	U
The Fracture Classification Manual	U
Current Procedural Terminology (CPT)	U
SAC operative codes	U
AAOS Orthopaedic Slide Management System	U
SNOMED	M
AO Classification of Fractures	M
Accident Compensation Commission of New Zealand – Injury Diagnosis	M
Departmental systems	
Belfast Orthopaedic Coding System (BOCS)	M
Edinburgh Coding System	M
Manchester Keywords	M
Windsor Codes	M

Heidenstrom's paper (1979) makes a compelling case for the modular approach and the conclusion bears repeating

> ...some apology is due the reader for imposing on his attention a system (i.e. modular) so elementary and obvious that a novice at statistics might have chosen it instinctively. Yet, it remains a fact that some statistical classifications that have been in use for over 50 years remain on an integral basis.
>
> This is perhaps not surprising when one considers that some written languages have existed for thousands of years without developing out of integral symbols (ideographs). These languages are known to be especially difficult and tedious to learn, uneconomical, lacking in versatility and prodigal in dictionary space. The analogy with coding systems is obvious, such systems being, after all, simply artificial languages.

The user interface

Once the terms for a lexicon have been defined and appropriate codes agreed, it is essential that a method of term and code selection is chosen that is usable in practice. The tedious search through two large volumes is harmful drudgery. It has been the root cause for inaccurate coding when this task has been delegated to doctors in training. A further confounding factor has been the lack of incentive for such doctors who have been unable to benefit from their efforts due to delays in the system. Most hospital systems are still forcing the end user to grapple with difficult text interfaces, operated by a standard keyboard. Errors in data entry are common in such circumstances.

There are a multitude of user interfaces (Figure 3.1) and design guidelines for human–computer interaction have been studied intensively (Shneiderman, 1987; Apple, 1992).

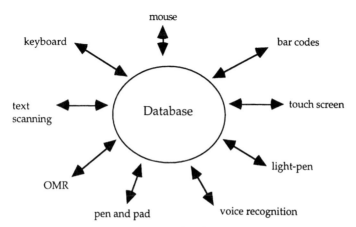

Figure 3.1 Illustration of possible computer-user interfaces

Nomenclature, classification and coding systems in use

ICD-9 (WHO, 1977)

The ninth edition of the World Health Organisation International Classification of Diseases has been in use since 1978 for diagnostic coding. It provides numeric codes to allow broad international comparisons to be made by WHO. ICD-10 has now replaced the ninth edition (WHO, 1992). Tables of equivalence allow data comparison between the two editions.

ICD-9-CM

CM stands for Clinical Modification. The National Centre for Health Statistics in the USA added a fifth digit to give a potential tenfold extension to ICD-9. The CM version has been used by the vendors of Diagnosis Related Groups (DRG) software [Commission on Professional and Health Activities (CPHA), 1988].

ICD-9-CM vol. 3 – procedures

This volume is an extension of ICD9-CM used for procedure coding. It is of very limited value for orthopaedic surgery and is largely used for compatibility with DRG grouper software systems.

Orthopaedic ICD-9-CM expanded

These codes are an extension of ICD-9-CM produced by the American Academy of Orthopaedic Surgeons Nomenclature and Coding Committee in 1986 (AAOS, 1988). The impetus came from the 'rapid advances in the understanding of pathological processes in all of the subspecialties which left the original document woefully lacking'. Increased detail has been achieved by the addition of two supplementary digits e.g.:

717.3   Other and unspecified derangement of medial meniscus.
717.333 Horizontal cleavage tear of medial cartilage or medial meniscus of knee, posterior.

ASSH ICD-9-CM

A similar approach has been taken by the American Society for Surgery of the Hand, with additional detail and supplementary digits (American Society for Surgery of the Hand, 1990).

ICD-10 (World Health Organisation, 1992)

The tenth version of ICD was introduced into the NHS in 1995 and has significant differences from ICD-9, particularly in structure. The introduction states '...conditions have been grouped in a way that was felt to be most suitable for general epidemiological purposes and the evaluation of health care'. As with previous editions, this approach is of limited value to the orthopaedic surgeon.

Read codes

The Read Clinical Classification is a computer-based thesaurus of clinical terms, each of which has a unique code. Currently at version 3.1, the Read codes are a super-set of ICD-9, OPCS, the British National Formulary. The Clinical Terms Project (CPT) has increased the detail of the Read lexicon. It has been expanded to include natural language descriptions but the system is constrained by being tied to the structure of ICD-9 and is not site based.

BOA trauma and elective lexicon (British Orthopaedic Association, 1993)

In 1993, the BOA Information Technology Committee published coding lexicons containing a terminology that reflects modern practice. However, compatibility of terms with those of ICD-9 and OPCS-IV on a one-to-one basis has constrained the usefulness of this exercise.

OPCS-IV (Office of Population Censuses and Surveys, 1987)

The fourth edition of the Office of Population Censuses and Surveys was released in 1987 and replaced the very limited OPCS-III which had been in operation since 1975. OPCS-IV offers more detail than OPCS-III. However, it still falls far short of a comprehensive description of modern orthopaedic operative practice.

Diagnosis related groups (DRGs)

A patient classification system developed in Yale in the 1960s, it assigns patients by diagnosis or procedure to one of 500 groups on the basis that the cases in each group are 'iso-resource', i.e. they should consume the same resources (Bardsley, 1987).

Healthcare related groups (HRGs) (Information Management Group, 1995)

Currently in version 2, HRGs have been developed for the NHS along similar, but more specific, lines to DRGs. It is intended that HRGs will be used by the NHS for contracting in the future. Whereas DRGs have 50 groups for orthopaedics, HRGs allocate 61.

The Fracture Classification Manual (Gustilo, 1991)

Published in 1991, and adopted by the Orthopaedic Trauma Association this system started with the work of Ramon Gustilo in the early 1980s. The aim was to produce a classification that was 'easy to learn, logical and have clinical relevance and application to orthopaedic practice and clinical research'. Existing fracture classifications that are generally accepted in clinical practice were incorporated and all are shown graphically. Separate trauma codes are allocated for procedures in addition to the ICD-9 CM procedure codes.

Current procedural terminology (American Medical Association, 1989)

Physician's Current Procedural Terminology (CPT) originated in the California Relative Value Scales. These were adopted and adapted by the AMA in 1966 and are now in their fourth edition. CPT-4 is revised annually and is the most widely used system of billing codes. It takes the form of 'think of a number – start at the top' with 5-digit codes ascribed to each procedure by region. Gaps are left in the sequencing to allow for new procedures.

Specialist Advisory Committee (SAC) operative logbook codes

These codes have been produced by the SAC of the Royal College of Surgeons in an attempt to standardise the format of logbooks, these codes are of the 'think of a number, start at the top' variety. In the main, they are based on anatomical region (Specialist Advisory Committee, 1989).

AAOS orthopaedic slide management system (Hamilton, 1990)

In 1990 the AAOS adopted an orthopaedic slide management system developed by James J. Hamilton. It is based on the surgical sieve approach with subdivisions for detail. As the author notes, 'current popular coding / classification systems such as CPT – Physicians Current Procedural Terminology, published by the AMA and ICD-9 - International Classification of Diseases published by WHO do not readily adapt to the classification of concepts, anatomy, principles or surgical techniques. Additionally, their codes are not sufficiently detailed to distinguish between different types of prostheses or even fracture types in the same bone.'

SNOP

The Systematized Nomenclature of Pathology, produced by the College of American Pathologists in 1965 derived from the 1928 Standard Nomenclature of Diseases and Operations. As the precursor to SNOMED, it used four axes to describe and code pathological diagnoses.

SNOMED (College of American Pathologists, 1987)

The Systematized Nomenclature of Medicine, first produced by the College of American Pathologists in 1976-7 extended SNOP to seven axes: Topology, Disease, Occupation, Morphology, Etiology, Function, Procedure. The editors of SNOMED contend that 'every concept in medicine and the health fields can be uniquely coded, stored and retrieved'.

AO classification of fractures (Muller, 1990)

A classification is useful only if it considers the severity of the bone lesion and serves as a basis for treatment and for evaluation of the results.

(Muller, 1990)

This work started in 1977 and resulted in a general classification of fractures based on the archives of 1 million X-ray films held in the documentation centre in Berne. The aim of the classification is to guide treatment. An alpha-numeric approach is used to denote anatomical location, morphology and severity. An attraction of the system is a 'pattern recognition' approach similar to that used in the clinical situation. However useful a classification may be, if it is difficult to use in practice, it will not find favour with hard pressed surgeons. The recent production of this classification as a stand alone, mouse-driven CD-ROM, may encourage its further use.

Accidental injury diagnosis codes (Accident Compensation Commission of New Zealand) (Heidenstrom, 1979)

This system modified ICD-9 with the addition of a *SITE* code to the *TYPE* of injury. The one-site-one-symbol approach is simple, concise and practical.

Departmental systems

A number of orthopaedic departments have developed their own homebrew coding systems in response to the deficits of official coding systems. These include a degree of detail that enables clinical, logistic and research information to be derived from a single system. The list below is not exhaustive but gives some illustrations of successful systems. Each of the units independently developed and now use their system.

Belfast Orthopaedic Coding System (BOCS) – an integral part of the Belfast Orthopaedic Information System (BOIS), this is a three axis system for detailed procedural coding based on anatomical sites developed by Beverland and his colleagues (1989). Anatomical location (site) is specified in detail, followed by broad procedural group and lastly details such as implant type are recorded. An alpha-numeric notation is used e.g.:

FG A5 15 = hip region, hip joint; arthroplasty; Charnley

Searching can be done on all or any of the axes independently.

Edinburgh Coding System – developed by Robin Strachan, this system uses numeric notation to record site, disease and procedure. It is used as the basis for the Princess Margaret Rose Hospital information system.

Manchester Keywords – developed by David Marsh, this is an information system that uses English (natural language) that is 'constrained', rather than codes. Agreed English terms are used for site, diagnosis, procedure, complication etc., for example 'THR' for total hip replacement. Data retrieval can be done using English terms. The system forms the basis for the Manchester Orthopaedic Database (Barrie, 1992).

Classifications are only relatively useful (E. A. Codman, 1917)

Nomenclatures, classifications and codes are of limited value in themselves. They must be part of a wider orthopaedic information system that extends far beyond the very basic details, to be useful. Despite the enormous recent technological advances in data processing, a limited situation still pertains with regard to orthopaedic information. The difficulty remains in the collection, storage and presentation of adequate clinical information. In the United Kingdom and elsewhere, this challenge has been sidelined whilst administrative and financial systems have received preferential funding.

Ellwood (1988) summarised this state of disarray in the USA in 1988, noting that payers, physicians and health care executives no longer share common insights into the life of the patient. Health care goals have been 'drowned out by the noise of commerce' and the wrong language, consisting of money, politics, goods and services is being used to describe medicine. Use of the wrong language leads inevitably to the wrong choices.

Similarly, selection and use of the wrong clinical language, nomenclature, classification or coding system also leads to wrong choices. Present national codes reflect only the tip of a much larger iceberg, with those aspects essential to orthopaedic clinical practice or research, largely below the waterline (Figure 3.2). Figure 3.3 shows the increasing detail needed to process clinical, pathological and biological information and how this diverges from the information required by those using the management end of the 'Orthoscope'. As a rule, those viewing at the management end control the budget available for the development of information systems.

Beyond diagnosis

In the United Kingdom clinical care can be classified into three areas:

1. Trauma
2. Post-trauma reconstruction
3. Elective orthopaedics

In addition to the 'bare bones' of diagnosis and procedure, it is important to note:

1. Place of work	Clinic, Accident and Emergency, Ward, Theatre, Office
2. Time of work	Working day, out-of-hours (85% of trauma cases can be safely undertaken on next day scheduled trauma lists. 15% of cases require to be done within 6 h).
3. Person working	Consultant, Career Registrar, SHO, Intern
4. Category of work	Operative, non-operative
5. Urgency (CEPOD)	Emergency, Urgent (i.e. unscheduled), scheduled, elective

Operative work should be graded in a quantitative sense using a system such as the British United Provident Association (BUPA, 1993). These gradings (Table 3.6) are generally accepted and provide a reasonably uniform inter- and intra-specialty grading scheme. The Harvard Relative Values data also has a section for degree of difficulty that can be used in a similar fashion (American Medical Association, 1995).

Outpatient consultations

The orthopaedic surgeon has struggled to evolve a precise language with which to describe but one of these areas – inpatient activity. Activity in outpatients, the

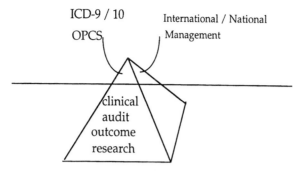

Figure 3.2 These areas 'below the waterline' appear largely invisible to those controlling the budget and investment is aimed at the tip of the iceberg for the management, as opposed to clinical information

accident and emergency department, the wards and in theatre must also be described and quantified. The complexity of orthopaedic outpatient consultations has been subject to limited study. Relative values from the USA have been suggested (American Medical Association, 1995) and the situation may yet arise where clinic time is classified and charged out on a time sheet basis accordingly.

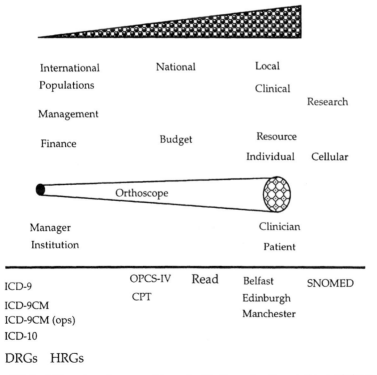

Figure 3.3 Available systems for nomenclature, classification and coding are shown relative to their ability to process the information needed for clinical assessment in orthopaedic surgery

Table 3.6 The British United Provident Association grading of operations (BUPA, 1993)

BUPA grade	IEV	Time taken
Minor	0.5	<30 min
Intermediate	1.0	1 h
Major	1.75	1–2 h
Major plus	2.2	2–3 h
Complex	4.0	>3 h

1.0 = Intermediate Equivalent Value (IEV)

Work by the British Orthopaedic Association (1995), published as a 'blue book', has clarified the volume of clinical work that orthopaedic consultants undertake. The recent emphasis on this type of study is clear when noting that all of the 17 references quoted in their document date from 1990 onwards.

Training and education

The welcome demise of an *ad hoc* approach to training requires a rigorous analysis of what each orthopaedic department can offer trainees. Clear evidence of the quantity and quality of departmental activity is now required for accreditation. Recent work to standardise the format, collection and presentation of *operative* experience, will set the standard for other areas of training such as ward work, outpatient activity, etc. These have been taken as read, in the absence of any objective way of describing, evaluating and assessing them.

Education requires ready access to the following:

i.   *Clinical cases of interest.* These records will require a system of nomenclature, classification and/or coding identical to that used for departmental activity.
ii. *Images.* Including plain X-ray films, ultrasound, CT, isotope and MRI scans. Also dynamic video-recordings of screenings, arthrograms, etc.
iii. *Photographs, slides and video-recordings.* These may include clinical, operative, arthroscopic or micro-surgical material.
iv. *References, reprints and bibliographies* on clinical, basic science and other topics.

Storage of such educational material generally uses the traditional methods of folders, ring binders and filing cabinets. Digital storage using scanned text and images offer increasing possibilities, at a cost. Modern software and hardware has solved many of the technical difficulties of storing text, graphics, sound and video-recordings together for use as an aid to teaching. Protocols to surmount the difficulties of incompatible hardware and software are now in wider use.

Retrieval of any of the above material in an accurate and repeatable method requires both a precise language of description and a comprehensive system of nomenclature, classification and coding. This should be an extension of that used for purely clinical material. The 'language of the orthopaedic workplace' should be integral to any system used by orthopaedic surgeons for education.

Audit and research

Audit and usually clinical research require an assessment methodology which involves data collection, retrieval and analysis. Audit is often a purely quantitative assessment of clinical activity, to go beyond this and undertake outcome studies is a qualitative exercise fraught with problems, not least because the information systems needed either do not exist or are not up to the task. Most of the current computerised information systems do not provide adequate data for research projects. Few enthusiastic young surgeons have been able to extract the data they need by interrogating the hospital information system. It should also be noted that clinical data must be owned by the clinician and confidentiality of this data is essential.

Administration, clinical budgeting and resource management

Waiting lists now require more than 'an eye to be kept on them'. Contracts must be monitored, theatre sessions utilised optimally and budgets managed. All these activities demand precise, timely and accurate information that extends well beyond the statutory coding produced for hospital activity analysis.

The need for an orthopaedic information system

We surgeons are a cottage industry – the best we seem able to do – and few even bother with this – is to keep an eye on waiting lists or assign dates of admission, work out some simple and not always logical priorities, and do one-off analyses of matters that interest us.

(Dudley, 1974)

Although said in the context of audit, the blame for the lamentable situation above was, and remains, a lack of adequate, timely, accessible information. How much things have improved in the last 20 years is debatable. The technology of information capture, retrieval and presentation has advanced more rapidly than could have been imagined, yet current coding systems will not provide answers to all the aspects of orthopaedic practice.

We need an information system that incorporates detailed clinical data and provides support for practice management, including audit, training, research, resource and contract management.

It is merely a plan for giving accurate, available, immediate records of each case which the hospital undertakes to treat.

(Codman, 1915)

Acknowledgements

I wish to acknowledge with gratitude the following colleagues and mentors: D. Beverland MD FRCS, F. D. Burke FRCS, G. Munroe BSc PhD, R.A.B. Mollan MD FRCSI FRCS and D. Marsh MD FRCS.

References

American Academy of Orthopaedic Surgeons (1986) *Technical Consulting Panel*. Harvard: School of Public Health

American Academy of Orthopaedic Surgeons (1988) *Orthopaedic ICD-9-CM*. Illinois

American Medical Association (1995) *Medicare resource-based relative value scale (RBRVS): the physician's guide*. Chicago

American Medical Association (1989) *Current Procedural Terminology*. Illinois

Apple Computer Inc. (1992) *Macintosh Human Interface Guidlines*. New York: Addison-Wesley

Ashley J, Aitken J (1988) *An Introduction to the Classification of Surgical Operations and Procedures*. Office of Population Censuses and Surveys

ASSH (1990) ICD-9-CM *Expanded coding*. American Society for Surgery of the Hand

Bardsley M, Coles J, Jenkins L (1987) *DRGs and health care*. King's Fund Publishing Office, London

Barrie J, Marsh D (1992) Quality of data in the Manchester Orthopaedic Database. *BMJ*; **304**: 159–162

Barton N (1986) *Terminology for Hand Surgery*. International Federation of Societies for Surgery of the Hand

Beverland DE, McKee WS, Barron DW, Murphy JSG, Mollan RAB (1989) Definition, computerisation and management of the Belfast hip waiting list. *Health Services Management*; **85**: 270–272

Blauvelt C, Nelson FA (1994) *Manual of Orthopaedic Terminology*, 5th edition. St Louis: Mosby Year Book

British Orthopaedic Association (1993a) *Coding Lexicon, Elective Volume*. London: BOA

British Orthopaedic Association (1993b) *Coding Lexicon, Trauma Volume*. London: BOA

British Orthopaedic Association (1995) *Consultant Staffing Requirements for an Orthopaedic Service in the National Health Service*. London: BOA

British Orthopaedic Association (1974) *Report of the Sub-Committee on Disease Indexing*. London: BOA

British United Provident Association (1993) *Schedule of Procedures*. London

Campbell E, Scadding J, Roberts R (1979) The concept of disease. *BMJ*; **2**: 757–762

College of American Pathologists (1987) *Systematized Nomenclature of Medicine*. Illinois

Codman EA (1917) *Study in Hospital Efficiency*. Massachusetts

Commission on Professional and Hospital Activities (1988) *International classification of diseases*, 9th Revision Clinical Modification, 9th edition. Michigan: Ann Arbor

Ellwood P (1988) Outcomes Management. A technology of patient experience. *New England Journal of Medicine*; **318**: 1549–1556

Engle R (1964) *The Diagnostic Process*. Ann Arbor: Mallory Lithographing

Fairbank HAT (1951) *Atlas of General Affections of the Skeleton*. Edinburgh: E and S Livingstone

Fraser P (1969) *Precision in Diagnosis: Numerical Taxonomy and Discriminant Analysis*. Ed. Sir Hedley Atkins, Oxford: Blackwell Scientific Publications

Gustilo R, Hanson M, Davis T (1991) *The Fracture Classification Manual*. St Louis: Mosby

Hamilton J (1990) *Orthopaedic Slide Management System*. Illinois: American Academy of Orthopaedic Surgeons

Heidenstrom PN (1979) Recording accidental injury diagnoses: an improved method. *Journal of Safety Research*; **11**: 156–161

Hensinger R (1986) *Standards in Pediatric Orthopaedics*. New York: Raven Press

Information Management Group (1995) *Healthcare Resource Groups*. Winchester: National Casemix Office

McManus G (1986) Orthopaedic office medical records using COSTAR. *Orthop. Clin. N. Am*; **17**: 581–590

Muller M, Nazarian S, Koch P, Schatzker J (1990) *The Comprehensive Classification of Fractures*. Berlin: Springer-Verlag

Office of Population Censuses and Surveys (1975) *Classification of Surgical Operations*, 3rd edition. London

Office of Population Censuses and Surveys (1987) *Classification of Surgical Operations*, 4th edition. London

Pynsent PB, Fairbank JCT (1990) Back pain a hierarchical nosology. In: Fairbank JCT, Pynsent PB (eds) *Back pain: Classification of Syndromes*. Manchester: Manchester University Press

Read J, Benson T (1986) Computer coding – comprehensive coding. *Br. J. Healthcare Computing*; May: 22–25

RNOH (1973) *Pocket Guide to Diagnostic Coding for Departments of Traumatic or Orthopaedic Surgery*. London: Royal National Orthopaedic Hospital

Specialist Advisory Committee (1989) *Log Book – Orthopaedic Surgery*. Royal College of Surgeons of England

Scadding J (1967) Diagnosis: the clinician and the computer. *Lancet*; October: 877–882

Schurman D (1985) Computerization of orthopaedic medical records. *Instructional Course Lectures* St Louis: C V Mosby Company, (pp. 469–474)

Scott-Samuel A (1978) Accuracy of data based on hospital discharge diagnoses. *BMJ*; **1**: 990

Shneiderman B (1987) Designing the User Interface. Reading, MA: Addison-Welsey Publishing Company, Inc.

Swanson AB, Goran-Hagert C, Swanson G (1987) Evaluation of impairment in the upper extremity. *J. Hand Surg.*; **12A**: 896–926

Wainwright D (1974) *Report on Disease Indexing*. British Orthopaedic Association

Wenger D, Rang M (1993) *The Art and Practice of Children's Orthopaedics*. New York: Raven Press

Whates P, Brizgalis A, Irving M (1982) Accuracy of hospital activity analysis operation codes. *BMJ*; **284**: 1857–1858

WHO (1977) *International Classification of Diseases*, 9th edition. Geneva

WHO (1992) *International Statistical Classification of Diseases and Health Related Problems*, 10th edition. Geneva

Windsor P (1986) *Introducing Körner*. Weybridge: Br J Healthcare Computing

Chapter 4

Decision analysis

PF McCombe

Introduction

Some clinical decisions are easy – should a displaced colles fracture be reduced? Most orthopaedic surgeons would have little trouble answering yes. There would also be little disagreement about the answer. The decision would be seen as non-controversial. However, some clinical decisions are difficult, with little agreement between clinicians, and are seen as controversial. Should a patient with back pain have a spinal fusion? Should arthritis of the hip in the young be treated by total hip replacement or arthrodesis? These questions do not have simple answers; moreover, when faced with the same information it is interesting that different clinicians may arrive at different conclusions. The discipline of decision analysis aims to:

- Help arrive at an optimal decision when faced with uncertainty.
- Help explain the reasons for the decision and focus on the cause of controversy.

Principles of decision analysis

The basic principle of decision analysis is 'divide and conquer'. Decisions need to be broken into manageable components of more simple choices. The appropriate choice for each of the components can then be combined in more meaningful and quantifiable ways to obtain the optimal solution to the whole problem. Even if numerical analysis is not used, the discipline of this process can lead to a clearer understanding of the problem and perhaps give the analyst new insights into the puzzle (Thornton et al.,1992).

The formal process of breaking the problem down into manageable components is that of construction of a *decision tree*. Numerical structure is then added to the tree by the allocation of probabilities to each possible outcome. These probabilities are then combined with measures of 'desirability' of outcome called *utility* to arrive at the optimal outcome. Finally, to try to explain how the various components of the model affect the result, *sensitivity analysis* is undertaken.

Decision trees

In virtually all clinical problems a complex interaction of events occurs. Some of these events are under the direct control of the surgeon (ordering a test, performing an operation) and others are beyond the surgeon's control (the results of tests, the outcome of an operation). The former *events* are the subject of choice and the latter *outcomes* are the subject of uncertainty.

The *decision tree* is a formal way of combining the three fundamental components of a decision.

- The alternative actions that are available to the decision-maker.
- The events that follow from each of these actions.
- The outcome of these events.

Figure 4.1 shows a typical decision tree for one of the simplest clinical problems – whether to operate or not. Let us consider, as an example, the question of whether to perform a spinal fusion on a patient with chronic back pain. The decision tree has one choice node (denoted by a square box) with two pathways – to perform the operation or not. We know that this form of surgery does not have a uniformly successful outcome (otherwise there would be no controversy and there would be no point in the analysis).

The decision analyst could assign three possible outcomes to each decision branch – the pain could be improved, it could be the same, or the pain could be worse. For another clinical problem the outcomes selected may, of course, be different. If the clinical problem was whether to operate on a patient with suspected acute appendicitis, the outcomes chosen may be recovery or death. While it may seem that the outcome nodes are the same for each branch of the tree, it is very important to understand that they are different. The improved outcomes, for example, could be more fully described as either *improved with surgery* or *improved without surgery*. The patient clearly would think that improvement without an operation would be preferable to improvement with an operation and hence would *value* the outcomes differently. The concept of valuation or *utility* of outcomes will be discussed later.

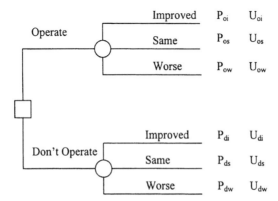

Figure 4.1 Decision tree for the value of an operation

Each of the outcome nodes now needs to have an estimate of the probability that this outcome will occur *given* that the decision in the previous decision node has been made. In Figure 4.1 these are labelled p_{oi} ..... p_{dw} and represent, respectively, the probability that improvement occurs with an operation (p_{oi}), that the pain is the same after the operation (p_{os}), that the pain is worse after the operation (p_{ow}), that the pain is improved without an operation (p_{di}), that the pain is the same without an operation (p_{ds}) and that the pain is worse without an operation.

Having assigned probabilities for each outcome, the analyst assigns utility values for each outcome. Utility, by definition, is a number with an arbitrary range (usually 0–1 or 1–100, though any range can be used). It has the property that it represents, in some way, *value of outcome* to the *patient*. If a scale of 0–1 is used, a utility of 0 represents the least desirable outcome and a utility of 1 represents the most desirable outcome. In Figure 4.1 the utility values are labelled $U_{oi}, U_{os}, U_{ow}, U_{di}, U_{ds}, U_{dw}$. To complete the analysis, the probability for each outcome is multiplied by the utility of that outcome and the results summed for each *branch* of the decision tree. This summation is called the *expected value* of each branch. In Figure 4.1 the expected value of the operate branch would therefore be $p_{oi}U_{oi} + p_{os}U_{os} + p_{ow}U_{ow}$. The branch with the highest *expected value* is the choice that the patient will prefer.

Decision trees can have more than one decision node. When this is the case the calculation begins at the end or *leaf nodes*. The expected value of the alternatives are calculated and the most valuable course of action is retained in the tree (representing the rational decision to choose the course of action with the highest expected value). The alternative branches are now discarded or *pruned* and the *expected value* of the remaining preferred branch is used as the utility for the more proximal outcome branch. The process of pruning all but the most valuable terminal branches, and using the *expected value* as *utility* for more proximal branches, continues until the root node is reached (c.f. Figure 4.7 and the example at the end of this chapter).

Probability

By definition, probability is a number in the range of 0–1. If an event has a probability of 0, its occurrence is impossible. An event with a probability of 1 will occur with certainty. A probability of 0.5 means that it is equally likely to occur as not to occur.

Probability can often be inferred from observed *frequencies, proportions and rates.*

If it is observed that 51% of a population is female, it can be assumed that the probability of an unknown individual in *that* population being female is 0.51. It cannot be assumed that the probability is the same, however, for being female in any other population. In the search to provide values to the probability figures for decision trees one often has to rely on results of published data describing frequencies of events. For the most part this is often reasonable; however, the important caveat is that to do this requires the assumption that the patients come from the same population. The notion of differing populations can be defined as populations with different *prevalence* of the condition or outcome in question. In probability terms this notion is called the *prior probability* of a condition.

If one knows the prior probability of occurrence of a trait of interest, it is often possible to revise this probability as new information becomes available (such as the result of a test). To understand how to revise probability requires a knowledge of the relationship of the 2×2 contingency table and Bayes' theory of probability.

The 2 × 2 contingency table and probability

The 2×2 contingency table is a deceptively simple device. Imagine that on an island a census of the population shows that 60% are women. Further, imagine that a study of the islanders heights shows that, as may be expected, 75% of the men and 10% of the women are over an arbitrary height (defined as tall). The population of the island is 1000. A 2×2 contingency table of frequencies is shown in Table 4.1.

If we now observe that an individual is tall, we may want to know the probability that that individual is male. Examination of the frequencies of Table 4.1 suggests that the answer is 300 ÷ 360 (0.83) or the ratio of the number of tall males divided by the total number of tall people. This value is often called the *positive predictive value* of the test of 'being tall' as a predictor of being male. In probability terms this is known as the *conditional probability* that the individual is male *given* that 'tallness' has been observed. This is usually denoted a $P[M|T]$, the $|$ sign is read as *given that* and this notation is read as the probability of M *given that* T has been observed. This particular form of conditional probability is usually called the *posterior probability* of a test. As we shall see, both the positive predictive value and the posterior probability of a positive test vary with the prevalence of the condition in the community. The *sensitivity* of the test in Table 4.1 is the proportion of males who are seen to be tall (0.75). The *specificity* of the test is the proportion of non-males who are not tall (short females). Sensitivity measures the ability of a positive test to predict the test condition is present. This ratio is the same as the *true positive* rate. Specificity measures the ability of the test to exclude the condition if the test is negative. This ratio is the same as the *true negative* rate. The sensitivity in probability terms is the conditional probability $P[T | M]$,or the probability that an individual is tall *given that* he is a male. The *specificity* is the same as the conditional probability $P[\bar{T} | \bar{M}]$, or the probability that the individual is not tall given that he is not male (the negation being indicated by the bar over the T and M). Table 4.2 shows the relationship between these measures.

Imagine now that on the island in question the ratio of males to females is quite different. Suppose that there are only 5% males and 95% females, the *prior probability* or the *prevalence* of being male is now 0.05. It is fair to assume that the proportion of males and females who are tall has not changed (The sensitivity

Table 4.1 Contingency table for hypothetical population. With a prevalence of males of 40%, the sensitivity of the test 'tallness' as a predictor of sex is 0.75. The specificity is 0.9 and the positive predictive value is 0.83 (300/360)

	Male	Female	
Tall	300	60	360
Short	100	540	640
	400	600	1000

Table 4.2 Relationship between contingency table and probability

Test	Condition +	Condition −	
+	a	b	a + b
−	c	d	c + d
	a + c	b + d	

Sensitivity or true positive rate	$\dfrac{a}{a+c}$	$P[T\,|\,D]$
Specificity or true negative rate	$\dfrac{d}{b+d}$	$P[\bar{T}\,|\,\bar{D}]$
Positive predictive value	$\dfrac{a}{a+b}$	$P[D\,|\,T]$
Negative predictive value	$\dfrac{d}{c+d}$	$P[\bar{D}\,|\,\bar{T}]$
Prevalence	$\dfrac{a+c}{a+b+c+d}$	$P[D]$

of the test of 'being tall' is unchanged). If the cell frequencies are now recalculated we see that the results for the positive and negative predictive values (and hence $\mathbf{P[T\,|\,M]}$ and $\mathbf{P[\bar{T}\,|\,M]}$) are changed. In fact the positive predictive value of the test has changed from 0.83 to 0.28 (see Table 4.3).

Bayes' theorem

The relationship between prior probability, posterior probability and conditional probability is the same as between sensitivity, specificity and prevalence. In probability terms Bayes' theorem describes how the observation of a piece of information changes the prior probability of a condition.

$$P[D\,|\,T^+] = \frac{P[T^+\,|\,D] \bullet P[D]}{P[T^+\,|\,D] \bullet P[D] + P[T^+\,|\,\bar{D}] \bullet P[\bar{D}]}$$

where

$P[D\,|\,T^+]$ = revised posterior probability that disease **D** is present given that test **T** is positive.

$P[T^+\,|\,D]$ = conditional probability that test **T** is positive in those individuals with disease **D.**

$P[D]$ = prior probability that disease **D** is present.

$P[\bar{D}]$ = prior probability that disease **D** is not present.

$P[T^+\,|\,\bar{D}]$ = probability that test **T** is positive given that disease **D** is absent.

In diagnostic applications, Bayes' theorem has been used successfully in the domain of acute abdominal pain by de Dombal *et al.* (1972), Horrocks *et al.* (1972), Adams *et al.* (1986) and in the diagnosis of dyspepsia by Knill-Jones

Table 4.3 Contingency table for hypothetical population. With a prevalence of males of 5%, the sensitivity of the test 'tallness' as a predictor of sex is 0.75. The specificity is 0.9 and the positive predictive value is 0.28 (37.5/132.5)

	Male	*Female*	
Tall	37.5	95	132.5
Short	12.5	855	867.5
	50	950	1000

(1987). Given a prior probability, each time a symptom or sign is observed, a new posterior probability is calculated and used as the prior probability for the next calculation. The assumption, however, that is implicit in the use of Bayes' theorem for this purpose is that each of the symptoms or signs must be *independent* of each other. Thus, if two tests really measure the same facet of the problem, then inclusion of both test results using Bayes' theorem will result in an overestimation of the posterior probability. The inclusion of both a positive myelogram and a positive CT scan for the diagnosis of prolapsed intervertebral disc will overestimate the probability that the disease is present. If it is thought that the assumption of independence cannot be made then the usual statistical solution is to use the technique of *logistic discrimination* (Spiegelhalter, 1984; Albert, 1987). This statistical solution attempts to reduce the values of the conditional probabilities of tests that are dependent on each other.

Utility

As already described, utility is a numerical way of defining the value of an outcome. In most clinical situations, utility is a value that the patient may attach to a particular outcome; however, in others, namely in public health planning, the value may be to the community. How, then, is a reasonable utility value arrived at for a particular clinical problem?

Assessing utility
A number of different approaches have been used to assess utility of outcome.

The standard gamble
This approach is patient based. The patient is asked to imagine that he is presented with two doors that he *must* go through. Behind the first door is a certainty (say that he will stay in the health state that he is now) behind the second door (the gamble) he will find uncertainty with two potential outcomes. In the spinal fusion example used above he would be told that there was, say, a 1% chance of being cured of his pain (without surgery) and a 99% chance of being no better or worse after an operation that *will* be performed. The patient is then instructed to choose a door. The probability values for the two outcomes are now adjusted and the patient is asked to choose again. The process is repeated until a probability is found at which the patient is indifferent and he would be unable to choose between doors. This situation is depicted in Figure 4.2.

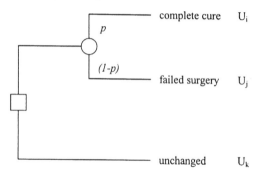

Figure 4.2 The standard gamble technique. The value of p is varied until $U_k = pU_i + (1-p)U_j$. If $U_i = 1$ and $U_j = 0$ then $U_k = p$

The relationship between the utility of the outcome behind the certainty door can now be related to the utilities of the outcomes behind the gamble doors. If the outcomes behind the gamble doors are both the best and the worst outcomes (with utilities of 0 and 1, respectively) then it follows that the utility of the outcome behind the certainty door is the same as the probability of the best gamble outcome. In the spinal fusion example, the utility of remaining with pain but by avoiding surgery is the same as the threshold p value for a complete cure (without surgery). For the standard gamble to work the utility of the certainty door must be intermediate between the utility of the two chance outcomes behind the gamble door. The other unknown utility in the spinal fusion problem is the value of successful surgery. This must be placed behind the certainty door and again contrasted with variable P values of the same two outcomes behind the gamble door.

The time trade-off method

This method (described in Llewelyn *et al.*, 1993) asks patients to consider how much time in a state of perfect health they would be willing to trade for a longer period in the state of health in question. For a chronic disease state the patient is asked to consider how much time (life expectancy) he is willing to trade in order to return to perfect health compared to remaining in this state for the rest of his life. In the case of temporary health states, the patient is again asked to choose the value of an intermediate health state i, between the best state h (completely healthy) and the worst state (temporary state j). The patient is now offered two alternatives.

- Temporary state i for time t (a specified duration of time to be in intermediate state i), followed by healthy.
- Temporary state j for time $x < t$, followed by healthy.

The value of x is now varied until the patient is again indifferent about the choice. Reference to Figure 4.3 shows that at this stage the area under the curve for each option is equal. It can be shown therefore that.

$$U_i t = U_j x + (t - x)$$

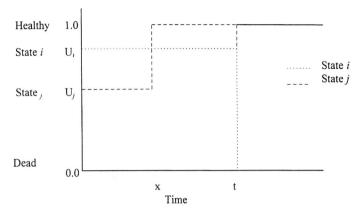

Figure 4.3 Time trade-off diagram to determine the utility of an intermediate temporary health state *i*

and that if $U_j = 0$ then

$$U_i = 1 - \frac{x}{t}$$

Direct measurement

A direct rating scale may be used. Using this approach a line on a page (or other similar device) with clearly defined end points is offered to the patient. The most preferred health state is placed at one end of the line and the least preferred health state, which may or may not be death, is placed at the other end of the line. Given a set of health states, the patient is then asked to place a mark on the line for each state, such that the distances between points is proportional to the patients preference for each state. The utility can be thus calculated by direct measurement of the relevant distances. This method is thus very similar to the visual analogue pain scale.

Utility and time

In the financial world it is well recognised that a sum of money that is available today is more valuable than the same sum that becomes available in the future. Bankers *discount* future cash flows by an *interest rate* to determine the *present value* of a future cash flow. In the same way it is clear that an individual may value more time spent in a particular health state *now* than time spent in that state in the future. The value of a 'year' can be discounted by a similar 'interest rate' (Fisher, 1989). Thus, in a decision tree that involves outcomes that will happen in the future, the patient may be willing to reduce the present value of that outcome by a certain amount. An example might be the value of conversion of an initially successful total knee replacement to a knee arthrodesis in 15 years time. The patient might assess the utility of conversion of a total knee replacement to an arthrodesis *now* as being 0.55. He discounts this by an 'interest rate' of 5% over 15 years to obtain a present value of 0.26.

The discount formula is:

$$T_p = \frac{1}{(1+r)^n}$$

where T_p = present value of time.
  r = discount 'rate' (expressed as a decimal value, *not* a percentage).
  n = number of years.

Utility and risk

Consider that a patient is indifferent about the outcome of a standard gamble between the certainty of accepting a life expectancy of 15 years, or the gamble of a 50% chance of a 50-year life expectancy or a 50% chance of a 0-year life expectancy. Fifteen years is said to be the *certainty equivalent* of the gamble. In this case this is not equivalent to the *expected value* of the gamble, which is 25 years. Such an individual is said to be *risk averse*. If the *certainty equivalent* of a gamble is more than the *expected value* of the gamble the individual is said to be *risk seeking*. Experience has shown that most patients are naturally *risk averse*, particularly when it comes to decisions about surgery.

Thus in the common situation of whether to accept the certainty of the current health state or accept the gamble of surgery, most people will define a utility for avoidance of surgery that would be *higher* than would be expected given the expected value of the surgery.

Quality-adjusted life-years

In circumstances where time affects the outcome of a decision it is often useful to consider the notion of *quality-adjusted life-years (QALYs)*. A *QALY* is simply arrived at by multiplying the time spent in any health state by its utility. Thus a clinical outcome after arthrodesis of the hip in a young patient of 25 years relief of pain (with a utility of U_a) followed by conversion to a total hip replacement (with a utility of U_r) for the remainder of his life (say 15 years) may be expected to have a *QALY* of $25U_a + 15U_h$.

Despite the attractiveness of this device, there are some assumptions that must be made about *QALYs* before they can be used – these are dealt with fully elsewhere (Weinstein *et al.,* 1980) but include the assumptions of *utility independence, proportional trade-off property* and *risk neutrality*. For most purposes, however, the use of *QALYS* can provide a useful insight into the value of an outcome.

Outcome and future uncertainty – the Markov process

Prognosis can often be described as a series of chance events for which the patient is at risk. For example a patient who has had successful spinal stenosis surgery is subject to an increasing risk of re-stenosis (Caputy *et al.,* 1992) as time elapses. Furthermore, repeat surgery is often successful in this circumstance. Further still, the patient is likely to be elderly and the natural forces of mortality due to age will cause an increasing chance of death as time progresses. To this natural risk of death must be added any *extra* risk of death associated with further surgery. It would be possible to model this state of affairs with a decision tree with a set of chance nodes for each possible event that might occur each year.

The tree would increase in width each year and rapidly become impossible to evaluate by hand or even by computer. With four outcomes possible each year, after only 10 years there would be 1.05×10^6 branches. Fortunately the vast majority of such a tree is repetitive, describing the same events year after year. It has become increasingly popular to model such problems using the Markov process (Beck and Pauker, 1983; Pauker and Kassirer, 1987; Fisher, 1989).

Markov models define a small set of allowable 'health states' that a patient may occupy in at any particular time. Allowable transitions between these states are specified and have a probability assigned to them in a *transition matrix*. The possible health states and their allowed transitions for the example given above is shown in Figure 4.4.

If one assumes that all transitions occur with equal probability each year, then the transition matrix remains constant each year, and the process can be modelled very elegantly using a *Markov chain* approach. Regardless of whether a constant or variable transition matrix is used, a vector of starting probabilities for each of the possible health states is required. In the example given above, health state no pain would have a probability of 1 and all others (pain, surgery, death) will have a probability of 0, if the starting condition was successful surgery for all patients.

The model can be 'run' by modifying the starting vector probabilities with each iteration according to the contents of the transition matrix and using this new vector of probabilities as the starting vector for the next iteration. At the end of each cycle the new probability distribution for each of the possible health states has been calculated. The model will need to be run for as large a number of iterations as is necessary to satisfy the requirements of either a *cohort* or *Monte Carlo* simulation. In the specific case where the transition probabilities do not change with time (the Markov chain) a precise algebraic solution is possible and no iteration is required. Table 4.4 shows an example transition matrix for the transitions possible in Figure 4.4.

Each iteration is accomplished algebraically by *matrix multiplication*[1] of the transition matrix by the probability vector representing the current state.

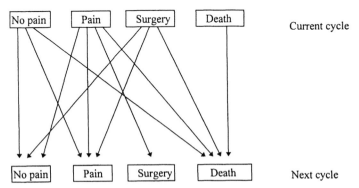

Figure 4.4 Health states in the successful post-spinal stenosis surgery patient. Arrows between states indicate allowable transitions between each cycle of the stimulation. The probability that each transition will occur is given in a separate transition matrix

[1] The Technique of matrix multiplication can be found in any introductory text on linear algebra. Tucker (1989) is an example. It should be noted that the order of multiplication is important.

Table 4.4 Hypothetical transition matrix for the prognosis of a patient having successful spinal stenosis surgery. A fixed death rate due to natural causes of 0.1 per year is assumed. Patients redevelop symptoms at a rate of 0.1 per year and are usually offered revision surgery that is usually successful, though this adds its own component to the natural death rate to increase it from 0.1 to 0.15. A small spontaneous resolution rate of pain is present. The column totals must add to 1.00 as each column represents the probability distribution in the next cycle of the health state in the current cycle represented by that column

| | Initial cycle | | | |
	No pain	Pain	Surgery	Death
No pain	0.8	0.05	0.65	0.0
Pain	0.1	0.05	0.2	0.0
Surgery	0.0	0.8	0.0	0.0
Death	0.1	0.1	0.15	1.0

The assumption of equal transition probabilities with time is often inappropriate. The natural death rate is an example. The death rate *increases* with age – values for instantaneous death rate can be obtained from life tables or by approximation by *Gompertz* functions (Strehler, 1960).

The age specific death can be approximated by the function (at least for over 30 years).

$$R_x = R_0 e^{ax}$$

where R_x is the death rate at age x, R_0 is the death rate at age 0 and a, the Gompertz coefficient, is the slope of the exponential term. Riggs (1990) has analysed mortality data for the United States and has expressed the results as a rate per 100 000 – using this format, the value for a is different though proportional to the above classic formula. Using 1986 data, Riggs has identified that for men, the relationship

$$log\ R_x = 0.036779x + 0.989557$$

holds true and that for women the corresponding relationship is

$$log\ R_x = 0.038911 + 0.604698$$

The Gompertz function gives an exponentially increasing mortality rate. Under some circumstances it may, however, be convenient to assume a constant death rate. Studies by Beck (1982a,b) have shown that when used with decision analysis techniques the optimal strategy is often not changed by this assumption. The DEALE (declining exponential approximation of life expectancy) approximation of life expectancy has the benefit of simplicity. Given the *average* population life expectancy of an individual of say 10 years, the *average* mortality *rate* can be calculated as the reciprocal of the average life expectancy –0.10. If that individual is exposed to extra risk from a disease or procedure of say 0.05, the disease specific mortality rate can be added to the population average mortality rate to obtain the patient specific average mortality rate –0.15. The reciprocal of this figure will give the new average life expectancy –6.7 years. This technique is used in Table 4.4 to add the risk of surgery to the underlying average mortality rate.

Simulation

The output of each iteration of a Markov process yields a table of probabilities corresponding to the likelihood that an individual will be in each of the health states for that period. Two further processes are now required to obtain a measure of *expected value* of the process.

Cohort simulation

In this method, a large (typically 100 000) number of patients are followed as a cohort. The cohort begins in an initial distribution of states and after each cycle the cohort is reallocated to states according to the transition matrix. The model is run until stability is achieved, typically by all patients being in the 'dead' state. At each stage, the number of patients in each state is multiplied by the utility value of that state to represent the quality-adjusted life-years spent in that state. The Total *QALYs* for that period can be summed and if necessary multiplied by a discounting function (described above). The *QALY* figures in all periods are now summed and divided by the total number in the cohort to give the *expected value* of the outcome.

Table 4.5 shows an example cohort simulation for the above hypothetical spinal stenosis prognosis. The transition matrix in Table 4.4 has been modified to include a Gompertz age dependent function for population mortality rate. The starting condition was that of a fit 60-year-old male having just undergone successful spinal stenosis decompression.

Monte Carlo simulation

In this approach, patients traverse the Markov process one by one. At each transition phase the next state is determined by the transition matrix and the output of a random number generator. Each patient therefore changes state

Table 4.5 Hypothetical Markov cohort simulation for the outcome of successful spinal stenosis decompression in a 60-year-old male. A time discount factor of 0.05 was used

Time (years)	No pain	Pain	Revision surgery	Death	Discount factor	QALY
0	100 000	0	0	0	1.000	100 000.0
1	78 210	8690	0	13 100	0.952	78 623.8
2	61 237	7468	5974	25 321	0.907	60 555.9
3	50 950	7344	5072	36 634	0.864	48 499.2
4	41 997	6153	4923	46 927	0.823	38 297.1
5	34 566	5193	4066	56 175	0.784	30 073.9
.	.	.	.	.	.	.
.	.	.	.	.	.	.
.	.	.	.	.	.	.
15	1 631	250	198	97 920	0.481	873.5
16	1 019	157	124	98 701	0.458	519.6
17	609	94	74	99 223	0.436	295.7
18	346	54	42	99 558	0.416	160.2
19	186	29	23	99 762	0.396	82.0
20	94	15	11	99 880	0.377	39.4
Utility	1.0	0.5	0.3	0.0		

Total quality adjusted life years for cohort **440 632**

Quality adjusted life years per patient **4.41**

according to the laws of chance. When the patient enters the state 'dead' the simulation ends for that patient. The cycle count for that patient represents his remaining lifetime. Along the way he has occupied various health states and has accumulated *quality-adjusted life-years* in much the same way as in the cohort approach. The *QALYs* can also be discounted or adjusted for risk aversion. After a sufficiently large sample (say 1000) has been modelled the mean *QALY* score can be calculated. While this method is computationally more expensive than the cohort method, it does allow calculation of measures of variability about the mean.

An example

Consider now the problem posed at the beginning of this chapter – whether a patient should have a spinal fusion for chronic back pain. There is, of course, no right or wrong answer to this, though formulation of the question in a decision analysis form may give one some useful clinical insight. Meta-analysis studies by Turner *et al.* (1992, 1993) of the reported literature have shown that the average estimate of good outcomes following spinal fusion is 68% with a wide range (16–95%). What has actually been reported is the positive predictive value of fusion in each of the individual study populations. As we have seen, one possible explanation for the large range in outcomes is that the *prior probability* of a successful outcome varied in those papers. It may not immediately be obvious what this statement means, however it has to do with the prevalence of whatever condition it is that *does* respond to spinal fusion in the sample populations.

Figure 4.5 shows a possible set of probabilities and utilities for the simple decision of whether to perform spinal fusion for chronic back pain. Two simple outcomes have used – success or failure. Probability values for the non-operative option have been selected based on the natural history of back pain as described by Frymoyer (1988) and Andersson (1983), showing that the majority of episodes of low back pain settle conservatively in about 12 weeks. If an individual's back pain has not settled in this time it is unlikely to settle, and that after 3–6 months there is only about a 0.05 probability of settling. Hence the probability of *failure* (staying the same) of no treatment is 0.95. A reasonably

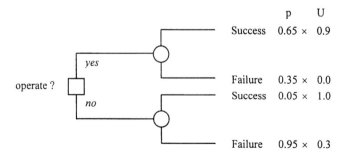

Figure 4.5 Decision tree for spinal fusion for back pain

average probability of successful surgery of 0.65 has been chosen based on the above meta-analysis.

Clearly the least attractive patient outcome is failed surgery – this would attract a utility value of 0. The most favourable outcome for a patient would be successful avoidance of surgery (i.e. spontaneous resolution of pain), this therefore would have a utility value of 1. The intermediate utility values have been chosen arbitrarily for this example, though in clinical situations the patient would be asked to assess these values using one of the methods outlined above. Using these figures the expected value of the decision to operate is 0.585 compared to the non-operative value of 0.335; hence the rational patient, given these probabilities of outcome and having chosen these utilities, would choose surgery. How, though, would his decision differ if he were presented with different probabilities of outcome, or chose different utility values?

Sensitivity analysis

Patients are naturally risk averse, and the probability of a successful outcome following spinal fusion has been shown to vary widely. Sensitivity analysis aims therefore to examine the effects of varying these parameters. Figure 4.6 shows a graph of the value of the decision 'to operate' when compared to various values of the utility of failed conservative treatment. Increases in this utility value indicate risk aversion when compared to failed surgery. Three graphs are displayed, each for differing probability values of successful surgery. The value of the decision has been defined as the expected value of the surgical branch of the tree minus the expected value of the non-surgical branch. Thus positive values favour surgery and negative values favour no surgery. Similar analysis can be carried out for all variables compared to all other variables. The value of sensitivity analysis is that it often leads to insights into what *threshold* values variables need to exceed before a decision will change. In Figure 4.7 the patient can tolerate an increasing utility of failed conservative treatment up to a level of

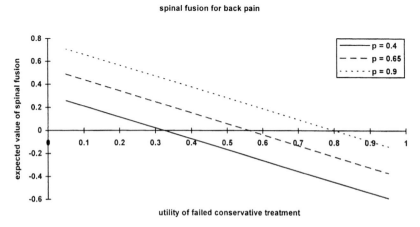

Figure 4.6 Sensitivity analysis of the expected value of spinal fusion for back pain based on the decision tree in Figure 4.5. The different p values are for probability of successful surgery

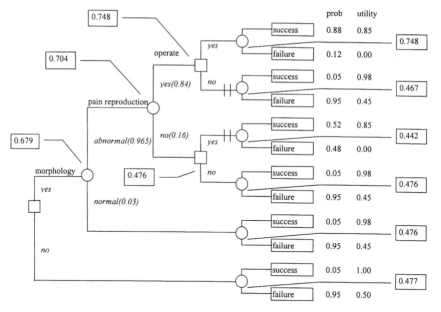

Figure 4.7 Decision tree representing the whether to perform a discogram on a patient with chronic back pain. Probability data from Colhourn (1988). The values in boxes represent the intermediate value of each node. A decision node takes on the highest value of its alternative (representing a rational decision). Paths from decision nodes marked with double vertical lines represent non-preferred alternatives

0.56 before surgery would be rejected, given that the assumed probability of successful surgery is 0.65.

A more complex example

How does the performance of a test change the outcome of a decision? In the assessment of patients being considered for spinal fusion, a discogram is often performed. If the morphology of the disc is abnormal (torn or degenerative) *and* there is typical pain reproduction then fusion is offered. Colhourn *et al.* (1988) have published the results of a highly selected group of patients with chronic back pain in whom spinal fusion had been successfully achieved. For the purposes of this discussion, patients with isolated disc resorption have been excluded from that data. Information is available for the success or failure of spinal fusion for patients with positive or negative discograms, both with and without concordant pain reproduction. Thus values for both positive and negative predicative value, sensitivity and specificity are available for the test of discography as a predictor of success of spinal fusion. The positive predictive value of 0.89 is one of the highest reported. Further evidence that this population is a highly selected one is shown by the very low incidence of normal disc morphology (0.03). Figure 4.7 shows the appropriate decision tree using the data of Colhourn *et al.* It can be seen that the tree has two extra decision nodes for choices about surgery based on the results of the discography. With the arbitrary utility values that have been assumed for this exercise, it can be seen that surgery is preferred if a painful *and* degenerative disc is identified, but not if the disc is only degenerative. At each of these two decision nodes the value of the *preferred* action is taken as the utility value for the more proximal outcome node. It can be seen, however, that varying some of the utility values will change the choice at each of the more terminal decision nodes. Thus with low values for utility of failed conservative treatment (an increasing gap between failed surgery and failed conservative treatment, representing patient risk aversion) the patient will initially have surgery regardless of pain provocation on discography, at intermediate levels he will choose surgery only with pain provocation and at higher values still he will reject surgery under all circumstances and there would be no value in doing the test.

Conclusion

Decision analysis, in its simplest form, can almost be used at the bedside. For this purpose the surgeon can estimate probability values of alternative outcomes for a particular patient based on his experience, knowledge of the literature and the individual patient. Where relevant literature is not available to obtain these probabilities, the judicious use of probability theory and in particular Bayes' theorem may be used to *revise* probability obtained from other, though not entirely applicable literature. For individual clinical decisions, it would be unusual for anything more than the simplest of decision trees to be constructed, though the clinician could encapsulate quite a complex series of events in each outcome.

More formal decision analysis techniques are appropriate when analysis of populations is undertaken – for example, when asking generic questions about the value of a particular procedure. In such circumstances more complex decision trees may need to be built. If the value of a particular outcome has time related uncertainty then simulation with a Markov process may prove useful. In orthopaedic practice, outcomes in the elderly are usually altered by the natural death rate and hence are ideal candidates for this method. It would appear that assessment of the outcome of joint replacement surgery may also be suited to this method, particularly as it is common to report results of such procedures with survival analysis.

Current public and Government opinion is such that as clinicians we are being increasingly asked to justify some of the decisions we make. Decision analysis is one tool that may allow us to achieve this goal.

References

Adams ID, Chan M, Clifford PC, de Dombal FT *et al.* (1986) Computer-aided diagnosis of acute abdominal pain: a multicentre study. *Br. Med. J.*; **293**: 800–804

Albert A, Harris E (1987) *Multivariate interpretation of clinical laboratory data.* New York: Marcel Dekker Inc.

Andersson GB, Svensson O (1983) The intensity of work recovery in low back pain. *Spine*; **8**: 880–884

Beck RJ, Pauker SG (1983) The Markov process in medical prognosis. *Med. Decis. Making*; **3**: 419–458

Beck JR, Kassirer JP, Pauker SG (1982a) A convenient approximation of life expectancy (the 'DEALE') I. Validation of the method. *Am. J. Med.*; **73**: 883–888

Beck JR, Pauker SG, Gottlieb JE, Klein K, Kassirer JP (1982b) A convenient approximation of life expectancy (the 'DEALE') II. Use in medical decision-making. *Am. J. Med.*; **73**: 889–897

Caputy AJ, Luessenhop AJ (1992) Long-term evaluation of decompressive surgery for degenerative lumbar stenosis. *J. Neurosurg.*; **77**: 669–672

Colhourn E, McCall IW, Williams L, Cassar Pullicino VN (1988) Provocation discography as a guide to planning operations on the spine. *J. Bone Jt Surg.*; **70-B**: 267–271

de Dombal FT, Leaper DJ, Stainland JR, McCann AP, Horrocks JC (1972) Computer-aided diagnosis of acute abdominal pain. *Br. Med. J.*; **2**: 9–13

Fisher WS (1989) Decision analysis: a tool of the future: an application to unruptured arteriovenous malformations. *Neurosurgery*; **24**: 129–135

Frymoyer JW (1988) Back pain and sciatica. *N. Eng. J. Med.*; **318**: 291–300

Horrocks JC, McCann AP, Stainland JR, Leaper DJ, de Dombal FT (1972) Computer-aided diagnosis: Description of an adaptable system, an operational experience with 2,034 Cases. *Br. Med. J.*; **2**: 5–9

Knill-Jones RP (1987) Diagnostic systems as an aid to clinical decision making. *Br. Med. J.*; **295**: 1392–1396

Llewelyn H, Hopkins A (eds) (1993) *Analysing How We Reach Clinical Decisions.* London: Royal College of Physicians of London

Pauker SG, Kassirer JP (1987) Decision analysis. *N. Eng. J. Med.*; **316**: 250–258

Riggs JE (1990) Longitudinal Gompertzian analysis of adult mortality in the U.S., 1900–1986. *Mechanisms of Ageing and Development*; **54**: 235–247

Spiegelhalter DJ, Knill-Jones RP (1984) Statistical and knowledge-based approaches to clinical support systems with an application in gastroenterology. *J. R. Statist. Soc. (Series A)*; **147**: 35–77

Strehler BL, Mildvan AS (1960) General theory of mortality and ageing. *Science*; **132**: 14–21

Thornton JG, Lilford RJ, Johnson N (1992) Decision analysis in medicine. *Br. Med. J.*; **304**: 1099–1103

Tucker A (1989) *A Unified Introduction to Linear Algebra.* New York: Macmillan

Turner JA, Ersek M, Herron L, Haselkorn J, Kent D, Ciol MA, Deyo R (1992) Patient outcomes after lumbar spinal fusions. *JAMA*; **268**: 907–911

Turner JA, Herron L, Deyo RA (1993) Meta-analysis of the results of lumbar spine fusion. *Acta Orthop. Scand. (suppl. 251)*; **64**: 120–122

Weinstein MC, Fineberg HV (1980) *Clinical decision analysis.* Philadelphia: W.B. Saunders

Chapter 5

Informed consent and the practical ethical issues

P Alderson

Introduction

Clinical trials are an important means of assessment though they raise practical difficulties. This chapter reviews some of the ethical problems which trials, in particular, raise. The means of resolving these problems will be considered. One central concern of ethics is patients' consent; this chapter begins by defining informed and voluntary consent to treatment and to research. Research is based on uncertainty, the ethics and means of sharing uncertainty, information and decision-making with anxious patients are considered. Problems and benefits of respecting patients' consent to various types of assessment, ranging from assessment as a routine part of treatment to assessment in audit and research, are reviewed. There are sections on the use of written information, with the basic information which patients require if they are to be able to give informed consent, and on the role of research ethics committees.

The development of consent

International support for consent was first stated in 1947 in the *Nuremberg Code*, which begins: '1. The voluntary consent of the human subject is absolutely essential'. The 'voluntariness' of a freely made decision is stressed, without any 'force, fraud, deceit, duress, overreaching or other ulterior form of constraint or coercion'. The first aspect of consent is that it is a choice; the person can freely say 'yes' or 'no' – or 'maybe later'. Secondly, the *Code* says that any competent person can make an 'understanding and enlightened decision'. People can use their own wisdom and discretion. Thirdly, the *Code* lists the details doctors should explain, to enable people to make an informed decision.

In this chapter 'consent' means a freely made, wise and informed decision, though the phrase needs qualifying. Someone might feel forced into giving consent through fear of disease, pain or disability. These are unavoidable pressures; 'freely made' therefore means free from avoidable pressures which health professionals and others might exert. 'Wise' means in the patients' own interests as they perceive them; other people might think a decision foolish, but competent adults have the right in Anglo-American law to refuse or consent to proposed treatment as they choose. Decisions about children have to be clearly not against their best interests (Nicholson, 1985). 'Informed' does not mean 'fully informed'; it means reasonably informed about the main issues, which will be summarised later.

The *Nuremberg Code* set high standards for consent to 'non-therapeutic' research. For years, consent to treatment and to research associated with it attracted less interest. In 1964 the Medical Research Council stated that because of 'the willingness of the subject to be guided by the judgement of the medical attendant' if the doctor is satisfied that the procedure being researched will benefit the patient 'he may assume the patient's consent' as he would assume consent to 'established practice' (MRC, 1964). However, over the past 30 years, attitudes have changed, and standards of consent to treatment have gradually become closer to the standards required for research.

The British government does not legislate on consent to clinical treatment or research, instead it issues guidance (such as Department of Health, 1990 and 1991a). *The Patient's Charter* (DH, 1991b) states that 'Every citizen has the right:

- to be given a clear explanation of any treatment proposed, including risks and any alternatives before you decide whether you will agree to the treatment;
- to choose whether or not you wish to take part in medical research'.

The Charter and other guidance do not have the force of law and only describe voluntary standards. However, the 'carrot' of official guidance is supplemented by the 'stick' of the law courts, and case law on consent. If a dissatisfied patient sues a doctor for not giving enough information, the court would want to be assured that high standards had been observed. The court would regard a signed consent form as necessary but not sufficient evidence, and would be more concerned to see that the patient actually had been given reasonable information and had not been deceived or coerced. Yet the court's standard of required information is what a 'reasonable doctor' would decide to tell (*Bolam v Friern HMC* [1957] 2 All ER 118). British courts very much rely on medical advice. In contrast, the North American standard is more exacting; it is based on what the 'prudent patient' might want to know.

Consent to treatment and to research

It is thought that British courts would require higher standards for consent to research than for consent to treatment alone. Though there is so far no case law on consent to research, lawyers advise researchers to take extra care over consent (Royal College of Physicians, 1986, 1990). There has been a long debate over 'therapeutic' and 'non-therapeutic' research and whether different standards of consent should apply. Part of the confusion, I suggest, arises through use of the term 'therapeutic'. It is a vague, unscientific word, expressing future hopes, but seldom present realities. If the treatment turns out to be useless or harmful, it is scarcely therapeutic. Research itself, as systematic investigation and data collection and analysis, is not therapeutic, even if the findings eventually benefit countless future patients. 'Non-therapeutic' research can bring equal or greater benefits, for example, in studies when surgery is withheld and is demonstrated to be unnecessary. Spinal fusion is no longer routine for most scoliotic curves between 20 and 40°.

One way to clarify the debate about levels of consent is to look at consent to research in sections. Does the research investigate treatment? If so, might it directly benefit the patient? Or are the effects too uncertain to promise direct benefit? Is the patient in a non-treatment, such as a control or placebo, group? Are people simply donating samples or other information? If the research does involve treatment, this can be explained in detail. Then the extra questions which the research itself raises can be discussed. The details to give on treatment and on research will be summarised later, but first here is an example about unravelling the overlap between treatment and research.

Mrs A, aged 72, will have her second hip replacement next week. She understands the treatment and its likely effects from her surgeon's explanations, her experience of her first operation, the differing results for some friends who have also had hip replacements and a magazine article written by a surgeon. The surgeon invites Mrs A to join a randomised trial of two slightly different types of hips, and to attend extra hospital appointments for assessment annually. Mrs A understands that the surgery is intended to benefit her directly. The idea of research causes her some worry, and she does not relish the prospect of long extra journeys to hospital. Yet she considers that if, in future, she needs another replacement and more is known about the optimal type of hip she might benefit. When Mrs A's younger sister, Mrs C, visits her after her operation, the surgeon tells Mrs C about some research investigations into the early stages of arthritis. Mrs C agrees to help with the research. She knows that she will not benefit directly, and might feel some discomfort, but she hopes that progress will be made in the treatment and prevention of arthritis which affects many of her friends.

Uncertainty and equipoise

Research starts from uncertainty. People appreciate the need for research when they accept that current knowledge is uncertain, and there are questions waiting to be answered. Mrs A was startled at first to find that her surgeon did not know which was the optimal hip replacement. She worried that she might be in the less fortunate group, though she came to terms with her fears and agreed that the research was worthwhile.

Yet recognising and tolerating uncertainty can be hard for patients and professionals. For example, Dr M, a general practitioner who was also an osteopath, wanted to demonstrate that osteopathy was more effective than orthodox methods in treating certain conditions. He was already convinced and felt unable to ask his patients for their consent to be randomised, as he expected them all to refuse and to opt for osteopathy. He decided to randomise them without informing them of the alternative options. However, before patients can give reasonably informed consent, they need to know about the research programme, the treatment alternatives, and that they can reject each option and refuse to enter the trial.

Dr M's convictions made it unethical for him personally to offer his patients what he believed to be a less effective treatment. Yet his certainty about the results would then appear to prevent him from doing ethical research. However, equipoise offers a way through this impasse, as a means towards high scientific and ethical standards in research. Equipoise is the belief that no arm in a particular trial is known to offer greater harm or benefit than any other arm. This belief enables clinicians sincerely to recommend to their patients that they enter a randomised trial. The problem remains as to how doctors can conduct trials when they do not personally have this equipoise. Freedman (1987) advises researchers to accept collective or clinical equipoise, based on current unresolved disagreement among the medical profession. Some researchers cite this collective uncertainty as an ethical imperative to treat patients through trials, instead of basing clinical decisions on opinion or on 'biased' personal experience (Collins *et al.,* 1992). However, 'trialists' have been criticised for over-stating their claims to uncertainty, since phase III trials have to be based on partial knowledge gathered from earlier phases. This knowledge can help clinicians and patients to make partly informed choices (Botros, 1990).

Dr M could achieve equipoise in several ways. He could accept that, until comparative outcomes have been demonstrated scientifically and statistically through trials, there is room for reasonable doubt. Apparently improved outcomes may result from placebo or halo effects or from other 'contaminating variables'. He could also accept that more needs to be known about which types of cases respond best to which treatments, or agree that the trial might provide answers to other important questions. Dr M could accept that, though he personally has no doubts, many other doctors do have doubts, and he could explain this to his patients. He could rely on his patients' own equipoise or uncertainty, offer them the options, explain the clinical uncertainty and, if asked to, his own opinions, and see how many people agree to be randomised. He might find that some people support the research, some definitely prefer one option and refuse to be randomised, and some people feel very anxious when told that the doctor they thought to be omniscient is not. If many patients refuse to enter the trial, he could decide to redesign it to satisfy his own and his patients' standards. This is beginning to happen in some cancer trials which have had very disparate treatment arms. Patients are now being more fully consulted during the design stages to help to plan research which is more widely acceptable. Finally, Dr M might decide that his own certainties prevent him from doing ethical research on this question, and he should leave the work to more sceptical colleagues.

The doctor's roles as clinician and as researcher complement one another in the responsible search for optimal care. Yet they can also conflict, when patients feel that they have been 'used as guinea pigs in research', or when patients are very shocked to be informed about clinical uncertainty. Whereas the clinician tries to provide the best care for the individual concerned, the researcher risks randomising people to sub-optimal treatment in the hope of benefiting many future patients. There can be a conflict of loyalties to present and to future patients. In the Hippocratic tradition, doctors have assumed that their advice, optimism and reassurance are as valuable to patients as the actual treatment. In contrast, modern scientific medicine demands that, when treatment has not yet been systematically evaluated, doctors should temper optimism with impartial information, caution and the courage to tolerate and test uncertainty. Reassurance and the placebo effect 'I will please you' or the 'feel-good factor' play a crucial part in much healing and palliative care. Yet scientific research demands that the 'contaminating' placebo effects are reduced, such as by double blind placebo controlled drug trials, or in trials with no placebo arm, but when everyone is honestly told, 'We do not yet know which is the best treatment for you'.

Sharing information and decisions

Honesty can undermine trust and hope. Some patients still expect to trust their doctor's judgement entirely and to have little information or share in deciding about their treatment. However, uninformed patients can later feel betrayed if the treatment has a poor outcome, if they hear about alternatives which they would have preferred, or if they find that, unknowingly, they have been in a trial (Faulder, 1985). People also report increased trust in doctors who inform them honestly (Alderson, 1990). A teenager waiting for spinal surgery described how she fainted when informed about the risk of paralysis, but that during the weeks of waiting for her operation she came to terms with the knowledge and preferred to know. Some surgeons consider that children as young as 7 or 8 years can understand the risks of paralysis, and that if these are significant these must be explained; nurses report finding well-informed and well-prepared patients less distressed and more co-operative (Alderson, 1993).

Blind faith in medicine is challenged by aspects of modern society such as consumer and rights movements, and public education about science. When people receive a serious diagnosis and alarming news about proposed treatment, inevitably they are shocked and distressed. Many clinicians are reluctant to increase distress by warning patients about uncertainty. The United States doctrine of therapeutic privilege allows discretion to doctors to withhold information from people who are likely to be extremely distressed. However, repeated research shows that most patients say they wanted more information than they were given (King, 1986). Research with children shows that they very much want to be informed about their serious treatment including details about risk and uncertainty (Bearison, 1991; Ellis and Leventhal, 1993), so how much more do adults wish to know?

On sharing in decision-making, a study of 120 experienced young patients aged 8 to 15 years having major orthopaedic surgery (on average their fifth operation) found that just over one in ten thought they were 'the main decider' about consenting to the surgeon's recommendation; over one-third thought they shared the decision with adults, and half thought that the adults had decided. When they were asked who should be the 'main decider', just over one in six said it should be the child concerned, well over one-third wanted to share decision-making with adults, and almost as many wanted to leave the adults to decide (Alderson, 1993, p. 164).

Some surgeons consulted children when there were 'grey areas', borderline cases of scoliosis or uneven leg lengths, or when assessments of pain or mobility included the child's estimations. When doctors were asked the age at which certain mature children could begin to make complex, informed and wise decisions about major surgery their responses varied. Replies ranged from respecting the decision of 7-year-olds, to, 'Never. They take my advice. If they do not like it, they can go elsewhere'. However, two surgeons who initially said 'never' were asked when they began to take children's agreement to surgical leg lengthening seriously, and they both replied, 'At 7 or 8 years'. Another surgeon who said, 'At 16 or 18 years' later agreed that he had just asked a 14-year-old to consider the surgery options which he had explained to her, and write to him with her decision. Sometimes, surgeons' actual practice appears to be more liberal than their beliefs about involving patients (Alderson, 1993, pp. 146–158).

Research with women having breast cancer surgery found a similar range of desires about sharing in making decisions on proposed surgical treatment: 16% wanted to 'decide for themselves', 34% to share decisions with their surgeon or other professionals, 20% preferred others to decide for them, and 30% gave complicated and qualified replies, such as 'there was no choice'. However, they were clearer about their wish to share in making decisions on whether to take part in research: 47% wanted to decide for themselves, 21% to decide with their doctor, 24% to leave others to decide, and 9% gave other replies (Alderson et al., 1994, p. 171).

Consent to research has only begun to be widely debated in recent years. Expectations among health professionals and the general public are changing towards informing and involving patients and research subjects more fully. Yet there are warnings that this can distress and anger, for example, some cancer patients (Fallowfield et al., 1994), and reduce enrolment into trials (Tobias and Souhami, 1993; Baum, 1994). Clinicians need to develop further their skills in discovering how much patients want to be informed, and in sharing clear information.

Patient information leaflets

To translate clinical information into clear lay terms can be extremely difficult. Some clinicians argue that lay people cannot understand clinical concepts; others blame poor communication rather than patients' abilities, and say that even young children can grasp complex and distressing knowledge when it is carefully presented. There is growing use of written information to explain surgical treatment and research. When writing information, a question and answer format is helpful. Start by thinking about what the patients might want to know, rather than what the surgeon may want to say. For example, some surgeons simply explain the nature and purpose of the planned operation. Yet many patients are far more concerned about many details of the likely after-effects on them and on their daily life. Whereas the surgeon thinks of consent relating to a few hours in the operating room, consent is actually being requested for a whole package of possibly months of multi-disciplinary care from admission to the follow-up clinics. With research and assessment, lay people want to know: What is the point of the project? Whom might it help and how? How could it affect me?

Well-written leaflets serve several purposes. They can help people to talk over the project with the researchers and back at home with their relatives or family doctor. This enables them to know more clearly which questions to ask, in order to give informed consent or refusal. For those who do consent, a leaflet to keep can help them to recall the agreed details – doing exercises or attending clinics – and why these matter. When people are well informed in advance, then mistakes, problems and complaints are less likely to arise, and there is less risk of wasted time and money over failed projects. The use of plain English, diagrams and drawings help people with low reading levels and those with learning difficulties to understand. Such leaflets are also easier to translate accurately into other languages for people who speak little or no English. Written explanations cannot replace spoken ones, but they can complement and enrich them. Whereas some people find leaflets very helpful, others do not, so that giving a leaflet should not be confused with assuming that the person has been fully informed.

Ethics committee members, funding bodies and other assessors can quickly gain an overall view of the project from a patient information leaflet. Sometimes these show up strengths or faults in the research design more clearly than a long protocol does. Leaflets help to ensure that all the staff affected by a project are informed. Nurses, junior surgical staff and technicians can then respond to patients' enquiries using clear terms from a well-written leaflet. Well-informed staff are more likely to give informed and efficient support to the project.

Content

The main points to include as the basis of informed consent are drawn from decades of guidelines such as the *Declaration of Helsinki* (World Medical Association 1964/1987). These have been summarised into a short booklet about writing and designing patient information leaflets (CERES, 1994a). Leaflets on treatment should explain:

- the problem or condition to be treated;
- the purpose of proposed treatment;
- the nature of the treatment, such as the investigations, surgical technique, types of anaesthesia and pain relief, follow up care and tests, use of adjuvant treatment, physiotherapy and any mobility aids to be used;
- the likely time to be spent in hospital, in bed, in plaster, away from work or school, and before full recovery;
- the likely benefits, and the chances of complete or partial success;
- the risks, how serious and how likely they are to occur;
- the harms, such as inevitable pain, needles, drips, drains, or scarring;
- possible alternative treatments, and the likely outcome if treatment is withheld or deferred.

There are some common objections to leaflets. For example:

Details will vary for each patient. Yes, so the leaflets can give only the range of likely events, leaving the staff to give more specific data, and to add details such as likely waiting times before elective surgery.

Patients get angry if, for instance, they have to stay in plaster or in bed for weeks longer than the leaflet states. Yes, so it is vital to use phrases like 'about', 'roughly', 'in most cases', 'to give you some idea...' Some information is better than nothing; it has been known for people to go home to spend weeks in bed in heavy plasters, without first realising that they would need to obtain a bedpan. It is not helpful to leave them to read this in a discharge leaflet on the way home.

Details keep changing and leaflets get out of date. They do, as when success rates rise or day surgery is introduced, so the leaflets need to be reviewed every few months, and checked with all the relevant staff. This takes time but is also a means of helping the staff as well as the patients to keep up to date.

Leaflets on research, besides explaining the treatment being researched, should also state:

- the purpose of the research, the questions it addresses and why;
- the research methods, the tests and treatments involved, each different treatment arm, if relevant, with its pros and cons;

- the hoped-for benefits of the research and whether these are likely to benefit the research subject directly;
- the risks or harms to subjects of additional research interventions;
- costs and inconvenience such as time needed off work or school to attend extra clinics;
- details about reimbursement and indemnity;
- names of the project sponsors and director/co-ordinator;
- the name and 'phone number of a researcher to contact when needed;
- details of respect for privacy and confidentiality, such as using anonymous records or means of limiting access to named records.

Each of these topics involves further details, such as the meaning of relevant terms, like 'randomised trial' or 'placebo'. Many people assume that 'consent' means doctors telling patients what they plan to do. It is helpful to include a note on consent, such as:

Do I have to say 'yes'?
No. You can refuse to take part in research. No one should feel forced to agree.
Can I change my mind?
Perhaps you have agreed to take part in the research but later change your mind. You can opt out at any time, even if you have signed a consent form. You do not have to give a reason, though giving a reason might help the researchers.
What will happen if I say 'no'?
You may worry that if you refuse to take part in research, this will affect your medical care. The researchers should explain that you will have the best possible care as a patient, whether or not you agree to help with the research. You may want to ask what kind of care you will have if you are not taking part in the research (from CERES, 1994b).

The list of topics may look daunting, and guaranteed to elicit 100% refusal rates. Yet people are willing to take part in research despite considerable risk and inconvenience, and the details can be fitted into two or four sides of A4 paper.

Research ethics committees – RECs

This section considers the part played by research ethics committees in assessing research and standards of consent. In the United States, hospitals have ethics committees to review research and also to review contentious treatment decisions. In Britain, the relevance of ethics committees to surgical research is still often questioned. These are some of the main objections to RECs.

- REC members tend to be ignorant about surgical research methods and their task is mainly to review drugs trials.
- RECs are under-funded and rely on many hours of unpaid work. This makes them inefficient and poorly administered.
- One effect is that RECs do not have members who are expert in assessing the potential harms and benefits of research.

- They do not guarantee that good research is supported and poor research prevented.
- RECs can be dominated by a few members who are determined to accept or reject certain protocols.
- RECs waste vast amounts of researchers' time and money through costly review procedures, especially when multi-centre research has to be submitted to many committees.
- RECs delay projects, which can cause havoc with employment contracts. In some cases, researchers have to move to a new post before they can complete, or even begin, their work. New staff may have to be recruited and trained.
- Funders do not cover the high costs of applications to RECs; some RECs now charge for reviewing protocols. How can these costs be met?
- There is a danger that researchers pass on ethical responsibility to RECs and conduct research which they privately believe is useless or harmful, arguing in public that 'it must be all right it's been approved'.
- RECs nit-pick over small points and disagree with one another's decisions about protocols. This shows that REC review is inefficient and unscientific.

Arguments in favour of RECs include the following.

- RECs can help to prevent poor and harmful research and to raise standards of promising protocols.
- They help to protect research subjects and to act as a buffer between the interests of subjects and of research when these conflict.
- They help to safeguard standards of informed and willing consent and of respect for confidentiality.
- RECs can challenge researchers who overestimate the supposed benefits of their work and under-play the costs.
- They help to raise awareness and serious concern about ethical standards of research.
- One effect is that many researchers now consider ethical aspects as a basic part of research design, rather than adding on these aspects as an afterthought.
- By involving lay members, RECs encourage researchers to take more account of lay views of research and to be accountable to them.
- RECs help to raise standards of clear information for research subjects.
- RECs can check that the research suits their area, when they see that too many protocols are proposed for under-staffed wards or clinics, or that leaflets in other languages and link-workers should be included in the research plans.
- Review by several local RECs is a safeguard, as errors and harms overlooked by some RECs are noticed by others.
- Disagreement among RECs is an important means of working towards higher ethical standards through practical debate about actual protocols.

An international survey found that two countries with very little debate about medical research, with rigid, centralised review systems dominated by researchers, and with recent reports of abusive research, are Germany and Japan (McNeill, 1993). The author contends that ethical review of research is not primarily scientific or moral; it is political – a process of different factions arguing for different values. REC review attempts to balance the conflicting interests of rigorous scientific enquiry with compassion and respect, and the interests of research subjects against those of potential future beneficiaries of research. This is partly why RECs differ in their conclusions, which depend on their various memberships. There is not necessarily a correct balance of conflicting values and the process of discovering reasonable solutions can evolve ways of combining higher ethical and scientific standards.

Consent is frequently presented in clinical journal papers and letter columns as a nuisance, a legal disruption to the smooth course of clinical treatment and research. However, growing numbers of surgeons agree that working with patients' consent has advantages. Informed patients who are committed to their treatment are more likely to benefit than those who feel ignorant and unwillingly coerced. People who understand the purpose of research and assessment can co-operate more fully and may contribute valuable insights, which the researchers had not considered, concerning the process and the outcome of treatment. Adequate assessment of the main tasks of orthopaedic care, to relieve and prevent disability, deformity and pain, has to take account of patients' own estimations and experiences. Their reports are more likely to be useful and relevant when they are informed and willing partners in the assessment. Surgeons who respect and inform their patients help to increase public understanding of, and support for, the value of well-planned assessment and research.

References

Alderson P (1990) *Choosing for Children: Parents' Consent to Surgery.* Oxford: Oxford University Press

Alderson P (1993) *Children's Consent to Surgery.* Buckingham: Open University Press

Alderson P, Madden M, Oakley A, Wilkins R (1994) *Women's Views of Breast Cancer Treatment and Research.* London: Social Science Research Unit and Cancer Research Campaign

Baum M (1994) Medical ethics: the four principles may clash. *B. M. J.*; **309**: 1159

Bearison D (1991) *'They Never Want to Tell You': Children Talk About Cancer.* London: Harvard University Press

Botros S (1990) Equipoise, consent and the ethics of randomised clinical trials. In Byrne P (ed.) *Ethics and Law in Health Care and Research.* London: King's Fund

CERES (1994a) *Spreading the Word on Research or Patient Information, How Can We Get It Better?* London: Consumers for Ethics in Research (CERES PO Box 1365, London N16 0BW, £2.50 each)

CERES (1994b) *Medical Research and YOU.* London: CERES (free leaflet)

Collins R, Doll R, Peto R (1992) Ethics of clinical trials. In: Williams C (ed.) *Introducing New Treatments for Cancer: Practical, Ethical and Legal Problems.* Chichester: Wiley

Department of Health (1990) *Patient Consent to Examination or Treatment.* (HC(90)22)

Department of Health (1991a) *Local Research Ethics Committees.* London: HMSO

Department of Health (1991b) *The patient's charter.* London: HMSO

Ellis R, Leventhal B (1993) Information needs and decision-making preferences of children with cancer. *Psycho-oncology*; **2,4**: 277–284

Fallowfield L, Hall A, Maguire P, Baum M, A'Hean R (1994) Psychological effects of being offered a choice of surgery for breast cancer. *B. M. J.*; **309**: 448

Faulder C (1985) *Whose Body Is It?* London: Virago

Freedman B (1987) Equipoise and the ethics of clinical research. *N. Engl. J. Med.*; **317**:141–145

King J (1986) *Informed Consent.* London: Bulletin of Medical Ethics Supplement 3

McNeill P (1993) *The Ethics and Politics of Human Experimentation.* Cambridge: Cambridge University Press

Medical Research Council (1964) *Annual Report 1962–3: Responsibility in Investigations on Human Subjects.* London: HMSO

Nicholson R (1985) *Medical Research with Children: Ethics, Law and Practice.* Oxford: Oxford University Press

Nuremberg Code (1947) Reprinted in: Duncan A, Dunstan G, Wellbourn R (eds) (1981) *Dictionary of Medical Ethics.* London: Darton, Longman & Todd

Royal College of Physicians (1986) *Research on Healthy Volunteers.* London: RCP

Royal College of Physicians (1990) *Research Involving Patients.* London: RCP

Tobias J, Souhami S (1993) Informed consent can be needlessly cruel. *B. M. J.*; **307**: 1199–1201

WMA (1964/1987) *Declaration of Helsinki.* Fernay-Voltaire: World Medical Association

Chapter 6

Economic appraisal

R Brooks

1 Introduction

This chapter discusses economic appraisal in health. There is no set of techniques specific to orthopaedic surgery, the methods treated have general applicability where resource allocation is concerned. In the United Kingdom (UK) and elsewhere, there has been increasing use of markets in the provision of health care, so it is important to explain why economic appraisal is still required in this environment. The second section outlines the relevant economic considerations. Section 3 starts with the measurement of costs, and this is followed by an examination of a number of economic appraisal methods: cost analysis, cost-minimisation analysis, cost-effectiveness analysis, cost-benefit analysis and cost-utility analysis. Most emphasis is placed on cost-benefit analysis and cost-utility analysis: the latter has been increasing in popularity in recent years, especially in the form which involves the construction of quality-adjusted life-years (QALYs). The opportunity is taken to raise a number of general issues concerning economic appraisal alongside a brief critique of QALYs. Finally, a short guide to the appraisal literature is presented.

2 Economic analysis

Scarcity, choice and opportunity cost

Economics as a discipline is concerned with the analysis of choice in the face of scarcity. Unless, a rare occurrence, there simply is no alternative to a particular action or, just as rare, there are such abundant resources that we can have all we want (imagine an unlimited hospital budget!), then choice or rationing is forced upon us. All choices have costs. Economists work with the concept of *opportunity cost,* defined as the value of the next best use of a set of resources. Think of time: as you read this book you will be aware of the alternative use of your time. If you would otherwise be playing tennis, then the opportunity cost of your present time use is the lost pleasure of your tennis match. If you have foregone an income-earning opportunity, then the income you have given up is a measure of the opportunity cost.

Social opportunity cost

For *social* choice, we require to measure social opportunity cost. The social costs of unemployment would appear to be the costs of unemployment benefit, other social transfers, and the lost tax revenue. Of more importance, economists would say, is the lost productivity of those out of work. The next best alternative use of most unemployed persons' time would be to employ them in productive activity, the value of which represents the opportunity cost both to the individuals concerned and to society, which is missing out on the benefits that would otherwise accrue. Similarly, someone with ill-health or disability may be prevented from working: the individual and society 'lose out' accordingly. By the same token, a social *benefit* will be created by returning the person to partial or full work.

Markets

How are scarce resources and limited budgets allocated? Perhaps more important analytically, how *should* they be? One answer to both questions could be 'by markets'. Let individuals make their own unfettered choices as producers and consumers. Demand and supply will rule and a price will prevail in each market. These ('equilibrium') prices will act as signals to all the players. There is every incentive for producers to be 'efficient' by meeting the demands of consumers in the least costly manner, especially in 'competitive' markets, thus maximising profits. Any firm making excessive profits will find these competed away by other firms. Consumers will thus face the lowest prices possible, consistent with the patterns of production and their associated costs. Markets minimise costs and maximise choice with the whole system orchestrated by a set of prices. Hence, resources are allocated optimally.

Markets in health

Would such a system be appropriate in the health sector? If so, then the optimal allocation of health-sector resources would require that the various markets for health services and products be competitive. Health-sector projects would have to be appropriately priced and decisions on expenditure would have to meet market tests. This need not, in principle, be a privately funded set of markets. The present UK government has embarked on the dual framework of publicly funded health services combined with 'internal' or 'producer' markets where purchasers (largely using public money derived from taxes) are separated from providers and the system is contract driven. A system of contract prices develops. Anyone or any organisation operating inefficiently will be driven out of the market and it follows that health care will be optimally provided. Note that this procedure leads to the pricing of, say, surgical operations. If the price is not 'right' this would mean no contract for the unsuccessful contractor hospital and the resources (e.g. orthopaedic surgeons) are now required to go elsewhere in the market or be made redundant.

If social choice in the allocation of resources was as straightforward as this, the role of the economist would largely be to analyse the workings of the health markets, with particular emphasis on how competitive (or not) these markets are proving to be. Meanwhile finance personnel would undertake all the necessary pricing and contracting arrangements. Consider, however, such phrases as 'health needs', 'value for money', and 'quality of care'. Market advocates would argue that health needs will be met and that the appropriate quality of care will be delivered within a value for money framework. What happens if markets 'fail'? Economic analysis points to a number of considerations here.

Difficulties with the market framework

(i) Private actions may not accord with social considerations: the more of us who become inoculated against an infectious disease, the less likely is this disease to spread. But what incentives are there for an individual to undertake the expense of inoculation? There is every incentive for the individual to misrepresent his or her true preferences and try to pay as little as possible, thus leading to under-provision of the service. The provision of 'public health' may require the public finance of such activities as immunisation, sewerage provision, etc., if not necessarily the public provision of such services. Some aspects of health provision, therefore, relate to the notion of 'collective' goods where consumption cannot simply be parcelled out to each individual and where the benefits are enjoyed collectively.

(ii) Health as an entity may be 'different'. Competitive markets depend for their smooth working on the free flow of information and knowledge. What happens when we cannot be sure about the outcomes of our actions? If I buy a refrigerator I expect to obtain certain 'results' from its use. If I 'buy' medical care I can be nowhere near as certain of the outcome. Indeed, there are many instances where the medical profession is uncertain about outcomes, with large variations evident in medical practice (Andersen and Mooney, 1990).

(iii) Consider the complexity of a market where the doctor will often act as an 'agent' for the patient. The patient presents himself or herself initially to a doctor but it is often the doctor's actions which then determine the pattern of demand. Are doctors then demanders, suppliers or both? The neat split between demand and supply sides of the standard market analysis then seems altogether less elegant. The consequences for the pricing of health services are not clear-cut.

3 Social appraisal

Necessity for social evaluation

If there is any reason for believing that a system of markets may not be the appropriate mechanism by which to deliver health care, then we need to turn to the techniques of social appraisal or social evaluation. Indeed, a case could be argued that where public money is involved, some form of social appraisal *ought* to be employed to assess how well scarce public resources are being used in the health sector, whether or not the actual provision is through markets.

Social appraisal in health

Social appraisal means the balancing of social costs and benefits. A framework for economic appraisal in health is illustrated in Table 6.1. Economic evaluation compares the inputs into a project or programme with the resultant outputs. The

Table 6.1 Types of economic evaluation. *Source*: **Adapted from Drummond** *et al.* **(1987)**

Type of evaluation	Cost measurement	Outcome measurement	Outcome valuation
Cost-minimisation	Pounds (£)	Assumed equivalent	No valuation
Cost-effectiveness	Pounds (£)	Outcome common to alternatives being evaluated, but achieved to different degrees	Common units, e.g. number of lives saved, days of disability avoided
Cost-benefit	Pounds (£)	Any effects produced by the alternatives	Pounds (£)
Cost-utility	Pounds (£)	Single or multiple effects, common or unique to the alternatives and achieved to differing degrees	QALYs, well years, other utility measures

term 'output' brings to mind physical things like cars or washing powder and seems out of place when dealing with human beings and their health, so the term 'outcomes' will be used instead. Defining what constitutes outcomes, however, can be a tricky task, one which has proved controversial. Indeed, economic appraisal recognises the possibilities of alternative outcome scenarios: this is evident from Table 6.1, where the (social) costs column remains the same for each appraisal approach whilst substantial differences can be observed in the outcomes columns. We shall consider first what is involved in the calculation of costs.

Costs

Social appraisal requires three main categories of cost be assessed (Robinson, 1993): health service costs, costs borne by patients and their families and external costs borne by the rest of society. Health service costs include staff time, medical supplies, e.g. drugs, hotel services and overheads such as heating and lighting. These items may be divided into *variable costs* which vary according to activity levels (e.g. staff time) and *fixed costs* which apply whatever the activity level (e.g. heating and lighting). All these health service costs are entitled *direct costs*. Patient and family costs include out-of-pocket expenses such as travel associated with health care, costs of family care and such items as drugs expenditure if incurred by the patient or family. These are also part of the direct cost calculations. *Indirect costs* include income losses to patients and family (which, as argued above, constitute the monetary representation of social opportunity costs) and the psychological stress experienced by patients and families. External costs may not amount to a large proportion of costs but may be important in particular health programmes such as the implementation of new environmental health regulations which could involve organisations in substantial costs of implementation.

Most of the costs just itemised are *current, recurrent* or *revenue costs* (the jargon varies but they essentially amount to the same entity). *Capital costs* comprise investments in buildings, plant and equipment – any asset yielding a flow of services over time. Investment appraisal techniques are used to analyse such expenditures. We shall consider aspects of these techniques in the context of cost-benefit analysis below. It should be noted that in the UK a formal system of capital charging is being introduced in which all NHS health service providers are required to keep registers of assets valued in excess of £1000 and to calculate interest and depreciation charges on these assets. This should help in the process of investment appraisal by providing the requisite information on capital costs.

One other important aspect of costs needs to be addressed. Economic analysts stress the requirement to look at margins. *Average cost* (unit cost), e.g. cost of an outpatient visit, can be calculated by dividing the number of patients into the total costs of running a clinic. There will be a significant difference in the cost of treating a patient who arrives at a less-than-busy clinic with staff in place than handling a patient in a congested clinic (necessitating additional staff). In the first situation the *marginal cost* (of treating the additional patient) is likely to be very small and almost certainly less than unit cost. In the second case, the marginal cost will clearly be somewhat higher. These differences must be recognised in appraisal. The retrieval and calculation of marginal costs can, unfortunately, pose considerable difficulties: use of average costs is common but clearly must be done with care.

Cost analysis

A form of appraisal using costs only is possible. If the outcome of alternative resource uses is clear-cut and known, then a comparison of costs of the alternatives will suffice. A good example is alternative forms of heating for a hospital. A contract specification would be drawn up for installation of the system and bids would be tendered. A gas-fired system may turn out to be cheaper than an oil-fired one. Unless there is some reason for judging that the social costs differ from the contract costs, then the cheapest alternative will be the socially 'correct' one.

Cost-minimisation analysis

Cost analysis is best applied for 'technical' decisions of the sort illustrated in the previous paragraph. Cost-minimisation is applied in situations where the outcome is not in debate but where programmes directly affect patient care. In maternity services live births would be regarded as the outcome. There are alternative forms of delivery, e.g. at home or in a hospital, so the evaluation would turn on the alternative social costs of achieving a given number of live births. Note that, as we saw above, the calculation of social costs is not simply a matter of assessing those costs incurred by the health services (e.g. midwives' salaries) but also those incurred by mothers and relatives (e.g. travel costs).

Cost-effectiveness analysis (CEA)

Suppose there is an agreed type of outcome but one for which a series of alternative programmes are available, some of which may be more costly (from a social point of view) but may also be more effective. Now it is necessary to compare the costs *and* effectiveness of alternative scenarios. The resultant decision criterion could still bear the flavour of a cost-minimisation. To illustrate: suppose the outcome is lives saved from a particular disease and there is a given target, e.g. 1000 lives saved over a specific time period, then the least costly of a set of alternative programmes would be the most (socially) cost-effective. Consider another version of CEA. Suppose a budget-holder has a given sum of money to spend within a specified time period on saving lives: now the criterion for choice is the way of spending the budget which *maximises* the number of lives saved. Clearly, the effectiveness of alternative programmes is a key component of this method. Examples of outcomes commonly employed in CEA include: lives saved, life years gained and cases handled. In the orthopaedic area if a surgical procedure has a known (medical) outcome, then this method can evidently be used.

The term 'cost-effective' has been used in a multiplicity of settings, some of which are not amenable to the approach. Some studies invested with the term 'cost-effective' simply compare the private costs and effects of alternative scenarios. This is not 'wrong' but extrapolation of private results to social policy must be done with care and would, in some cases, be quite inappropriate.

There are two major difficulties in the use of CEA. One is the lack of comparability of outcomes if we take a broader approach than that indicated above. How can programmes be compared which have differing types of outcomes? Further, how can the 'one-off' project be handled: by what criterion can a single project be judged in relation to its impact on social welfare? There is little point in describing such a project as cost-effective when there is no basis for comparison. And yet one-off projects may be quite common.

Cost-benefit analysis (CBA)

These limitations of CEA can, in principle, be overcome in the application of CBA. In CBA the costs and benefits of a project are compared in terms of a common unit, usually monetary. Table 6.1 shows the £ sign in both the cost and outcome columns. The use of a monetary unit does not imply that money has to change hands, simply that the pound, for example, is to be used as the 'unit of account'. An immediate implication is that 'one-off' projects can be assessed using CBA. If a project is expected to deliver a surplus of benefits over costs, then social welfare would be increased by implementing the project. Clearly, alternative projects can also be ranked using the CBA approach.

The comprehensive approach of the CBA approach can be illustrated using the following formula from Evans (1984):

$$\sum_{i,k,t} \left[\frac{P_{ikt} B_{ikt}}{(1 + R)^t} \right] - \sum_{j,k,t} \left[\frac{V_{jkt} C_{jkt}}{(1 + R)^t} \right] \gtreqless 0$$

If a particular project gives a positive result, then a social surplus is predicted. If the result is negative, then the social costs of undertaking the project would exceed the social benefits and the project would be rejected on economic grounds. The B and C symbols are the benefits and costs of the project. Table 6.2 gives a list of examples of the types of costs and benefits that can be assessed. The further down the table we proceed, the more comprehensive the evaluation. Different types of benefit are indicated by the i subscript, and different types of cost by the j subscript. Similarly, the k subscript refers to the recipient of the

Table 6.2 Types of cost and benefit. *Source*: **McGuire, Henderson and Mooney (1988)**

Costs: examples	*Benefits: examples*

Capital used
  land
  buildings
  vehicles
	Capital released for uses
	  land
	  buildings
	  vehicles

Revenue used
  labour
  supplies
  support services
	Revenue released for other uses
	  labour
	  supplies
	  support services

More work for staff	Less work for staff

Fewer staff training
  possibilities
	More staff training
	  possibilities

Patient/relatives/staff costs
  ignorance
  dissatisfaction
  decision-making burden
  time lost
  inconvenience
  expense
	Patient/relatives/staff benefits
	  information
	  satisfaction
	  relief of decision-making
	  time saved
	  convenience
	  less expense

Unhealthier patients
  less cure
    (more pain, disability; worse prognosis, etc.)
  less care
    (more discomfort, boredom; worse
    environment, etc.)
	Healthier patients
	  more cure
	    (less pain, disability; better prognosis, etc.)
	  more care
	    (less discomfort, boredom; better
	    environment, etc.)

Lost output (outside health service)	Increased output (outside health service)

benefit (individual or group) or to the person or agency incurring the cost. All projects have a time dimension, sometimes a project will be in place for decades. The subscript t allows for this. Time is often sliced into yearly intervals but this is not a requirement. The expression C_{jkt} thus indicates C units of cost of type j incurred in time period t by person or agency k.

Note should be taken of how comprehensive this approach is: benefits and costs are being assessed wherever, whenever and to whomsoever they may accrue or by whom they may be incurred. One of the arts of CBA is to categorise all the benefits and costs that might be associated with a project. It should be evident that we are not simply dealing with the budgetary arrangements of health agencies: in terms of Table 6.2 we do not stop halfway down the table.

Two further aspects of the above equation remain for contemplation. The P and V symbols refer to the *social* valuations of the benefits and costs respectively. In some cases 'market' prices will suffice for social valuations, for example salaries are often assumed to represent the social cost of employing people. In other cases, the analyst may need to determine social valuations, e.g. the valuation of changes in risks to human life. In many countries, government departments have been involved in preparing social valuations so that official guidance and recommendations are available.

This is often the case for the final aspect of the formula, namely the *social discount rate,* represented by R. This rate allows adjustments to be made for the time value of the benefits and costs. This time value arises because the use or accrual of a resource within one time period is not equivalent to that in another time period. We all have *time preferences*: most of us would rather enjoy the use of something this year than next year. If we were to postpone our consumption of a resource until next year, we would require some sort of premium to do so. In addition, there is usually an opportunity cost of holding on to money or resources. Rather than keep our savings in a box under the bed, most of us would prefer to earn interest on the moneys involved. Or a capital good (e.g. a piece of equipment) could be created using present resources which would enhance future productivity. Thus, the concept of the interest rate is of crucial importance. The discount rate is the interest rate used to discount future sums back to the present (i.e. the obverse of compounding present values into future values). The discounting procedure is shown in the equation by $1/(1 + R)^t$.

There has been fierce controversy on the determination of the social discount rate, especially over the relative merits of time preference and opportunity cost considerations, not to mention the complications of the treatment of risk and uncertainty in what is essentially a forecasting situation. Fortunately, for our purposes, the aforementioned official guidelines can be brought into play here. In the UK, the 'standard rate of discount' is set at 6%, so this rate should be used in health projects involving public money (HM Treasury, 1991). The 'mechanics' of discounting are not formidable: discount tables are readily available, as are standard statistical packages for computer use.

More generally, advice on economic appraisal recommends the use of *sensitivity analysis*. Alternative assumptions should be made about the flows of costs and benefits and their valuations. If a project is predicted to give a surplus of (discounted) benefits over (discounted) costs for a wide range of such assumptions, then there is a strong presumption that this will be a 'robust' project, well worth undertaking. And *vice versa* for a social 'loss-making' project of course. What of those projects that are sensitive to the assumptions made? Then the CBA analyst should at least present the decision-maker or sponsor with the relevant range of results. In summary, the CBA approach involves:

- Definition of the objective(s) of a project.
- Enumeration of the costs and benefits to be considered.
- Evaluation of these costs and benefits.
- Discounting the costs and benefits to obtain the discounted social value of the project.
- Application of sensitivity analysis.
- Presentation of the results to the decision-maker.

Doubts about the CBA approach have focused on the use of monetary measures, with critics especially unhappy that health outcomes be viewed in monetary terms. Cost-benefit analysts would argue that the £ sign is simply a monetary representation of social welfare which enables costs to be compared with benefits using a common unit. Partly in reaction to this criticism, but also by making use of the burgeoning work accomplished on the development of health status and health-related quality of life measures, analysts developed the cost-utility analysis method.

Cost utility analysis (CUA)

Costs are part of this approach, as ever, but health outcomes are to be viewed in terms of such entities as 'utility' (happiness, satisfaction, etc.), health status, or health-related quality of life. Utility as a concept has had a long history in moral philosophy and economics, amongst other disciplines. Some attempts have been made to assess utility changes from health programmes by the direct application of utility functions, but CUA has become most associated with the conjunction of costs and QALYs (quality-adjusted life-years).

The key to the QALY approach is the proposition that one life-year is not necessarily equivalent to another: a year in a 'poor' health state is not the same as a year in 'full health'. The inverted commas are used because clearly we need criteria by which to make such judgements about health status. Much of the work on health status measurement has concerned the choice of such criteria and the implications of this choice. If we accept for the moment that 'quality adjustment' is feasible, how is a QALY constructed? By providing a scale, usually normalised to zero to one values, on which to place assorted health states. The endpoints of the scale are, typically, 'full health' and 'dead' (hardly a health state: the treatment of death is controversial). Should a person be in a health state of, say, 0.5 prior to treatment (for example, a surgical operation) and be restored to full health by the treatment then for each subsequent life-year a gain of 0.5 QALYs would be achieved. Clearly the method requires good prognostic data. The method allows for aggregation – if 1000 people benefit in this way then 500 annual QALYs would be created. A nice picture of the approach is shown in Figure 6.1. An assortment of scaling (measurement) methods has been applied in health status measurement and reviews of these are available (see, e.g. Brooks, 1995).

The next step in CUA is to place the social costs of health programmes against the quality gains, thus allowing a *cost per QALY* to be estimated for each programme. The similarity with CEA will be evident here, if the QALY is taken as the given outcome measure. This method has given rise to controversy,

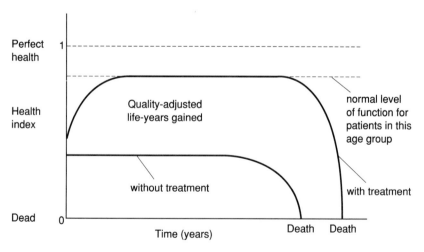

Figure 6.1 Quality-adjusted life-years added by treatment. *Source*: Drummond (1989)

especially concerning the construction of cost/QALY league tables, with the potential implication that decisions be taken on health expenditures according to the ranking of procedures in such league tables. An example of such a table is provided in Table 6.3.

Some issues in economic appraisal

The QALY concept has been subject to criticism from economists and non-economists alike. The flavour of the debate can be captured by considering some of the criticisms of cost/QALY league tables. This will also provide a convenient framework to raise a number of more general issues concerning economic appraisal in health.

(1) *The mortality and morbidity data on which the QALY calculations are based are not sufficiently precise.* This criticism is not specific to QALY measurement and if the criticism is correct, then the data requires improvement. In this connection it is worth making the point that economic appraisal in health is only as good as the medical and epidemiological evidence on which it is based. The impression is sometimes created that economic appraisal has a life of its own, with the economist viewed as a species of 'expert' who considers health projects armed with a set of techniques which are somehow detached from their

Table 6.3 Quality-adjusted life-year (QALY) of competing therapies: some tentative estimates. *Source*: **Maynard (1991)**

	Cost/QALY (*£ Aug 1990*)
Cholesterol testing and diet therapy only (all adults, aged 40–69)	220
Neurosurgical intervention for head injury	240
GP advice to stop smoking	270
Neurosurgical intervention for subarachnoid haemorrhage	490
Anti-hypertensive therapy to prevent stroke (ages 45–64)	940
Pacemaker inplantation	1 100
Hip replacement	1 140
Valve replacement for aortic stenosis	1 180
Cholesterol testing and treatment	1 480
Coronary artery bypass graft (CABG) (left main vessel disease, severe angina)	2 090
Kidney transplant	4 710
Breast cancer screening	5 780
Heart transplantation	7 840
Cholesterol testing and treatment (incrementally) of all adults 25–39 years	14 150
Home haemodialysis	17 260
CABG (1 vessel disease, moderate angina)	18 830
Continuous ambulatory peritoneal dialysis	19 870
Hospital haemodialysis	21 970
Erythropoietin treatment for anaemia in dialysis patients (assuming a 10% reduction in mortality)	54 380
Neurosurgical intervention for malignant intracranial tumours	107 780
Erythropoietin treatment for anaemia in dialysis (assuming no increase in survival)	126 290

medical contexts. No amount of fancy economic footwork will produce a sound appraisal if a project's aims are unclear, if aspects of the project are mis-specified, or if the medical and/or epidemiological evidence is equivocal or even misleading.

(2) *Summary data of the cost/QALY type is dangerous because it suggests quick and easy solutions to the decision-maker.* This is an important point and again it leads to a more general issue, that of the temptation to use available techniques as substitutes for thought rather than as aids in decision-making. It is incumbent on economists to stress that economic appraisal is an aid to decision-making and not simply a set of rules to be applied uncritically whatever the circumstances. A related criticism is the view that a quantitative algorithm of the QALY type glosses over the essentially arbitrary nature of the judgements being made concerning the values being placed on health status. (We have noted this above in the criticism of CBA as being 'mercenary'). Economists have countered that the process of QALY quantification *does* explicitly bring out the value judgements that are being made, and thus *can* be subjected to analysis and criticism.

(3) *Broad comparisons across widely differing fields are unwise.* Such choices have to be made anyway, so the exclusion of the QALY approach for this reason would seem to be unfair. Furthermore, cost/QALY information has been used within given clinical fields and could also be used to allocate budgets amongst specific care groups such as the elderly. Some analysts have also argued the case for programme-specific QALYs (Donaldson *et al.,* 1988).

(4) *Strict application of cost/QALY league tables would imply that those whose treatment has a high cost/QALY would receive no care.* Implicit in this criticism is that the approach is not explicitly concerned with equity or justice or, for that matter, 'need' in the distribution of health care resources. Apart from assuming that a QALY is a QALY, no matter to whom it accrues, advocates for QALYs have deliberately eschewed any formal ethical approach concerning equity or justice, a position that has caused considerable debate (Harris, 1987; Kawachi, 1989; Broome, 1993).

QALY users vary in the strength of their advocacy for the approach in the decision-making context, a context which is highly likely to involve the rationing of scarce resources. The QALY, as we have seen, is part of one approach (CUA) to economic appraisal: it can only be reiterated that this method be critically considered, along with all others, for its potential to inform decision-making.

4 Recommended reading

This chapter has tried to show how economic appraisal can be applied to health expenditures and given some indication of the issues which arise from this endeavour. There is plenty of published guidance available concerning economic evaluation. The excellent series of short articles by Robinson (1993) is as good (and accessible) an introduction as any. A detailed article-length treatment is that of Drummond *et al.* (1993). A full text is that of Drummond *et al.* (1987): this contains practical advice on everything from how to allocate overheads in costing exercises to the methods available for scaling health states in cost-utility analysis. An overview of the field of health status measurement is provided in Brooks (1995). The comprehensive treatment of this area by Patrick and

Erickson (1993) is likely to prove the standard text for some time to come. A substantial literature on QALYs and CUA has developed: the field of CUA has been usefully surveyed by Gerard (1992). 'Official' guidance on economic appraisal in the UK is provided in an HM Treasury booklet (1991). Two detailed bibliographies on economic evaluation in health, containing thousands of references, are Backhouse *et al.* (1992) and Elixhauser (1993).

Unfortunately, despite all the available advice, the application of economic appraisal as reflected in the published results has been very uneven. The article by Udvarhelyi *et al.* (1992) makes for salutary reading in this respect. It is important, therefore, that the users of economic appraisal methods keep to the standards required of such methods. Poor economic appraisal is the enemy of good practice where resource allocation in health is concerned.

References

Anderson TF, Mooney G (eds) (1990) *The Challenges of Medical Practice Variations.* Basingstoke: Macmillan Press

Backhouse ME, Backhouse RJ, Edey SE (1992) Economic evaluation bibliography. *Health Econ.*; **1** (Suppl): 1–236

Brooks RG (1995) *Health Status Measurement: A Perspective on Change.* Basingstoke: Macmillan Press

Broome J (1993) QALYs. *J. Pub. Econ.*; **50**: 149–167

Donaldson C, Atkinson A, Bond J (1988) Should QALYs be programme-specific? *J. Health Econ.*; **7**: 239–257

Drummond MF (1989) Output measurement for resource allocation decisions in health care. *Oxford Rev. Econ. Pol.*; **5**: 59–74

Drummond MF, Brandt A, Luce B (1993) Standardising methodologies for economic evaluation in health care. *Int. J. Technol. Assess. Health Care*; **9**: 26–36

Drummond MF, Stoddart GL, Torrance GW (1987) *Methods for the Economic Evaluation of Health Care Programmes.* Oxford: Oxford University Press

Elixhauser A (ed.) (1993) Health care cost benefit and cost effectiveness analysis from 1979 to 1990: a bibliography. *Med. Care*; **31** (Suppl): JS1–JS149.

Evans RG (1984) *Strained Mercy: The Economics of Canadian Health Care.* Toronto: Butterworth

Gerard K (1992) Cost-utility in practice: a policy maker's guide to the state of the art. *Health Policy*; **21**: 1–31

Harris J (1987) QUALYfying the value of life. *J. Med. Ethics*; **13**: 117–123

HM Treasury (1991) *Economic Appraisal in Central Government: A Technical Guide for Government Departments.* London: HMSO

Kawachi I (1989) QALYs and justice. *Health Policy;* **13**: 115–120

McGuire A, Henderson J, Mooney G (1988) *The Economics of Health Care.* London: Routledge and Kegan Paul

Maynard A (1991) Developing the health care market. *Econ. J.*; **101**: 1277–1286

Patrick DL, Erickson P (1993) *Health Status and Health Policy: Allocating Resources to Health Care.* New York: Oxford University Press

Robinson R (1993) Economic evaluation and health care. *Br. Med. J.*; **307**: 670–673; 726–728; 793–795; 859–862; 924–926; 994–996

Udvarhelyi IS, Colditz GA, Rai A, Epstein AM (1992) Cost-effectiveness and cost-benefit analysis in the medical literature: are the methods being used correctly? *Ann. Int. Med.*; **116**: 238–244

Chapter 7

Questionnaire design

R Fitzpatrick

This chapter is intended to be of use primarily for someone who is faced with the task of drawing up and using a questionnaire and wants guidance on the principles involved. As with many aspects of research, assessment and measurement, methods of questionnaire design can be outlined but the reader should not expect a set of explicit rules which, if followed, will automatically result in perfect questionnaires. Both the development of experience in design and use of questionnaires and consultation with recognised experts in survey design will be of advantage to build upon the broad themes outlined here. This chapter can only outline principles of good practice endorsed by the very substantial social scientific literature on questionnaires and identify major pitfalls to avoid.

The chapter will pre-suppose that the reader has come to the correct conclusion by deciding that a questionnaire is the appropriate tool to solve a problem. It does not, for example, address alternative solutions that may be more relevant to many problems, such as varieties of qualitative methodology that are increasingly used in the field of health care (Fitzpatrick and Boulton, 1994). Nor can it address another important question that faces the potential author of a new questionnaire, namely whether to use an existing instrument 'off the shelf' instead. For many problems, particularly aspects of patients' experience of pain, disability, health status or satisfaction with treatment, the option of using what is already available needs to be considered seriously as investigators always underestimate the time and effort involved in developing new instruments. Decisions about the validity and appropriateness of the plethora of existing health care questionnaires are beyond the scope of this brief chapter and are dealt with elsewhere (Wilkin *et al.*, 1992). The choice between using an existing instrument and designing a new one does raise clearly at the outset the need to be clear-minded about one fundamental issue: 'what exactly is the problem to which a new questionnaire is the solution?'

Concepts and indicators

The significance of the rather general question just expressed needs to be underlined. If one were restricted to enunciating just one principle of good practice in questionnaire design it would have to be the importance of being as clear and precise as possible about the purpose of a new questionnaire. Put at its most simple, *never* start a questionnaire in the way it is most tempting to do, that is 'brain-storming' on good questionnaire items. One should begin by clarifying the ideas about the phenomena to be examined by means of a questionnaire. The social scientific literature has a useful framework for addressing this issue. It distinguishes between 'concepts' and 'indicators'. Concepts are the cognitive tools whereby the world is mapped; a conceptual guide as to how and why events occur. Indicators are the operational measures (such as specific questionnaire items) which are relied upon to measure concepts.

An artificial and simplistic illustration may be used to clarify the distinction. It may be interesting to investigate whether patients find the routine follow-up in outpatient clinics helpful to their problems. It is decided, therefore, that patient satisfaction is a subject of interest. This is the starting concept. However, a moment's thought would suggest that satisfaction with outpatient clinics is likely to be multi-dimensional: patients may have quite distinct views about the ease with which they can attend clinics on the one hand, and, on the other hand, regarding therapeutic benefits of attendance. The initial concept has become two concepts. After discussions within the clinic, exploratory interviews with patients, it is suggested that patients' views regarding the value of clinics will depend, amongst other things, on their state of health. Quite different patterns of views regarding the clinic amongst those whose health problems are relatively resolved can be expected compared to other patients. The conceptual framework thus expands to a clearer view of the object of enquiry and why it is of interest. In this hypothetical example three concepts have emerged: satisfaction with access, satisfaction with benefits of treatment and health status and a reasonably clear view about why they have been selected has emerged (in grandiose terms we have 'a model'). Only at this stage should the need for operational measures be addressed (of which, questionnaire items might be one solution).

Interview versus self-completed questionnaire

One important decision is always faced by investigators embarking on a survey, whether to collect data by means of a self-completed questionnaire or by interview. This decision is often determined by practicalities but a summary of the advantages and disadvantages of the alternatives can guide choices.

The interview

The interview is likely to result in fewer questionnaire items being omitted because of the face-to-face nature of data collection. Completion of the questionnaire to the end is also enhanced by the interviewer. Interviews also enable clarification of the meaning of items and additional flexibility in the case of particularly complex content.

The main disadvantage of the interview is cost. Interviewers need to have specialised general training as well as guidance and supervision in the conduct of the survey at hand. There is also evidence of subtle biases in answers to questionnaires produced by attributes of the interviewer, although training may be expected to overcome the majority of such effects (Streiner and Norman, 1994). Increasingly telephone interviewing has been used because it reduces costs. There may be some sampling bias associated with telephone ownership.

The growing use of unlisted numbers has resulted in random digit dialling as a technique to obtain representative telephone samples.

The self-completed questionnaire

The main advantages of the self-completed questionnaire are low costs of administration and processing data. It avoids biases associated with attributes of the interviewer. Disadvantages should be obvious from the discussion of the interview: lower response rates, more omitted items, less flexibility to address complex material.

Several studies have directly compared the results of health surveys obtained by both methods. There is some evidence that patients are more prepared to report problems of ill-health in a self-completed questionnaire than in face-to-face interview (Cook *et al.*, 1993). By contrast, respondents were more prepared to report problems of alcohol consumption in a face-to-face interview (Cutler *et al.*, 1988). To date, there is insufficient evidence to determine which method generally produces more valid results, and much probably depends on the subject of the survey, its context and the skills and training of investigators (Cook *et al.*, 1993).

Principles for selecting questionnaire items

It is assumed that the reader has now gone as far as possible in teasing out the model and relevant concepts. Later in the chapter, the formal requirements of a questionnaire will be dealt with: reliability, validity and other measurement properties that are universal to all measuring instruments, whether obtained from a laboratory or from the self report of a human subject. This section deals with the technical considerations of questionnaire development that are ultimately intended to improve measurement properties. There are three over-riding aims behind the following list of pieces of advice: (i) that information conveyed by respondents in questionnaires should accurately reflect their views, attitudes and behaviour; (ii) that information conveyed should as much as possible be in a form that can be clearly used by the investigator and (iii) that the data-gathering process should not generate negative feelings on the part of the respondent (irritation, embarrassment and other forms of distress) that lead to non-completion of the survey at hand or deterioration in future potential relations between respondents and service providers.

Avoid technical jargon

Questionnaire items need to be expressed as much as possible in the language of the respondent so that technical terms, such as 'hypertension', that have either no meaning to respondents or different meanings from their medical scientific usage (Blumhagen, 1980) are avoided. Some authoritative statements recommend that the vocabulary used in questionnaires should not be beyond the reading skills of a 12-year-old child (Streiner and Norman, 1994). This may seem unnecessarily low, but is intended to ensure that surveys capture in responses, the substantial minority of adults who are functionally illiterate. Technical solutions, that ensure a text is readable, include the elimination of words with large numbers of syllables as calculated by Flesch scores (Flesch, 1948). In practice, it is more realistic to test this dimension with pilot studies.

Avoid lengthy items

Questionnaire items should not include sentences that are too long. They will have poor response rates. Oppenheim (1992) suggests avoiding sentences with more than 20 words. Surprisingly, the research evidence on the effects of the overall length of questionnaires upon response rates are more equivocal, as longer instruments can be acceptable if the subject matter is of particular importance to the respondent.

Avoid ambiguity and complexity

Even the simplest of phrases can be ambiguous. 'Have you been to the doctor in the past year?' may be interpreted by some as referring to the 12-month period prior to interview and by others as referring to the current calendar year. Language needs to be based on short and simple phrases. Two common forms of unnecessary ambiguity and complexity are the 'double barrelled' question and the 'double negative'. An example of the former would be: 'Have you had pain or difficulty sleeping in the last week?' An example of the latter would be: 'I do not have difficulty in moving around'. Respondents find it difficult to decide whether to agree or disagree with such negative propositions. Although it is preferable to maintain positively worded items, occasionally questionnaires will insert a negatively expressed item to address the problem of acquiescent response set, where respondents assume similar meaning in similarly formatted items and give their content less thought in selecting answers.

Even the simplest of words can, in a particular context, become ambiguous. For example, depending on the context of the questionnaire, in the item – 'how often has a doctor visited you at home in the last year?', the 'you' may be taken to refer not just to the respondent but to the whole family.

Avoid value-laden questions

It makes great sense to avoid questions in which one answer appears to be preferred or more positively valued than another. An obvious example is the question: 'Do you often bother the doctor with trivial problems' (Streiner and Norman, 1994). The wording of the question has made it quite unlikely to elicit a positive response. However, while it is easy to express the principle, in practice words or phrases that are largely neutral in meaning may subtly shift to more loaded significance by their context.

Some subjects may be expected to be sufficiently sensitive that respondents are unlikely to report socially undesirable views or behaviours. The wording of questions may, in these circumstances, be modified to 'give permission' for the expression of deviant responses. For example, the wording may imply that the apparently deviant experience is more common: 'Some people find caring for a very disabled family member so distressing that they feel bitter about that individual. Have you felt this way at all in the last month?'

Avoid excessive demands on respondents' memories

There is substantial evidence that individuals have difficulty in recalling even quite recent events, such as, for example, episodes of ill-health (Allen *et al.*, 1954). One should not, therefore, overestimate individuals' memories as there is the risk of obtaining highly inaccurate data. Furthermore, the task of trying to recall distant details will add to the sense of irritation or incompetence felt by the respondent.

Response categories

In fixed choice questionnaires, not only are the questions but also the range of possible answers predetermined. As much care is required in choosing response categories. Some basic principles can again be set out.

Response categories must be logical

Options need to be mutually exclusive and cover the likely range of options. A common mistake in questionnaires is to include response options that overlap; for example respondents may be offered options for a question of frequency that include '10–20 minutes' '20–30 minutes'.

A potential problem in statistical analysis of survey data is that responses are skewed, to an extent that is unavoidable, since human views and behaviours are not necessarily normally distributed. However, a somewhat different problem can be anticipated: the extent to which the range of questionnaire responses artificially skews data. For example, in asking patients with functional limitations how far they can walk, if we offered patients six response options, five of which were distances in excess of 5 miles, we would have skewed responses to the one low distance response category. Response categories need to reflect the likely range of responses.

Select appropriate number and type of response categories

There are many questions concerned with factual matters in which response categories are almost entirely constrained by reality; gender being an obvious example. However, for the majority of topics, especially regarding views and subjective experiences, a large range of alternative formats of response is possible. At one extreme individuals could be constrained to binary choices: 'yes' or 'no'. At the other extreme, the visual analogue scale (VAS) presents respondents with a line, usually 100 mm long, with anchors at either end, such as 'no pain' and 'worst possible pain' and no intermediate words. In between such extremes, questions can be presented with a finite number of explicitly worded response options, typically four to seven.

The psychometric literature regarding the appropriate number of response categories is substantial and difficult to summarise (Streiner and Norman, 1994). Binary options ('yes' or 'no') are increasingly falling out of favour for subjective phenomena such as views, beliefs and subjective experiences such as pain and satisfaction. They do not permit shades or degrees of views to be expressed. Investigators tape-recorded the informal responses of respondents asked to complete a health status questionnaire which comprised only binary response categories (Donovan *et al.*, 1993). Respondents frequently reported difficulties and frustration in trying to force their experiences of pain, disability and problems into 'yes' or 'no' responses and often reported arbitrary selection.

At the other extreme, the visual analogue sale is a widely used method of eliciting responses. Again the literature is inconclusive, partly because there are a large number of possible criteria with which to compare VAS with alternatives: reliability, validity, responsiveness (Guyatt *et al.*, 1987). Supporters of the VAS point in particular to the precision it permits compared to all alternatives. Such precision may make the VAS particularly sensitive to small but important changes over time in clinical trials. Guyatt and colleagues (1987) assessed patients views' of their respiratory problems before and after a respiratory rehabilitation programme by both VAS and a seven-point Likert scale. They concluded that neither method demonstrated superior responsiveness but the seven-point scale was easier to administer and interpret.

In between these two extremes are questionnaire items which offer a finite range of usually four to seven response options. There is little evidence to suggest that more than seven points increase the true rather than apparent precision of items (Cox *et al.*, 1992). A study of patients with heart-related problems examined the reliability over 2 weeks and construct validity of two alternative and randomly allocated formats of quality of life questionnaires, with either five or seven point response categories (Avis and Smith, 1994). The seven point scale consistently produced more satisfactory reliability and validity than the five point scale version.

Details of the wording of response categories may make a difference to results. Patients attending medical clinics were randomly allocated to express level of satisfaction with their care to formats of questionnaire either expressed in terms of a 'very satisfied' to 'very dissatisfied' or 'excellent' to 'poor' range of responses (Ware *et al.*, 1988). Tests of reliability did not differ between formats but the 'excellent' to 'poor' format showed greater response variability and construct validity.

The open-ended question

A questionnaire may include open-ended questions as well as those with predetermined response options. The advantage of such a format is that one can get a little closer to the 'real' range of views a population may have because one has not so obviously constrained their range of answers. It is also possible to elicit some of the logic or rationale behind respondents' answers by leaving space on the questionnaire that invites a more expansive answer. Another advantage is that on certain topics investigators may simply not be confident of the nature or full range of views on a particular issue, and an open-ended question avoids having to identify all of the possible response categories. However, this is often a sign that investigators have not done sufficient exploratory background work, open-ended items should not be used as a short-cut to developing a questionnaire.

It is important only to use open-ended questions for positive reasons rather than 'because something interesting might come out of it'. This is because there are disadvantages to open-ended questions, the most important of which is that they are enormously time-consuming to process. Essentially, unless answers are used purely anecdotally or illustratively, the investigator has to develop a coding frame for the material and then code respondents' open-ended statements, tasks which are easily underestimated. All too often, because of the time and costs involved, investigators do not use the material gathered from open-ended items. The other disadvantage of open-ended questions is that they impose an additional burden on the respondent which may contribute to jeopardising compliance. In general terms, questionnaires should not have too many open-ended questions and they should be carefully justified in the logic of the survey.

Scales

In the social sciences and, increasingly, in health care research it is normal practice in questionnaires to measure more complex personal experiences by means of a number of items rather than a single question. The items form a scale and an essential prerequisite of such a scale is that it is homogeneous and internally consistent. For example, to develop a 'patient satisfaction with communication' scale to assess patients' views of this aspect of outpatient clinics, all of the items would be expected to measure different aspects of a relatively unitary view: satisfaction with information given by surgeon, satisfaction with opportunities to explain patient's own concerns and similar items. The advantages of a scale over individual items are four-fold.

1. Many aspects of human subjective experience such as pain, disability and satisfaction are quite complex and multifaceted and therefore cannot be captured by single questionnaire items.
2. Measures comprising multiple items are more likely to be valid because they sample different aspects of a problem and are less prone to distortion or bias inherent in single observations (items).
3. Scales have repeatedly been shown to be more reliable than single items (Streiner and Norman, 1994).
4. Scales actually simplify analysis. If one has a single score from a scale it is easier to analyse and interpret statistically than a series of separate items, where in addition to practical problems of multiple comparisons, the risk of chance statistical significance is increased.

There are a number of different forms of scale, each with its own method for identifying items. This section describes the simplest and far the most commonly used type, often associated with Likert scales. There are two basic stages in the development of such a scale. The purpose of the first stage is to generate a large number of questionnaire items that address the domain in which we are interested, pain, disability or whatever. The second stage involves the statistical analysis of the pool of items to identify the scale or scales of interest. Many questionnaire items are lost at the second stage because they do not fall within a scale. These two stages are briefly described in turn.

Generation of scale items

At this first stage the objective is to generate a large number of items that address the different aspects of the subject of concern. Ideally this should be done by means of in-depth unstructured interviews conducted by trained interviewers, although other methods may be used such as focus groups (Fitzpatrick and Boulton, 1994). Content analysis of such material will provide a wide range of relevant experiences reported by participants which then need to be turned into questionnaire items. This stage can be supplemented by use of available literature and expert opinion to generate items. Sometimes such sources are used as a short-cut alternative to exploratory in-depth interviews when available skills and resources are insufficient.

Development of scales

Stage one has generated a large number of items. In some studies, this pool is trimmed by means of an intermediate survey in which a relevant sample completes a questionnaire containing the full list, redundant or difficult items are identified and dropped at this stage. More often investigators omit this intervening step and proceed to the second stage of administering a questionnaire containing the full pool of items, the results of which are then subjected to statistical analysis. Most commonly factor analysis is used, the principle of which is to identify items that go together in terms of statistical correlation. Thus a hypothetical pool of items administered to patients about to undergo hip replacement surgery might be expected to produce one list of items concerned with pain, another with mobility, and so on. The items that go together in this way are termed candidate scales.

The final step is to establish that scales identified in this fashion actually do have the necessary measurement prerequisites. Above all, a scale must be internally consistent. This can be assessed by means of statistical expressions of internal reliability. Cronbach's alpha (Cronbach, 1951) summarises the overall pattern of correlations between items to the total scale score that is produced by summing items. In addition to internal reliability, we would expect the scale to have other desirable measurement properties for it to be useful. It is therefore essential to examine test–retest reliability and validity (as discussed below).

As indicated, it is usual to adopt a simple method of scoring in which items contribute equally to a summed scale. However, it may be argued that some items should have greater weight in a scale. Such weightings can be derived by statistical techniques beyond the scope of this review (Streiner and Norman, 1994). There is substantial evidence that such weighting methods may have surprisingly little effect in improving the measurement accuracy of scales. Lei and Skinner (1980) examined a well-known scale for the assessment of life event stress – The Social Readjustment Rating Scale. This scale assigns weights to such very different events as death of spouse and getting a parking ticket. They found almost complete agreement between results in a sample of respondents whether their answers were scored by the panel-derived original weighted version, random assignment of weights or simple additive scoring of equally weighted items. In the same way, Jenkinson and colleagues (1991) found the sensitivity to change over time of health status scales in patients with arthritis was no greater with original weighted items or a simple additive score.

Alternative scaling techniques

There are alternative methods of developing scales. Guttman scales are homogeneous and individuals' scores are cumulative in a way that it is possible to estimate accurately which items an individual has affirmed from knowledge of the total score. This idea has received particular attention in relation to disability. Katz and colleagues (1963) argued that functional capabilities are lost in a particular order, and then regained during rehabilitation in the same order reversed. For example, more complex activities such as dressing are lost before simpler activities such as continence. This principle of Guttman scaling has been extended to other areas of disability such as shopping and transportation (Spector et al., 1987). However, Guttman scaling remains a problematic method because, in reality, a large proportion of respondents in studies of disability and other fields of application give answers inconsistent with the required cumulative pattern expected (Wilkin et al., 1992).

Thurstone scaling is based on the principle of equivalence and equal appearing items. Panels of judges are presented with large numbers of questionnaire items that have been developed to address a particular domain. They rate the items on a scale of, for example, 11 points, from 'most favourable' to 'least favourable'. It is the average scores of panels that are the basic elements used to create item scores. The Nottingham Health Profile, a commonly used health status scale, was devised by use of these methods (Hunt et al., 1985).

As already argued, scales are particularly appropriate for many of the dimensions of experience of concern to orthopaedics. It is not surprising to find their increased use in recent studies in this field. Scales have been used in several studies to examine outcomes of total hip replacement surgery (Liang et al., 1985; Johanson et al., 1992; Cleary et al., 1993). A particularly good example of scale development and testing can be found in an instrument to assess symptoms and function in carpal tunnel syndrome (Levine et al., 1993).

The pilot study

An essential step in the development of any questionnaire is the need to pilot draft forms prior to actual use in a survey. The value of a pilot survey cannot be over-emphasised. Many of the errors built into a questionnaire will emerge from piloting. In a pilot survey one is testing all aspects of a questionnaire, not only the wording of items and the overall layout, but also details such as the letter of explanation and methods of processing results. The most rigorous method of piloting a questionnaire is to adopt a randomised design. If it is not clear whether two alternative formats are appropriate both can be tested. This is not realistic in many questionnaire-based studies. Errors in questionnaire design are more often detected in other ways. Pilot surveys may identify questionnaire items which unusually large numbers of respondents leave blank, suggesting difficulties in comprehension or acceptability. Another common problem that is picked up by means of a pilot survey is where answers are excessively skewed, suggesting that the item is not informative or has a bias in wording. One can also more directly involve respondents in improving the quality of a questionnaire. Respondents in a pilot can be asked if any items caused particular difficulties or whether any topics or issues have been neglected in the questionnaire as a whole.

Measurement properties

It may initially seem strange to assess the measurement properties of a questionnaire but even for the simplest of questionnaire-derived information about its accuracy should be of concern, as with any other health data. In other words reliability, validity and, in some instances, responsiveness are the important issues.

Reliability

Reliability is dealt with extensively in Chapter 1 and has also been addressed as an important prerequisite of scales. A reliable questionnaire is one in which we obtain the same result on repeated occasions, provided no change has occurred in the subject addressed. With scales, as already argued, it is most readily and most commonly addressed via internal reliability, that is whether different indicators of a single concept produce similar results. This cannot be done where single items are used to elicit information. Test–retest reliability can be used for both single items and scales, provided that not too much time elapses between administrations so that true changes have occurred.

Validity

A valid measure is one which measures what it is intended to measure (see also Chapter 1). A questionnaire, and indeed any measuring instrument, can only be shown to be valid *for a particular purpose*. It is quite erroneous to regard an instrument as valid *per se*. There are three methods of establishing the validity of an instrument.

1. Content validity. This is the most informal method of validating an instrument but the one most relevant to a questionnaire. Content validity is established by examining the content of a questionnaire to ensure that items cover the relevant aspects of concepts of concern. This process can be enhanced by (i) exploratory interviewing to gain insights into the subject (ii) piloting (see above) and (iii) involving a wide range of expertise and experience in the process of development.
2. Construct validity. This addresses whether an instrument produces results consistent with theoretical expectations. For example, items in a questionnaire intended to address mobility should correlate more with a hip score than do items to address psychological mood.
3. Criterion validity. Here the questionnaire is expected to correlate with what is currently viewed as a 'gold standard' measure of a phenomenon. In reality, this is unlikely to be a way of testing a questionnaire, simply because we are unlikely to have such 'gold standards' in the first place.

Responsiveness

Questionnaires are increasingly used to assess change over time in patients' experiences of pain, disability or some other dimension of experience. In circumstances where observations at different time periods are used to assess change (for example before and after surgery), we then need to assess responsiveness. It is quite possible for a questionnaire to be valid but not responsive to change (Guyatt *et al.*, 1989). Questionnaires may systematically vary in their sensitivity especially to more subtle changes in the patient's health status (Fitzpatrick *et al.*, 1992). However, it is important to remember that in addition to repeating measures of pain or disability and calculating the degree of change between measures, it is possible directly to ask patients to assess retrospectively the degree of change they have experienced and, in some circumstances this direct approach has substantial validity (Fitzpatrick *et al.*, 1993).

Presentation and layout

There are a number of general principles in the layout and presentation of questionnaires that are rather general in form and draw on common sense but are vital to the success of a survey. Investigators often make the mistake of considering the following matters of detail to be left to the secretary or computer software (de Vaus, 1986; Oppenheim, 1992).

1. Explanations. Questionnaires must always have clear and accessible explanations of at least the following: (i) why the survey is being conducted, (ii) how the respondent has been selected (iii) what he or she is requested to do (iv) how information obtained will be used, including clear statements of confidentiality and anonymity (if true). These are usually conveyed in an accompanying letter.
2. Clarity. Tasks within the questionnaire should also be made clear and easy to follow. Do not simply state the questions; the respondent must know whether to tick, ring or otherwise indicate the answers and whether multiple answers are appropriate.

   Clarity is also aided by good use of spacing. Space has to be left for open-ended questions and for fixed choice items that include an 'other' response with the invitation to explain or describe. Space should neither be too little, conveying the sense that answers are not actually of value, nor too large, thereby increasing the apparent scale of the task.

   If filter questions are used (for example 'if no, go to question 3'), the route of the respondent through the questionnaire can be aided by arrows or directions.

   Only use one side of a page, as respondents may miss pages presented double-sided.

3. Attractiveness. It is particularly difficult to give explicit advice on attractiveness of layout but attention is needed to the overall appearance.
4. Politeness. This is also an obvious prerequisite but often overlooked. Every opportunity should be taken to ask for information politely (for example, by avoiding repeated use of blunt requests such as 'marital status'). Similarly respondents should be properly thanked for participation.
5. Logical order. The consensus view is that respondents should be asked easier and more factual questions early on and more difficult material later in the questionnaire. Early questions should have an obvious relevance to the stated aim of the questionnaire. Demographic questions are normally placed at the end.

Conclusion

Many of the principles presented in this chapter are expanded upon in more detail in the variety of excellent textbooks available on questionnaire design and survey research (de Vaus, 1986; Oppenheim, 1992; Streiner and Norman, 1994). It has only been possible to offer general principles which should assist the reader in obtaining accurate responses from survey participants. Every questionnaire poses unique challenges.

References

Allen G, Breslow I, Weismann A, Nisselson H (1954) Interviewing versus diary keeping in eliciting information in a morbidity survey. *Am. J. Pub. Hlth.*; **44**: 919–927

Avis N, Smith K (1994) Conceptual and methodological issues in selecting and developing quality of life measures. In: Albrecht G, Fitzpatrick R (eds) *Quality of Life in Health Care*. Greenwich, Connecticut: JAI Press

Blumhagen D (1980) Hypertension: a folk illness with a medical name. *Culture Medicine Psychiatry*; **4**: 197–227

Cleary P, Reilly D, Greenfield S, Wexler L, Frankel F, McNeill B (1993) Using patient reports to assess health-related quality of life after total hip replacement. *Quality of Life Res.*; **2**: 3–11

Cook D, Guyatt G, Juniper E, Griffith L, McIlroy W, Willan A, Jaeschke R, Epstein R (1993) Interviewer versus self-administered questionnaires in developing health-related quality of life instrument for asthma. *J. Clin. Epidem.*; **46**: 529–534

Cox D, Fitzpatrick R, Fletcher A, Gore S, Jones D, Spiegelhalter D (1992) Quality of life assessment: can we keep it simple? *J. R. Stat. Soc.*; **155A**: 353–393

Cronbach L (1951) Coefficient alpha and the internal structure of tests. *Psychometrica*; **16**: 297–334

Cutler S, Wallace P, Haines A (1988) Assessing alcohol consumption in general practice patients – a comparison between questionnaire and interview. *Alcohol Alcohol.*; **23**: 441–450

de Vaus (1986) *Surveys in Social Research*. London: Allen and Unwin

Donovan J, Frankel S, Eyles J (1993) Assessing the need for health status measures. *J. Epidem. Comm. Hlth.*; **47**: 158–162

Fitzpatrick R, Ziebland S, Jenkinson C, Mowat A, Mowat A (1992) Importance of sensitivity to change as a criterion for selecting health status measures. *Quality in Health Care*; **1**: 89–93

Fitzpatrick R, Ziebland S, Jenkinson C, Mowat A, Mowat A (1993) Transition questions to assess outcomes in rheumatoid arthritis. *Br. J. Rheumatol.*; **32**: 807–811

Fitzpatrick R, Boulton M (1994) Qualitative methods for assessing health care. *Quality in Health Care*; **3**: 107–113

Flesch R (1948) A new readability yardstick. *J. Appl. Psychol.*; **32**: 221–233

Guyatt G, Townsend M, Berman L, Keller J (1987) A comparison of Likert and visual analogue scales for measuring change in function. *J. Chron. Dis.*; **40**: 1229–1233

Guyatt G, Deyo R, Charlson M (1989) Responsiveness and validity in health status measurement: a clarification. *J. Clin. Epidemiol.*; **42**: 403–408

Hunt S, McEwen J, McKenna S (1985) Measuring health status: a new tool for clinicians and epidemiologists. *J. R. Coll. Gen. Pract.*; **35**: 185–188

Jenkinson C, Ziebland S, Fitzpatrick R, Mowat A, Mowat A (1991) Sensitivity to change of weighted and unweighted versions of two health status questionnaires. *Int. J. Health Sci.*; **2**: 189–194

Johanson N, Charlosn M, Szatrowski T, Ranawat C (1992) A self administered hip-rating questionnaire for the assessment of outcome after total hip replacement. *J. Bone Jt. Surg.*; **74A**: 587–597

Katz S, Ford A, Moskowitz R, Jackson B, Jaffe M (1963) Studies of illness in the aged: the Index of ADL: a standardised measure of biological and psycho-social function. *JAMA*; **185**: 914–919

Lei H, Skinner H (1980) A psychometric study of life events and social readjustment. *J. Psychosom. Res.*; **24**: 57–65

Levine D, Simmons B, Koris M, Daltroy L, Hohl G, Fossel A, Katz J (1993) A self administered questionnaire for the assessment of severity of symptoms and functional status in carpal tunnel syndrome. *J. Bone Jt. Surg.*; **75A**: 1585–1592

Liang M, Larson M, Cullen K, Schwartz J (1985) Comparative measurement efficiency and sensitivity of five health status instruments for arthritis research. *Arthr. Rheum.*; **28**: 542–547

Oppenheim A (1992) *Questionnaire Design, Interviewing and Attitude Measurement.* London: Pinter Publishers

Spector W, Katz S, Murphy J, Fulton J (1987) The hierarchical relationship between activities of daily living and instrumental activities of daily living. *J. Chron. Dis.*; **40**: 481–489

Streiner D, Norman G (1994) *Health Measurement Scales.* Oxford: Oxford University Press.

Ware J, Hays R (1988) Methods for measuring patient satisfaction with specific medical encounters. *Med. Care*; **26**: 393–402

Wilkin D, Hallam L, Doggett M (1992) *Measures of Need and Outcome for Primary Health Care.* Oxford: Oxford University Press.

Chapter 8

Gait analysis

HS Gill, EN Biden and JJ O'Connor

Introduction: putting gait analysis into context

Gait analysis: a definition

Gait analysis is the quantification of human movement. It seeks to evaluate the angles of flexion/extension, abduction/adduction and long axis rotation at the joints of the human locomotor system during walking. It also seeks to estimate the forces and moments transmitted across joints. Although walking has been the principle application for these techniques, they can be applied readily to other activities involving the whole of the musculo-skeletal system.

The analysis of human movement is practised informally in many situations. In clinical practice, a patient's patterns of movement can be a strong indication of state of health. It is not surprising that interest in how to quantify such observations has developed.

Development of modern gait analysis

The ability to quantify movement depends on some method of measurement and it has only been within the last 100 years or so that measurement techniques have been equal to this task. Optical methods using cine cameras or video have proved most practical in clinical gait analysis. Cine photography with manual measurements from successive frames laid the foundation for current methods but it took the combined development of video cameras and powerful computers to bring gait analysis into widespread use.

Winter (1974), Jarret (1976) and Whittle (1982) used video cameras to track the movement of markers attached to the separate limbs of subjects. Computers were used to calculate the values of the joint angles and to reconstruct simple images of the locomotor system during walking. These measures were augmented with measurement of the forces applied to the foot by the floor. These data were interpreted in the light of the phasic activity of the muscles detected by electromyography (EMG).

Many commercial companies have entered the gait analysis arena. Some of these provide relatively simple systems which collect data and leave the user to process it using their own techniques, others have developed 'turn key' systems which can collect data, analyse it and present the results in standard ways. A large number of systems have been installed. For example, a report at the East

Coast Clinical Gait Analysis Conference in 1991 (Sienko-Thomas, 1991) showed over 50 laboratories with significant clinical work in the United States alone.

The most extensive application has been in the gait analysis of children with cerebral palsy. There are many reasons for this. Children with cerebral palsy provide a challenge to the surgeon trying to address a variety of factors. Sutherland (1984) and Gage (1991) have provided examples of how their practices are influenced by gait studies.

Gait analysis as an outcome measure

The first volume of this series painted a rather bleak picture of gait analysis, concluding its section on gait with the comment: (Pynsent *et al.*, 1993, p. 260)

> ..gait analysis, in skilled hands, may provide useful adjunctive information regarding function but, at present, cannot be considered useful for routine outcome measurement.

It has certainly been the case in the past that gait analysis has been oversold, or perhaps it was the subject of over-expectation. The data produced by gait analysis are different in many ways from those which are familiar within medicine. Gait data involves measures of motion, forces and electrical activity, unfamiliar concepts in the more biology and chemistry based environment of medicine, requiring a somewhat different approach to assessment and evaluation.

The keys to linking such measures to outcome are:

1. to be able to compare individuals with appropriate normals.
2. to be able to compare measures made before and after treatment.

Most gait data are keyed to some sequence of events such as the *gait cycle* (*vide infra*). This means that, rather than comparing single values of measured quantities, one should compare curves. This is not a trivial task and the statistics can be somewhat daunting. The simple approach is to use assumptions which are commonly applied to single variables but these are not always appropriate.

The limitation of any statistical model of gait analysis is that one is comparing the subject under study back to either normals or some group of peers. Statistical techniques are needed for classifying individuals, detecting changes from one test to the next so as to record changes due to time or treatment.

Basics of gait analysis

Gait analysis has mainly focused on the measurement of the lower limb with limited regard for trunk movement.

The gait cycle

The basic concept in gait analysis is that of the gait cycle (Figure 8.1). The gait cycle represents a complete set of movement events for each leg, beginning and ending with successive floor contacts of one foot. Gait is a cyclic activity and for normal individuals it is symmetrical. Referring to Figure 8.1, the cycle is

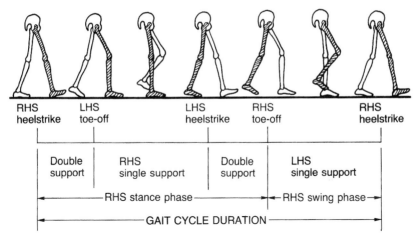

Figure 8.1 The gait cycle (see text for an explanation)

described in terms of the movement of the shaded limb (right-hand side). The start of the cycle, for the shaded leg, is the foot/ground contact event, or *foot-strike*, for that leg. Once the foot is in contact with the ground, the shaded limb enters its *stance phase* and there is an initial period of *double support*, i.e. both feet are in contact with the ground. During the double support period, the support of the weight of the body is transferred from the opposite foot to the shaded foot. The opposite foot then leaves the ground, termed *opposite toe-off*, and there is a period of *single leg stance*, when all the weight of the body is supported by the shaded foot. During this period of single leg stance the opposite leg is in the *swing phase*, i.e. is moving forward of the supporting foot. The opposite leg's swing phase is terminated by its contact with the ground, the **opposite foot strike**. There is then a second period of double support when support of the body's weight is transferred from the shaded foot to the opposite foot. Once this has happened, the *toe-off* event for the shaded foot occurs and the shaded leg enters its swing phase. The shaded leg's swing phase is terminated by its next foot strike and the cycle is complete. The stance phase for each leg represents about 60% of the cycle, and 24% of the cycle is spent with both feet on the ground. The left and right leg cycles operate in anti-phase.

The gait cycle provides a convenient time frame for measurement of limb movement, evaluation of the electrical activity of muscles (see later section on electromyography) and the kinetic variables such as the forces and moments applied to the limb.

Gait variables

Gait is characterised by the values of and trends in key variables. Only the important ones are mentioned here. For a more detailed account, the reader is referred to more specialised texts such as Sutherland (1988), Gage (1991) and Giannini (1994). The key variables are of two main types, *kinematic* and *kinetic*. Kinematics is the study of motion without reference to the associated forces. Kinetics is the study of the forces that produce motion.

Kinematic variables

Time/distance variables

The temporal variables *cadence* and speed may be considered as kinematic variables, as may the distance variables *step length* and *stride width.* Cadence is the number of steps per unit time, each step being a separate foot/ground contact event, thus one gait cycle includes two steps. Cadence is therefore connected by step length with speed in the direction of progression. Step length is defined as the distance between a point on one foot and the corresponding point on the opposite foot during the double support period, measured in the direction of progression. Stride width is similarly defined but is measured perpendicular to the direction of progression. *Stride length* is the sum of two consecutive steps, i.e. the distance covered in one complete gait cycle. The time/distance parameters are the easiest measurements to make in gait analysis. Some commonly measured variables are:

1. Walking speed
2. Cadence
3. Step length, right and left
4. Stride length = right step length plus left step length
5. Cycle time
6. Time of following events expressed as percentage gait cycle, for both left and right sides: opposite toe-off, opposite foot strike, toe-off, single leg stance

Directly measured/calculated kinematic variables

The following kinematic variables are derived from the direct measurements of the trajectories of markers attached to the subject, and are thus calculated variables.

Joint angles

The main kinematic variables generally considered are the joint angles in the sagittal and coronal planes. Two-dimensional analysis has traditionally focused on the sagittal plane due to the fact that it is much easier to make measurements in this plane. Commonly reported sagittal plane angles are the angles of the trunk and pelvis to the vertical and the angles of flexion of the hip, knee and ankle. The definitions of these angles are important and are related to the kinematic model used by the gait system. Kinematic and kinetic models are discussed later. Three-dimensional gait analysis extends the consideration of angles to the coronal plane and long axis rotations in the transverse plane. Figure 8.2 shows examples of kinematic gait variables plotted against time over a complete gait cycle.

Linear/angular velocity and acceleration

An important part of the kinematic data are the velocities and accelerations, both linear and angular, of the limb segments; these data are also required for the calculation of some kinetic variables. Modern gait systems produce spatial measurements of markers placed upon the subject. From these measurements the positions of the limbs may be determined at any point in time. To obtain velocity and acceleration data from the position data, numerical methods are used to differentiate the data. Numerical differentiation is a noise enhancing process, so the position data must be smoothed prior to differentiation.

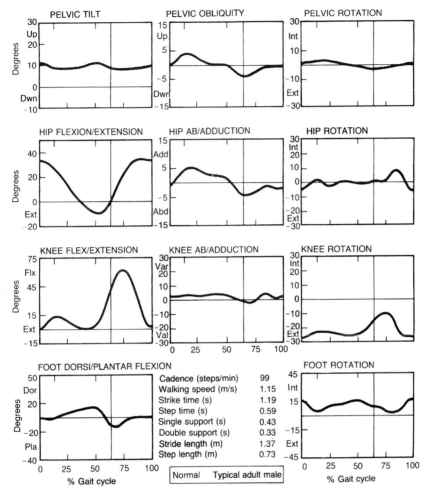

Figure 8.2 Typical kinematic variables for normal adult males, plotted against time base of the gait cycle and averaged between left and right limbs. The usual kinematic variables are the angles between the various limb segments in the sagittal, coronal and transverse planes. All angles are given as relative angles between the proximal and distal limb segments, except those for the pelvic angles which are defined relative to the laboratory axis system. The first column contains the sagittal plane angles, the second the coronal plane angles and the last contains the transverse plane angles

Kinetic variables

Force and moment

Kinetics is concerned with forces, moments and energy. Forces cause movement when they act upon objects. For an object not to move, either no forces are acting upon it or the forces acting upon it cancel out the effects of one another. Forces have both a magnitude and a direction, so two equal but opposite directed forces acting on the same object may cause no movement if they are co-linearly aligned. Forces are thus vector quantities. Vector quantities can be divided into

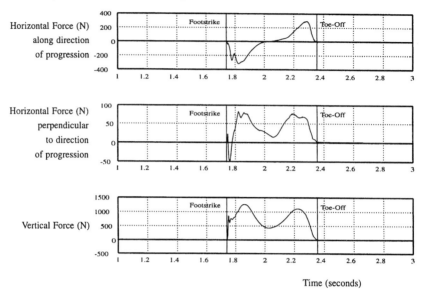

Figure 8.3 Typical ground reaction forces for a normal adult male, during stance phase of gait cycle with foot-strike and toe-off events indicated

component parts, oriented in different directions. Commonly a force may be decomposed into three perpendicular components; the combined effect of the components being equal to the effect of the total force. The main advantage of regarding a force in terms of its components is that the effects of each component are often simpler to understand than the effects of the total force. Commonly the forces in gait analysis are resolved into vertical, fore-aft and medio-lateral components.

A moment of a force about a particular point in space is equal to the magnitude of the force multiplied by the perpendicular distance between the point and the line of action of the force. A moment acting on a body about a particular point tends to rotate the body. The magnitude and direction of a moment depends upon the point about which it is defined, as well as the magnitude and direction of the force which gives rise to it.

Gait kinetic variables
Kinetic variables can be divided into two groups, directly measured variables and calculated variables.

1. Directly obtained kinetic variables
The directly obtained variables in gait analysis are usually the components of the ground reaction force, measured using a force platform. The ground reaction force is divided into components which are oriented in the direction of progression (fore/aft shear), perpendicular to the direction of progression (medio/lateral shear) and vertical to the floor. The force platform provides the three perpendicular components of the ground reaction vector (usually plotted against the time frame of the gait cycle, see Figure 8.3), the position in the plate of its centre of pressure and the associated spin moment about a vertical axis. The

position and the direction of the ground reaction vector in the laboratory is thereby obtained. The raw force measurements, direct from the force platform, have been used to characterise gait.

From Figure 8.3, considering the vertical force, there is an initial very fast rise (the *transient*), due to the impact of the foot on the floor, followed by a curve which is often referred to as an *M* curve. The height of this curve oscillates about body weight, with the middle section somewhat less than body weight and the two peaks somewhat higher. The oscillation represents the vertical force needed to produce oscillatory vertical movement of the centre of mass of the body. The time up to the first peak of the *M* is, at least approximately, the time during which load is being transferred from one foot to the other. The time from the second peak of the *M* to the end of the record at toe-off is the time during which load is being transferred back to the other foot.

The other two curves, fore/aft shear and medial/lateral shear, also have typical patterns, although they are of much lower magnitude than the vertical force. In the case of fore/aft shear, the overall shape of the curve is similar to a sine wave. In the initial portion, the foot pushes the floor forward or the floor pushes the foot backwards. At about midstance the direction of the force reverses and the foot pushes backwards on the floor, the floor pushes the foot forward, to propel the individual along.

The medio-lateral forces are usually directed laterally after foot contact after the transient, followed by a largely medial pattern. The medial acting forces are necessary to ensure that the line of action of the forces passes close to the centre of mass of the gravity during single leg stance.

2. Calculated kinetic variables

Calculated kinetic variables also require numerical processing of the kinematic variables, the processed data is then combined with the directly obtained kinetic variables to derive quantities such as joint moments. The calculation of such kinetic variables requires the use of a kinetic model (*vide infra*). The net joint moments acting about the hip, knee and ankle in the sagittal, coronal and transverse planes are the usual set of variables produced from such models (see Figure 8.4). The moments thus produced may be multiplied by the angular velocity to give joint power. Power curves for the hip, knee and ankle are also shown in Figure 8.4.

Electromyography

Electromyography is the recording of the electrical signals produced by muscle during activity. The recorded signal is known as an electromyogram (EMG). The signal is the summation of the motor unit action potentials in the localised area of the muscle from which the measurement is being made (Basmajian, 1985). The measurements may be made non-invasively, using surface electrodes attached to the skin over the muscle; or invasively using fine wire electrodes inserted into the muscle. Surface electrodes have the advantage that they are noninvasive, easy to apply and give good results for large muscles or muscle groups which lie fairly close to the surface. The invasive alternative uses fine wire electrodes, where a needle containing a pair of fine insulated wires is inserted into the bulk of the muscle. The needle is then withdrawn leaving the

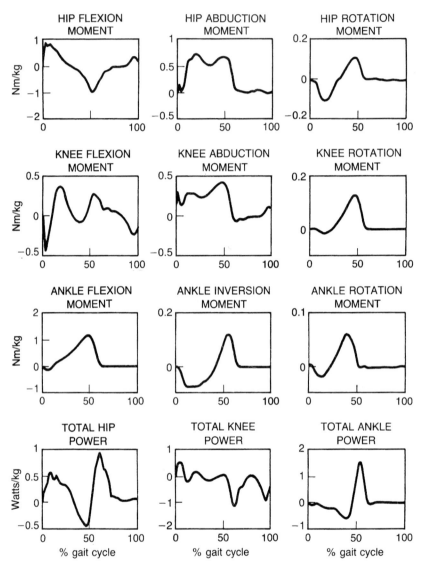

Figure 8.4 Typical kinetic variables for normal adult males, plotted against time base of gait cycle and averaged between left and right limbs. The moments given are the internal moments, which are the moments produced by the muscles acting about the joint and are normalised by the mass of the subjects. The moments acting in the sagittal plane are given in the first column, those acting in the coronal plane in the second column and finally those acting in the transverse plane are given in the last column. The last row of graphs show the total power for the hip, knee and ankle joints. The power is calculated by multiplying the joint moment by the angular velocity in each planar direction and the total power is the sum of the powers in all three planes for each joint

wires in the muscle and capable of recording the electrical activity. Although this procedure is invasive, it allows very high specificity in testing.

The measured signals are amplified and filtered. Two electrodes are commonly used. An earth reference voltage is also needed and can be taken from any point on the body of the subject. The filtering is used to distinguish low frequency movement artefacts from the EMG signal. A 3 Hz high pass filter is commonly used. Some systems incorporate further filtering to remove higher frequency components of the EMG signal and noise.

EMG signals are mainly used to indicate phasic activity of muscle in a gait analysis context, that is when the muscles are on or off during the gait cycle. To aid in determining phasic activity, further processing may be performed on the signal. Commonly the signals are (full-wave) rectified and smoothed (see Figure 8.5). The signal may be enveloped to reveal magnitude above an arbitrary threshold.

Gait variables from measurements

For measuring the variables mentioned above, different levels of complexity of equipment are needed. The time/distance variables can be measured very easily with rudimentary equipment. However, in a modern context, full gait analysis is usually performed using a commercial optometric measurement system. This type of system measures the movement of well defined markers attached to the

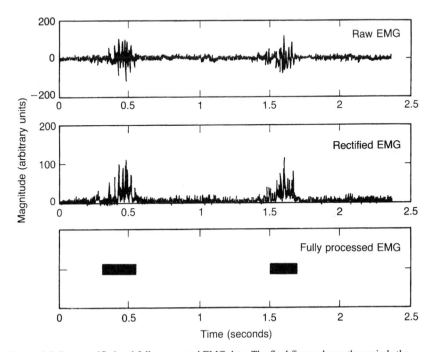

Figure 8.5 Raw, rectified and fully processed EMG data. The final figure shows the periods the muscle is active, indicated when the magnitude of the rectified EMG signal is above an arbitrary threshold

subject. Most systems incorporate the facilities for simultaneous force plate and EMG recording. The calculated gait variables are obtained by processing the recorded trajectories of these markers in combination with the force plate and EMG data. This processing relies upon the use of kinematic and kinetic models. From an engineering standpoint, any time that a particular set of rules or procedures is applied to manipulate data those rules and procedures are said to constitute a *model*. The model calculates the values of quantities which are not measured directly.

Kinematic models

A kinematic model is necessary, since the kinematic variables need to be derived from trajectory measurements of markers. The model is basically a set of rules for relating the movement of the markers to the motion of the individual limb segments. The models used rely upon a number of assumptions made about the nature of the locomotor system. Most models assume that the locomotor system is made up of rigid segments connected at spherical (ball and socket) or revolute (hinge) joints. The models also usually assume that the markers do not move relative to the segment to which they are attached. The model allows the orientation and location of each limb segment under consideration to be determined. The segment orientations are usually defined in terms of the orientation of a co-ordinate axis system fixed in the segment, defined relative to anatomical landmarks on the segment. For determining absolutely the position of a segment in space, measurements of three markers on it are needed. Once the positions and orientations of all the limb segments are known, the relative orientations can be derived and these lead to the kinematic variables required.

There are a number of models used by the various commercial gait systems. The marker placements are usually dependent upon which model is in use, as is the measurement procedure. Two main approaches are used in the measurement of kinematic information. The markers may be placed directly over anatomical landmarks and the position of the landmarks is continuously recorded during the measurement (Kadaba, 1990). Alternatively, arrays of markers attached to plates may be placed in an arbitrary position on each limb segment and the relationship between this array and the anatomical landmarks is determined from a static calibration procedure. In the subsequent measurement, only the positions of the marker array are continuously recorded and the position of the landmarks are deduced from these measurements (Angeloni, 1992). Joint angles are then calculated.

Kinetic models

For determining the resultant force and moment at each joint, additional information and processing is required; as well as some additional assumptions. The kinetic model encapsulates these assumptions and formalises the processing rules. Most kinetic models use the rigid body segment representation of the locomotor system as in the kinematic models discussed above. In addition, the kinetic model must define the distribution of the mass within a segment and the points about which moments are calculated for each segment.

The majority of commercial gait analysis systems use multi-link segment models which have either spherical or hinge joints connecting the segments.

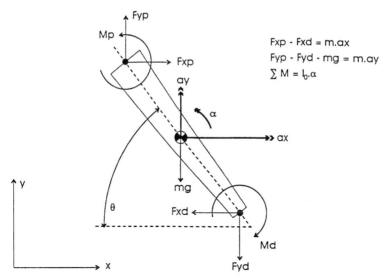

$$Fxp - Fxd = m.ax$$
$$Fyp - Fyd - mg = m.ay$$
$$\sum M = I_0.\alpha$$

Figure 8.6 Free body diagram of a segment. *Fxp* is the component of force in the x direction and *Fyp* is the component of force in the y direction, both acting on the proximal end of the limb segment. *Mp* is the moment acting about the proximal end of the limb segment. Similarly, *Fxd*, *Fyd* and *Md* are the force components and moment acting on and about the distal end of the segment. The linear acceleration of the centre of mass of the segment is given in terms of the components ax and ay, in the *x* and *y* directions respectively and α is the angular acceleration of the segment. I_0 is the moment of inertia of the segment taken about the centre of mass, *m* is the mass of the segment and *g* is the weight force per unit mass, sometimes referred to as the acceleration due to gravity; thus the product *mg* gives the weight of the limb segment

Thus in these types of models the joint rotation centres are fixed with respect to the co-ordinate systems embedded in each segment.

Each segment may be considered as a free body (see Figure 8.6). The linear accelerations of the centre of mass, the angular orientation, velocities and accelerations are known from the optometric measurement, its subsequent processing and use of the kinematic model. The resultant force and moment acting at the distal end of the segment are assumed to be known (from previous analysis of the more distal segment). Considering the six equations of dynamic equilibrium (for three-dimensional analysis), it is possible to determine the three components of the resultant force and the three components of the resultant moment acting at the proximal joint.

In this manner, the resultant joint forces and moments are calculated for the linked segment model in a step-wise process. Starting with the foot segment, upon which the known ground reaction acts at a known point, the resultant force and moment required for dynamic equilibrium at the ankle joint (the link between foot and shank segments) are calculated. Considering the shank segment, the resultant force and moment at the knee joint (the link between shank and thigh segments) are then determined. The process is repeated for the thigh segment. Thus resultant joint moments can be determined for the ankle, knee and hip joints as well as the resultant inter-segmental forces. This process is called *inverse dynamics*.

Quality of gait data

Resolution

Resolution defines the finest difference which can be measured by the system. Resolution is a function of the capability of the system used to gather the data and the techniques used in analysis of the data. In gait analysis, temporal and magnitude issues are of concern. The temporal aspects of gait measurement arise because human gait movements are periodic (but not simple harmonic) and each variable may have a number of harmonics. This means that a signal representing a movement (such as vertical displacement of the ankle versus time) is the sum of several signals of different frequencies. A digital computer system must be able to sample the analogue data at a rate which is at least twice as fast as the highest frequency component of interest. This minimum sampling frequency is known as the *Nyquist frequency*. Failure to adhere to this minimum will introduce aliasing errors (for further details see Lynn, 1973). Usually the force and EMG measurements need to be sampled at higher rates than the spatial data, since these measurements usually contain higher frequency components. Most motion events during gait typically contain frequency components up to 6 Hz, so an adequate sampling frequency would be 12 Hz. However, there are some events which have much higher frequency components, such as heelstrike. Most modern gait systems use sampling frequencies between 25 and 60 Hz for capturing spatial data.

Magnitude resolution is the finest measurement of the value of a quantity over the whole possible range of values. This issue arises particularly in digital measurement systems because of the nature of digital representation. Reality is continuous but digital representation of reality consists of a collection of discrete values taken at the sampling frequency. In order to sample a range of possible real continuous values, the range must be sub-divided into discrete steps, the number of such steps is directly related to the resolution of the system. The number of possible steps is a function of the hardware used for data capture.

Thus any measurements made by any digital system are subject to limits in temporal and magnitude resolution. Differences between measurements made using such systems can only be distinguished up to the resolution of the system.

Repeatability and accuracy

Reliable data is that which is both repeatable and accurate. Repeatable data is data which may be wrong in some sense, but which will be consistent from test to test. Accurate data are data which conform in some sense to truth. The objective in gait analysis is to provide data which are reliable, that is accurate to a reasonable degree and repeatable as well.

The various components of the gait analysis system are subject to various factors which affect both repeatability and accuracy.

Noise
The data gathered from gait analysis often contains an element of noise. If the noise is excessive, it may not be possible to extract the signal which is required. The noise may be of a single frequency, or a narrow band of frequencies, in which case it is possible to remove it using a filter (for further details see Lynn,

1973). However, if the noise contains a large number of frequencies or is of similar frequency to the required signal, it is a considerable problem and must be removed or reduced at source, rather than from the measurement. Random noise may lead to poor repeatability. Noise affects all the types of data measured in gait analysis, position, force and EMG.

Noise also determines the level of processing required to extract the desired quantities from the signal. For example, to obtain velocity data from position measurements, the data must be differentiated. Differentiation amplifies noise, so the signal must be smoothed before differentiation. Some of the actual signal may be lost in the smoothing process, the amount of smoothing depends upon the noise present in the measured data.

Skin movement artefact

A source of error in spatial data is skin movement artefact. This error arises from the relative movement of the skin-mounted markers to the bones of the segment to which they are attached, due to soft tissue displacements. All skin-mounted marker systems suffer from this problem. Reduction in this error is one of the rationales for using arrays of plate-mounted markers (Angeloni, 1992).

Cross-talk

Cross-talk is not usually a problem for spatial data, but can affect force and EMG measurements. Data from a force plate or EMG system are usually recorded on separate channels. For a force plate, the perpendicular components of force are usually recorded as separate signals on separate channels. If a force is applied to the plate purely along one of the perpendicular axes, there should be a signal only on the channel recording that component of force. Any signal on the channels recording the force components along the other two axes is cross-talk or due to cross-sensitivity of the platform.

Similarly, EMG electrodes placed on adjacent muscles may pick up signals from one another. Careful electrode placement is needed to reduce such cross-talk.

Processing

The manner in which the data are collected is not the only factor influencing its repeatability; its subsequent processing also plays a major role. The majority of the key gait variables are derived from measurements after a large amount of processing has occurred. The models used for kinematic and kinetic processing greatly affect the end result. A number of techniques exist for smoothing and differentiating signals. Also, there are a number of conventions for angular representation (Woltring, 1994). Some of these conventions are more accurate than others, in terms of representing reality in a non-ambiguous manner.

The calculated kinetic variables are extremely sensitive to the assumptions made about the location of the centre of the joints. Most commercial systems use a generic kinetic model, which may not be appropriate for all pathologies investigated.

Consider the following classes of variables:

1. Kinematic time/distance.
2. Kinematic angles.
3. Kinetic moments and powers.

Going from the first class of variables to the last, there is an increasing amount of processing needed to obtain them. As the amount of processing increases, the effects of the assumptions made are greater.

Use of gait data

Baseline data

The key to clinical gait analysis is the ability to compare an individual to normal and to before and after treatment, or over time. The establishment of some sort of baseline from which comparisons can be made is vital before gait data can be used for evaluation. When monitoring the change in an individual, the first set of data taken on that individual establishes the baseline. Comparison to normal requires an understanding of what normal means. Comparisons before and after treatment, or over a period of time require that the data collection, models and so on be consistent.

Normal data

When we say normal gait, we likely mean gait which falls within some generally typical range for people without overt orthopaedic or neurological problems. The harder we try to define it, the more conditions we place on the subjects who will be allowed to be normal. Murray (1964) described normal gait in men as they aged. She focused on the mean of the motions, possibly in large part because the computing required to develop descriptions of the variability would have been prohibitively expensive at the time. Winter (1974) has provided normative data for a number of conditions, using means and standard deviations as the basis for defining both the midline of the population and its variability. Sutherland *et al.* (1988) have provided normal means and variability for children up to the age of 7, and the gait of 7-year-old children can be taken to represent something very close to that of adults. His work, which entails a form of statistical analysis which had not been invented when Murray's work was done, described the variability in a somewhat different way than by simply using standard deviations. Nobody is really average. A subject who is near the mean at one point in the gait cycle may not necessarily lie near the mean at some other points. This is illustrated in Figure 8.7 which shows knee flexion for normal 7-year-old children, with examples of knee flexion for some typical children. Also shown in the figure are the curves for one and two standard deviations from the mean. Our usual assumptions that plus or minus one standard deviation from the mean contains roughly two-thirds of the population does not hold.

Generally, one finds that the width of the boundaries which really describe movement and other variables in gait are very wide. This complicates the problem to some extent, in that one cannot rely exclusively on testing for abnormal gait by checking to see if a person is within some arbitrary limit such as plus or minus two standard deviations, rather it requires that we use some statistical procedure to define the bounds.

A statistical method for addressing this problem has been proposed by Sutherland and co-workers (Sutherland *et al,* 1988; Olshen *et al.*, 1989), based on a technique known as the *bootstrap.*

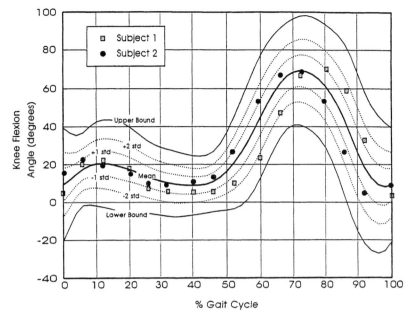

Figure 8.7 Knee flexion angle versus gait cycle for normal 7-year-old children. The upper and lower bounds enclose 95% of 46 subjects, the dotted lines show one and two standard deviations from the mean. Also plotted are the data points for two typical subjects

Cross centre comparison

A difficulty in making comparisons across centres has been the proliferation of different measurement systems. Up until the mid-1980s, there were few commercial gait analysis systems and those systems which were in use often had locally developed protocols for measurement and reporting of results. In principle, one complete set of measurements can be converted to different formats but, in practice, the data collected from two systems are seldom compatible. This is beginning to change, as the clinical users of such systems achieve greater awareness of the subtleties of data collection, processing and presentation. There is still some controversy about the angular representations of limb segments and no international standards have yet been agreed. Similarly, no agreed international standards exist for kinetic variable calculation and representation.

The end result of the differences between equipment and procedures in different centres is that each centre has effectively its own baseline, or set of baselines, for each patient group. As long as an understanding of the collection and processing effects on the data exists, it should be possible to make cross centre comparisons if both individual and baseline data from each centre is available. It should be easier to compare the results of two centres using equipment from the same manufacturer but the reliance of data on procedure must be appreciated.

Use of variables

Gait data consists of many different types, which can be grouped as follows:

1. Kinematic time/distance variables.
2. Calculated kinematic variables (segment angles).
3. Directly obtained kinetic variables (ground reaction force).
4. Calculated kinetic variables (resultant joint moments and powers).
5. EMG data.

For each set of variables there exist normative data, where normal has to be considered as discussed above. These groups can be divided into directly obtained variables and more abstract variables, obtained after significant processing.

Directly obtained variables

The first group is the simplest to deal with, since it contains variables which are described by single numbers for the whole of an individual's gait cycle. It is relatively simple to distinguish between an individual's left and right sides, as well as compare that individual to various groups of subjects, using familiar statistical tools. These variables can reveal a great deal about overall well-being. Change in walking speed, for example, is a sensitive measure of function.

Normal gait is highly symmetrical. Dissimilar step lengths or timing of events are indicators that the gait is asymmetrical and hence abnormal. Recording of such ratios before and after treatment can show whether changes have been toward or away from normal. The ideal ratio of any right to left comparison is one to one.

The proportion of the cycle spent in single stance is also an indicator. Immature walkers (Sutherland, 1988) have relatively short periods of time when only one foot is on the floor and the body is in a controlled fall (Inman, 1966). As the gait of the toddler matures, balance allows this time to increase until, in normal adults, single leg stance occurs for about 75% of the gait cycle. A reduction in this time or a change in right/left symmetry is an indication of abnormal gait. Once again, as an outcome measure, the measurement before and after treatment is key.

Considering the third group of variables next. These variables are time variant, the use of the gait cycle enables the time frame to be normalised. Over this normalised time frame the trends in the ground reaction forces are established for normals and the changes in them are indicative of problems or compensations.

The comparison of actual data to normals involves deciding whether both the pattern and the magnitudes are altered. For example, it is typical of above knee amputees, or others with a basically unstable knee, that they load relatively slowly after their foot hits the floor and the slope of the beginning part of the vertical force is reduced. The speed of walking will alter the amplitude of the M, with slow walking producing a much smaller change than fast walking.

The variables of group 5 can also be regarded as directly obtained variables. EMG signals are time variant. Use of the gait cycle normalises the time frame. Further processing of the raw data can reduce the signal to one of two values, indicating whether a muscle is active or not. Comparison with established patterns of activity during the gait cycle may indicate abnormal function.

Variables obtained after processing

The remaining two groups of variables (groups 2 and 4) are somewhat more abstract and their use has really developed from expert users' own practice. The changes in these variables over the gait cycle are not as intuitive as some of the variables in the first group. Deviations from normal patterns of activity are clearly visible on the series of two-dimensional charts that show them; the ability to reconstruct the gait of a subject from these representations requires intimate familiarity and extensive experience. The variables are time dependent curves, which cannot be reduced to simpler set of values. The dependence of these variables on the assumptions of the models and the processing involved also requires experience to understand; however, they can be powerful indicators of clinical problems or the success of clinical procedures.

The resultant joint moments and powers are indicators of the efficiency of gait, for satisfactory function reasonably efficient ambulation is required. However, due to the synergy of the body, great care is needed in interpreting the results from such an analysis. The interaction between the joints of the lower limb require that such analyses are performed for the whole limb and the results for the whole limb be considered together.

Clinical interpretation and use

The challenge in interpretation is how to balance all these data and to come to some conclusion. Clinicians are faced with this sort of challenge on a regular basis, when balancing the results of physical examination, laboratory tests, patient comments and other information. There is growing interest in means of summarising data to make it more meaningful for those who are not expert in the interpretation. Software such as that of Delp and others (Delp, 1990) allows the motions and muscle activity to be visualised by presenting an animation of the moving bones and muscles on a computer screen. Other systems have applied so-called expert systems or artificial intelligence techniques to do the initial screening of data (Lapham and Bartlett, 1995) so as to draw the important points to the attention of those who will use the results. These technologies, now in their infancy, will no doubt make the use of gait data easier as time goes on. Gait data should seldom be used in isolation. The data, much like X-rays, laboratory results, or other information, must be considered in the context of the individual being tested, other medical conditions and so forth. The ideal use of gait analysis is where it provides additional information which cannot be gathered by eye alone.

Documentation

At its very simplest, gait analysis provides a numeric record of a subject's walking function. Human memory provides, in general, a poor record of how movements change. The patients themselves have trouble remembering just what it was like before they were treated. At the most basic level, a video tape or other photographic record of the individual before and after their treatment allows a visual assessment of the individual in two different states without the intervening time for memory to fade. Combined with quantitative measures of movement, force, EMG and combined effects to get moments and other information, the gait study can paint a very complete picture of the differences before and after some event. Comparison of these two records can show whether or not the treatment had the desired effect. Gait analysis provides the clinician with a method of rigorous documentation. Although no unique convention exists for data representation, extensive use of well established engineering and physical methodologies can be used to provide an unambiguous record.

Function and pathology

Gait is a natural function, essential for a reasonable quality of life. Accurately measuring gait gives an indication of function. However, in gait there exits the complication of compensation mechanisms. Any measure of gait which is to be used to evaluate pathology and function should be carefully examined to establish whether the deviations from the normal patterns are due to the primary pathology or are adaptations to allow ambulatory function. This can currently only be established by users with experience and understanding of gait data.

Concluding remarks

Gait analysis provides a quantitative measure of walking function. It has provided the clinician with an unambiguous method of documentation and description. However, it is not without its problems, full interpretation of the data is still a specialised area. The increasing use of computer methods to facilitate data interpretation and presentation will allow more widespread use. It is critical that the measurements made remain stable over time. An X-ray taken today can be compared, more or less directly with one taken ten years ago. This has not been the case with many gait systems, where the underlying models and hence the form of the output changed from time to time with little consideration of how to map the older data to the newer.

We see a strong future for gait analysis. In an environment increasingly concerned with outcome measures, gait data provide tools to assess in a quantitative way how much has been achieved by treatments aimed at improving the ambulatory function.

References

Angeloni C, Cappozzo A, Catani F, Leadini A (1992) Quantification of relative displacement between bones and skin- and plate-mounted markers. *Eighth Meeting of the European Society of Biomechanics*, p. 279

Basmajian, JV, De Luca CJ (1985) *Muscles Alive: Their Functions Revealed by Electromyography.* Baltimore: Williams and Wilkins

Delp SL, Loan JP, Hoy MG, Zajac FE, Topp EL, Rosen JM (1990) An interactive graphics-based model of the lower extremity to study orthopaedic surgical procedures. *IEEE Trans. Bio. Eng.*; **37**: 757–767

Gage JR (1991) *Gait Analysis in Cerebral Palsy.* London: Mac Kieth Press

Giannini S, Catani F, Benedetti MG, Leardini A (1994) *Gait Analysis: Methodologies and Clinical Applications.* Amsterdam: IOS Press

Inman VT (1966) Human locomotion. *Can. Med. Assoc. J.;* **94**: 1047–1054

Jarret MO (1976) *A Television/Computer System for Human Locomotion Analysis.* PhD thesis, University of Strathclyde

Kadaba MP, Ramakrishnan HK, Wootten ME (1990) Measurement of lower extremity kinematics during level walking. *J. Orthop. Res.*; **8**: 383–392

Lapham AC, Bartlett RM (1995) The use of artificial intelligence in the analysis of sports performance: a review of applications in human gait analysis and future directions for sports biomechanics. *J. Sports Sci.*; **13**: 229–237

Lynn PA (1973) *An Introduction to the Analysis and Processing of Signals.* London: Macmillan Press

Murray MP, Drought AP, Kory RC (1964) Walking patterns of normal men. *J. Bone Jt Surg.*; **46A**: 335–360

Pynsent PB, Fairbank JCT, Carr AJ (1993) *Outcome Measures in Orthopaedics.* Oxford: Butterworth-Heinemann

Olshen R, Biden E, Wyatt M, Sutherland D (1989) Gait analysis and the bootstrap. *Ann. Statist.*; **17**: 1419–1440

Sienko-Thomas S (1991) *The Gait Analysis Laboratory.* Keynote Address, Session #4, Proceedings of the 7th Annual East Coast Clinical Gait Laboratory Conference, 31 Oct–2 Nov, Richmond, Virginia

Sutherland DH (1984) *Gait Disorders in Childhood and Adolescence.* Baltimore: Williams and Wilkins

Sutherland DH, Olshen RA, Biden EN, Wyatt MP (1988) *The Development of Mature Walking.* Oxford: Blackwell

Whittle MW (1982) Calibration and performance of a 3-dimensional television system for kinematic analysis. *J. Biomech.*; **15**:185–196

Winter DA, Quanbury AO, Hobson DA, Sidwall HG, Reimer G, Trenholm BG, Steinke T, Shlosser H (1974) Kinematics of normal locomotion – a statistical study based on T.V. data. *J. Biomech.*; **7**: 479–486

Woltring HJ (1994) 3-D attitude representation of human joints – a standardization proposal. *J. Biomech.*; **27**: 1399–1414

Chapter 9

Measuring joint range of motion and laxity

DP O'Doherty

Introduction

Loss of motion is a sensitive, but not specific, feature common both to injury and to disease of the musculo-skeletal system. Measuring the range of motion of joints is clinically useful because certain conditions are associated with more profound restriction of motion than others. For example, injury and infection tend to cause a greater loss of motion than do the chronic arthritides. In addition, serial measurements of joint range of motion over time may be helpful when monitoring the progression of a disorder such as rheumatoid arthritis (Parker *et al.*, 1988), or for monitoring the recovery from an injury (Rowley *et al.*, 1986).

There do, therefore, seem to be sound reasons for measuring the range of motion of joints, although these data will only be useful if they are accurate and reliable. On first inspection, measurements of joint range of motion appear to fulfil these criteria. Measurement tends to be straightforward and there is the added attraction of producing a number that can be compared to previous recordings in the same patient or to reference ranges for normal joints. Unfortunately, there are many potential pitfalls in the measurement of joint range of motion and, increasingly, orthopaedic surgeons are becoming aware that ease of application does not necessarily make a test accurate or reliable. Burnstein and Cohen (1993) have called for greater appreciation of the science of measurement in orthopaedic surgery, discussing as an example the measurement of joint motion. This section will discuss some of the problems one needs to be aware of when measuring joint motion and to offer guidelines that may help to optimise the accuracy and reliability of the data.

Difficulties in the measurement of joint range of motion

It is important to be aware when measuring joint range of motion that it is not a measurement of the true way that joints move. Normal functional activities require that joints move in three dimensions; however, measuring this sort of motion remains a research tool and has not been validated in clinical practice. The accepted approach is to describe motion as if it were uniplanar and occurring along one of the cardinal planes of the trunk (sagittal, coronal and transverse). Effectively, this breaks three-dimensional data into its component vectors and, most of the time, this is an acceptable compromise. In the presence of gross deformity, however, the reliability of the data may be greatly reduced.

Which instrument?

Numerous ways for measuring joint range of motion have been described for each joint and this makes comparisons of data between studies almost impossible. A consistent approach to examination is therefore very important for individual studies and, ideally, a consensus should be reached for all measurements.

There is general acceptance that visual inspection is an unreliable method for measuring joint movement (Hellebrandt *et al.*, 1949). Goniometric measurement is likely to be more reliable (Low, 1976) and is the preferred method at the fingers, wrist, elbow, foot, ankle and knee (Greene and Heckman, 1993). These joints allow palpation of bony landmarks and reasonably consistent alignment of the goniometer. Goniometers are also used at the shoulder and hip, although the soft-tissue coverage does not allow the same degree of repeatability when aligning the goniometer in these areas.

Few of the investigators who have studied the reliability of goniometric measurement have used the same study design, but nevertheless, there is consensus in several areas. It is generally accepted that goniometers are only accurate to approximately 5°, which implies a significant reduction in both the accuracy and reliability of measurement when the range of motion under test is small. The use of different goniometers does not seem to affect reliability, so long as the goniometers are of appropriate size for the joint examined (Rothstein *et al.*, 1983; Stratford *et al.*, 1984). The reliability of goniometric measurement varies from joint to joint, being least acceptable in small joints, such as those of the foot, where it is difficult to accurately identify the centre of motion, the axes of movement, and consistent surface landmarks. Stratford *et al.* (1984) comment that reliability of goniometric measurement is improved when only one arm of the goniometer is moved.

With consistent positioning the most accurate method of measuring joint motion is from radiographs, as it isolates the joint concerned thus removing error due to the use of surface landmarks (Backer and Kofoed, 1989; Bohannon, 1989). Under rigorous conditions the dose of radiation can be very small, but it remains difficult to justify radiography for routine usage (Backer and Kofoed, 1989).

More sophisticated measuring devices have been employed by some authors to improve accuracy and reliability. Electrogoniometers have been used in some laboratories to measure joint angles during walking. The accuracy of these devices, particularly those based on potentiometers, has been questioned (Whittle, 1991). Pendulum goniometers have been used at the foot and ankle, but their accuracy does not appear to be as good as simple goniometry (Clapper and Wolf, 1988). Fluid-filled inclinometers have been advocated for measuring spinal movement (Loebl, 1967; Mayer *et al.*, 1993) but Boline *et al.* (1992) found inter-examiner measurement error to be large compared to the scale of measurement. Others have found skin distraction methods more repeatable (Gill *et al.*, 1988; Williams *et al.*, 1993).

Sources of measurement inconsistency

Several sources of inconsistency in measurement have been described (Stratford *et al.*, 1984; Burnstein and Cohen, 1993). Error may arise through failure to measure the range of motion correctly, such as reading off the wrong side of a goniometer. This type of error occurs most frequently in inexperienced observers (Stratford *et al.*, 1984). In addition, observers are prone to end-digit preference whereby readings tend to be rounded up or down to values ending in zero. Expectation bias may occur in serial measurements where the previous reading may influence what is recorded at the next reading. Thus if one anticipates that treatment will improve the range of motion, one will tend to demonstrate change before it has actually occurred.

Biological variation may significantly affect recorded ranges of motion. Diurnal variations are observed in many normal individuals and are a characteristic feature of the chronic arthritides. In addition, maximum range of motion may vary from day to day. In serial studies such biological variation should be considered when changes in the range of motion are observed. Consideration should be given to carrying out testing at similar times of the day.

The instrument used to measure the range of motion must be evaluated for precision (the resolution of the instrument), accuracy (the degree to which the reading of the instrument correlates with the angle under study), reproducibility (the ability of the examiner to obtain similar successive results from repeated measurements) and bias (the systematic alteration of a measurement from the true value being measured). With goniometers, wear or damage to the instrument may result in sloppiness of the hinge, introducing measurement error. If the arms of the instrument are too long or too short interpretation of the reading may be difficult.

The environment of the test and the motivation of the patient may significantly influence the readings obtained when measuring joint range of motion. In particular, the role of pain in limiting joint motion should be recognised.

Measurement reliability

Relatively few studies have examined the reliability of measuring joint range of motion, and the statistical methods used have varied considerably, making their interpretation difficult. Nevertheless, there are some features observed consistently throughout the studies which need highlighting.

There is clear evidence that the reliability of measurement varies according to the joint under consideration (Low, 1976; Boone *et al.*, 1978) (Table 9.1). Reliability is also reduced with increasing complexity of joint movement (Gadjosik and Bohannon, 1987) and where the axes of motion are short and difficult to define, for example in the foot. When the arc of motion under test is small, such as at the subtalar joint, measurement error may sometimes be greater than the arc of motion being tested.

In all reported studies intra-observer reliability is consistently higher than inter-observer reliability. This implies that, in serial studies, the same investigator should perform all the measurements. It also implies that data from different studies cannot be directly compared. Boone *et al.* (1978) suggested that the inter-observer reliability was greater for upper limb motion than for lower. They stated that a change of 5° of motion in the upper limb and 6° in the lower

Table 9.1 The reliability of measurements for active joint range of motion, based on analysis of variance (after Boone et al., 1978). Only one motion was tested at each site: internal rotation at the shoulder, flexion at the elbow, ulnar deviation at the wrist, abduction at the hip, flexion at the knee, and dorsiflexion at the ankle. At least some of the variation between the joints may be due to the smaller ranges of motion tested at some sites. Note the higher intra-observer reliability at almost every site

	Inter-observer	Intra-observer
Shoulder	0.97	0.96
Elbow	0.88	0.94
Wrist	0.73	0.76
Hip	0.55	0.75
Knee	0.50	0.87
Foot	0.69	0.80

limb could be considered significant when more than one observer was taking measurements. In fact, these figures should be doubled to improve the likelihood that true change will be detected at the 5% level. Thus in the upper limb changes in the range of motion of less than 10° may reflect measurement error rather than true change of motion. The corresponding figure for the lower limb is 12°.

Reliability is increased by the use of standard methods for examination (Ekstrand et al., 1982), suggesting that written protocols should be used. This appears to be more important than the particular measurement technique employed. The use of the neutral zero position, which represents the normal anatomical position of the body, is widely recommended as the starting point for the measurement of joint movements (Cave and Roberts, 1936; Debrunner, 1982; Stratford et al., 1984; Greene and Heckman, 1993). Measurers should be aware of end-digit preference and expectation bias, and when studies are being reported the reliability of the measurements should be recorded.

General factors influencing normal joint range

Even when the range of motion is tested using standardised methods, great individual variation is recognised (Table 9.2). One must be cautious therefore of defining normality in terms of a specific range of motion for a given joint. This has been demonstrated, amongst others, by Boone and Azen (1979) and Roass and Anderson (1982). In random samples of normal males they demonstrated that for a given arc of motion under test the arcs varied considerably from person to person.

In population studies the range of motion of joints tends to diminish slightly with age, but the changes are small (Boone and Azen, 1979; Roach and Miles, 1991; Dvorak et al., 1992; Nigg et al., 1992). For most joints significant loss of mobility is more likely to be due to a pathological process than to ageing per se (Roach and Miles, 1991). The situation in neonates is complicated by the effects of intra-uterine packaging so that for the first few months of life there are contractures at most joints in the extremities (Forero et al., 1989). In later childhood ranges of motion are usually greater than those observed in adults and this is thought to reflect joint laxity (Wynne-Davies, 1971; Svenningsen et al., 1989; Cheng et al., 1991).

Table 9.2 Mean maximal ranges of motion (in degrees) and the 95% confidence intervals (CI) from three studies of joint range of motion in young adults (age 20–50 years). Note the wide confidence intervals for most measurements indicating both the considerable person to person variation and the differences between the studies. Ahlberg *et al.* (1988) and Roass and Andersson (1982) (data for left side only) measured passive range of motion whereas Boone and Azen (1979) examined active motion

	Ahlberg *et al.* (n = 50)		Roass and Anderson (n = 180–210)		Boone and Azen (n = 56)	
	Mean	95%CI	Mean	95%CI	Mean	95%CI
Hip						
Flexion	13.9	(3.1–24.7)	9.5	(–0.9–19.9)	12.1	(1.5–22.7)
Extension	130.8	(103.4–158.2)	120.4	(104.1–136.7)	121.3	(108.8–133.8)
Abduction	50.8	(38.8–62.8)	38.4	(24.5–52.7)	40.5	(28.7–52.3)
Adduction	30.1	(17.4–42.8)	30.5	(16.2–44.8)	25.6	(18.5–32.7)
Internal rotation	36.7	(12.8–60.6)	32.5	(16.5–48.7)	44.4	(36.0–52.8)
External rotation	72.9	(51.9–93.9)	33.7	(20.4–47.0)	44.2	(34.8–53.6)
Knee						
Extension	–6.7	(–12.0–1.4)	–1.7	(–7.4–4.0)		
Flexion	159.6	(142.9–176.3)	143.7	(131.1–156.5)	141.2	(130.8–151.6)
Ankle						
Plantarflexion	43.4	(23.8–63.0)	39.6	(24.8–54.6)	54.3	(42.7–65.9)
Dorsiflexion	32.2	(21.2–43.2)	15.3	(3.9–26.7)	12.2	(4.2–20.2)

No consistent differences have been noted between males and females for joint motion at any site (Greene and Heckman, 1993). In contrast, cultural differences may be important, with increases in hip, knee and ankle motion reported in Saudi Arabians compared to Scandinavians (Ahlberg *et al.*, 1988), and increased hip motion in Chinese compared to Caucasians (Hoaglund *et al.*, 1973).

Occupation may also influence joint range of motion with significant changes in hip and knee motion observed in ballet dancers (Reid *et al.*, 1987).

The consistent observation that ranges of motion in paired joints are virtually identical on the right and left sides of the body (Boone and Azen, 1979; Ahlberg *et al.*, 1988; Svenningsen *et al.*, 1989; Mallon *et al.*, 1991) is of major importance. This implies that where there is an uninjured limb it may be used as a control against which the injured or diseased limb may be tested.

Principles of goniometry

The principles of goniometry will be described as this is the most commonly used method for measuring joint movement (Green and Heckman, 1993). The key to measurement is consistency of technique, both in terms of what method of measuring joint motion is used and in how it is applied. Unfortunately, for every joint several different methods of examination have been described and each has its advocates. Thus at the ankle some clinicians measure active dorsiflexion and some passive, some measure dorsiflexion with the knee bent and some with the knee straight, and some measure dorsiflexion in the weight-bearing ankle (loaded active dorsiflexion) whilst others measure it in the unloaded foot. For each of these methods different reference ranges have been described. Generally speaking, passive range of motion will be greater than active, particularly in the presence of muscle weakness or arthritis. In practice, the precise method used is not critically important provided that the method has been documented and applied consistently. The best way of achieving this is to write a standard protocol to be followed at each measurement.

Cave and Roberts in 1936 laid the foundations of modern goniometry. They introduced the concept of measuring joint range of motion from a defined starting point, and advocated the use of goniometers. These concepts have been refined and form the basis of the protocols for measurement put forward by the American Academy of Orthopaedic Surgeons (Greene and Heckman, 1993).

The first aim in measurement is to define the starting position for measurement. This is termed the 'zero starting position' and for most joints is the extended anatomic position of the extremity, i.e. the patient is standing upright with the arms by the side, the elbows extended and the forearms supinated, the knees and hips extended and the feet pointing forwards. This position is designated 0° and the range of motion in a given plane is measured in degrees from this point. A distinction is made between extension (normal motion opposite to flexion but in the same plane) and hyperextension (atypical motion). A consistent starting point is critical for reliable measurement of motion but at certain sites (e.g. the subtalar joint) it may be difficult to define. This introduces a significant measurement error which may adversely affect reliability.

The next step is to locate the centre of rotation of the joint and to place the pivot of the goniometer over it. The arms of the goniometer are then placed along the longitudinal axes of the limb, one proximal and one distal to the joint. Ideally, the 'nought' mark should be positioned on the distal segment. The proximal end of the goniometer is held in place while the joint is moved and the distal arm of the goniometer rotated. At completion of the movement, the degree of joint motion can be recorded from the goniometer.

Specific regions

Rather than discuss the advantages and disadvantages of individual refinements of technique it is proposed to discuss the particular movements that consensus suggests can be usefully measured for each joint. For greater detail the reader is referred to *The Clinical Measurement of Joint Motion* from the American Academy of Orthopaedic Surgeons (Greene and Heckman, 1994) which should be required reading for all clinicians interested in measuring the range of motion of joints.

Upper limb

Movement at the shoulder allows the arm to sweep through more than a hemisphere of motion. This is achieved by a combination of movements occurring at the glenohumeral, scapulothoracic, acromioclavicular and sternoclavicular joints. For convenience motion is examined as a composite, and is recorded in relation to the cardinal planes of the trunk. The zero starting position is the neutral anatomic position with the arms by the side of the body, the elbows extended and forearms supinated. From this position, with the patient standing, one can measure flexion, extension and abduction. Rotation is measured with the elbow flexed to 90°, either with the arm at the side of the body or abducted to 90°. Posterior reach (internal rotation) is also commonly recorded, being the highest midline segment of the back that is reached by the hitchhiking thumb. There are no data on reliability for this measurement but examiners not infrequently have difficulty locating the midline landmarks suggesting that reliability is probably suspect.

Despite three articulations where motion can occur (ulnohumeral, radiohumeral and radioulnar joints), the elbow is effectively a uni-axial joint. The zero starting position is with the extremity straight. Natural motion is flexion and is centred on the ulnohumeral joint. Motion in the opposite direction is extension.

Forearm rotation occurs at the proximal and distal radioulnar joints, and the radiohumeral joint. The zero starting position is with the elbow flexed 90°, the wrist and fingers straight and the hand lined up with the humerus, i.e. standing upright on its ulnar border. Pronation attempts to turn the palm face down, and supination turns the palm face up. One arm of the goniometer is lined up with the thumb while the other remains vertical.

The wrist allows flexion (volar flexion) and extension (dorsiflexion), and radial and ulnar deviation. Circumduction does occur at the wrist but requires special techniques for measurement that are not of practical usage. The centre of motion lies in the proximal pole of the capitate, and this is where the goniometer should be centred. LeStayo and Wheeler (1994) found that the position of the goniometer which gave the most reliable results was when the goniometer lay on the dorsum of the wrist.

Finger joint motion is essentially uni-axial, being pure flexion or extension. Some abduction and adduction occur at the metacarpophalangeal joints but are not routinely measured. One should be aware that the position of the other joints in the hand can influence motion via the tenodesis effects of the long extensors of the fingers (Mallon *et al.*, 1991). It is important, therefore, that the wrist remain in the neutral position when measuring finger motion and the fingers not being evaluated should be allowed unrestrained motion. The dorsal position of the goniometer is recommended (Greene and Heckman, 1993). A summation of finger movements (i.e. for each finger the sum of their flexion at the metacarpophalangeal and interphalangeal joints minus their extension deficits) can be measured for both active and passive motion (ASSH, 1976). The difference between the total active motion and total passive motion is said to reflect tendon adherence. The attraction of this measurement is that it produces a single global figure for each finger that can be used for analysis. It should not be forgotten, however, that adding three measurements will significantly increase the error of measurement.

Reflecting its importance to hand function, motion of the thumb is complex. In practice only flexion and extension at the metacarpophalangeal and interphalangeal joints, and opposition are routinely measured. The zero position is the extended thumb with the phalanges in line with the thumb metacarpal, and the wrist in neutral. Opposition is a composite movement most easily measured by recording the distance from the tip of the thumb to the base of the little finger. Few reliability data are available for this measurement.

Lower limb

As at the shoulder, considerable three-dimensional movement is possible at the hip joint. Movement is tested with the patient lying down, and most movements are recorded in the supine position. All except flexion may be measured with the hips flexed or extended, and rotation can also be tested with the patient prone. In the supine position the zero starting position for flexion is achieved by flexing the opposite hip until the lumbar spine flattens onto the examiner's hand. For abduction and adduction the zero position is with the legs at right angles to a transverse line drawn between the anterior superior iliac spines. In infants and young children it is more usual to measure abduction with the hip flexed to 90°. Rotation can either be measured with the patient supine, the hips flexed 90° and the knees flexed 90°, or in the prone position with the knees flexed 90°.

For measuring purposes the knee is essentially uni-axial. Although three-dimensional components such as the screw home mechanism are measurable using skeletal co-ordinate data and Eulerian mathematics (Wei *et al.*, 1993), such techniques remain experimental. The zero starting position is with the knee straight.

Several methods have been proposed for measuring ankle motion. Active ankle motion with the knee flexed seems to provide the most reliable data (Greene and Heckman, 1993). The zero starting position is with the knee flexed to a right angle and the foot perpendicular to the tibia.

Subtalar motion is commonly measured but has poor reliability due to the difficulty in finding the landmarks and to the small range of motion. The zero starting position is with the patient prone, knees flexed 90° and the ankle gently dorsiflexed. This tends to line the subtalar joint perpendicular to the tibia. Inversion and eversion are measured from here.

Midfoot motion is subjective and cannot be measured with any accuracy. Lesser toe motion is seldom recorded. Hallux motion is not measured from the anatomic neutral position. The zero position has the proximal phalanx of the hallux aligned with the plantar surface of the foot.

The spine

The measurement of spinal movement is less straightforward than in the extremities. Movements occur at several joints simultaneously and this makes the use of a goniometer cumbersome. In consequence, alternative methods are used for at least some movements, although there remains little consensus on which method is best. There are few data on measurement in the thoracic spine, and most interest has focused on the cervical and lumbar spines. For both, the zero starting position is the erect posture, with the neck aligned with the trunk and the nose vertical and perpendicular to the axis of the shoulders. For neck motion it is important to stabilise the trunk so that motion only occurs at the neck.

For the cervical spine visual estimation is the commonly used method for estimating motion (Greene and Heckman, 1993) but better reliability is found using goniometry (Youdas *et al.*, 1991) and inclinometry (Alund and Larsson, 1990; Youdas *et al.*, 1991; Dvorak *et al.*, 1992). Rotation appears to be best measured using goniometry.

Several methods for measuring lumbar spine motion have been tested with most interest expressed for measuring flexion. The common fingertip-to-floor method has only poor reliability. The modified Schober method, a skin distraction technique, has consistently been shown to be the most reliable method for measuring lumbar spinal flexion (Moll and Wright, 1971; Williams *et al.*, 1993). In this technique a midline mark is made connecting the dimples of Venus, and further marks made 5 cm below and 10 cm above this mark. At maximum flexion the increase in length is recorded. Extension may be measured in a similar fashion (Williams *et al.*, 1993). Lateral flexion may best be measured by the distance the outstretched hand travels down the outside of the thigh when moving from the zero position to maximal lateral flexion (Mellin *et al.*, 1986). Spinal rotation is much more difficult to measure, and tests have poor reliability.

Joint laxity

Excessive joint laxity is a common finding in young children, in certain ethnic groups and in some gifted athletes and artistes. In addition, it is a feature of a number of medical conditions, such as the Ehlers–Danlos syndrome and osteogenesis imperfecta. It should be recognised, however, that the mobility of a joint is a continuously distributed variable with one end of the range being limitation of motion and the other being hypermobility. Where the cut-off point may be is uncertain. Interest in this field has spawned a number of methods for determining generalised joint laxity including visual methods examining laxity at one or several joints, or more sophisticated measurements from single joints using radiographic, photographic or mechanical techniques. In practice the reliability of simple clinical tests are satisfactory (Cheng *et al.*, 1991). The five point method of Carter and Wilkinson (1964) (Table 9.3), or its subsequent modification (Beighton *et al.*, 1973), is the most widely used method and examines finger hyperextension, thumb to forearm apposition, elbow and knee hyperextension and ankle dorsiflexion. Dijkstra *et al.* (1994) added an additional test of lumbar spine flexion and found good inter- and intra-tester reliability.

For individual joints testing for joint instability may be important for evaluating symptoms and disability. One should recognise, however, that detectable laxity may not signify dysfunction (Emery and Mullaji, 1991).

Only at the knee have serious attempts been made to quantify joint laxity, fuelled by the tremenduous interest in injuries to the cruciate ligaments. Clinical examination remains the most successful method for diagnosing ligamentous instability of the knee, but it can only grossly estimate the severity of the

Table 9.3 Criteria for measuring joint hypermobility (after Carter and Wilkinson, 1964). The presence of three or more features suggests hypermobility

- Thumb opposition to the volar surface of the forearm
- Hyperextension of the elbow >10°
- Hyperextension of the knee >10°
- Passive hyperextension of the fingers to lie parallel to the dorsum of the forearm
- Passive dorsiflexion of the ankle >45°

instability (Frymoyer, 1993). Instrumented measurement of tibial translation is said to provide more accurate quantification of instability, and a number of different devices are now available for this. These instruments are expensive, require proficiency in their use and are sensitive to the examiners experience. Several observers have questioned their reliability and accuracy (Graham *et al.*, 1991; Fleming *et al.*, 1992), and their relation to function is at best uncertain. They cannot currently be recommended for routine use, but may be of value in research protocols.

References

Ahlberg A, Moussa M, Al-Nahdi M (1988) On Geographical variations in the normal range of joint motion. *Clin. Orthop. Rel. Res.*; **234**: 229–231

Alund M, Larsson SE (1990) Three dimensional analysis of neck motion: a clinical method. *Spine*; **15**: 87–91

ASSH (1976) *Clinical Assessment Committee Report.* American Society for Surgery of the Hand

Backer M, Kofoed H (1989) Passive ankle mobility: clinical measurement compared with radiography. *J. Bone Jt. Surg.*; **71B**: 696–698

Beighton P, Solomon L, Soskolne CL (1973) Articular mobility in an African population. *Ann. Rheum. Dis.*; **32**: 413–418

Bohannon RW, Tiberio D, Zito M (1989) Selected measures of ankle dorsiflexion range of motion: differences and intercorrelations. *Foot Ankle*; **10**: 99–103

Boline PD, Keating JC, Haas M, Anderson AV (1992) Intra-examiner reliability and discriminant validity of inclinometric measurement of lumbar rotation in chronic low-back pain patients and subjects without low-back pain. *Spine*; **17**: 335–338

Boone DC, Azen SP, Lin C-M, Spence C, Baron C, Lee L (1978) Reliability of goniometric measurements. *Phys. Ther.*; **11**: 1355–1360

Boone DC, Azen SP (1979) Normal ranges of motion of joints in male subjects. *J. Bone Jt. Surg.*; **61A**: 756–759

Burnstein AH, Cohen J (1993) Editorial: measurements in the conduct of research. *J. Bone Jt. Surg.*; **75A**: 319–320

Carter C, Wilkinson J (1964) Persistent joint laxity and congenital dislocation of the hip. *J. Bone Jt. Surg.*; **46B**: 40–45

Cave EF, Roberts SM (1936) A method for measuring and recording joint function. *J. Bone Jt. Surg.*; **18**: 455–465

Cheng JC, Chan PS, Hui PW (1991) Joint laxity in children. *J. Paediatr. Orthop.*; **11**: 752–756

Clapper MP, Wolf SL (1988) Comparison of the reliability of the Orthoranger and the standard goniometer for assessing active lower extremity range of motion. *Phys. Ther.*; **68**: 214–218

Debrunner HU (1982) *Orthopaedic Diagnosis.* Georg Thieme Verlag. Stuttgart.

Dijkstra PU, de Bont LGM, van der Weele LTh, Boering G (1994) Joint mobility measurements: reliability of a standardized method. *J. Craniomand. Pract.*; **12**: 52–57

Dvorak J, Antinnes JA, Panjabi M, Loustalot D, Bonomo M (1992) Age and gender related nomal motion of the cervical spine. *Spine*; **17**: S393–S398

Ekstrand J, Witkorsson M, Oberg B, Gillquist J (1982) Lower extremity goniometry measurements: a study to determine their reliability. *Arch. Phys. Med. Rehabil.*; **63**: 171–175

Emery RJH, Mullaji AB (1991) Glenohumeral joint instability in normal adolescents. *J. Bone Jt. Surg.*; **73B**: 406–408

Fleming BC, Johnson RJ, Shapiro E, Fenwick J, Howe JG, Pope MH (1992) Clinical versus instrumented knee testing on autopsy specimens. *Clin. Orthop. Rel. Res.*; **282**: 196–207

Forero N, Okamura LA, Larson MA (1989) Normal ranges of hip motion in neonates. *J. Pediatr. Orthop.*; **9**: 391–395

Frymoyer JW (ed.) (1993) *Orthopaedic Knowledge Update 4.* American Academy of Orthopaedic Surgeons. Rosemont.

Gadjosik RL, Bohannon RW (1987) Clinical measurement of range of motion: review of goniometry emphasizing reliability and validity. *Phys. Ther.*; **67**: 1867–1872

Gill K, Johnson GB, Haugh LD, Pope MH (1988) Repeatability of four clinical methods for assessment of lumbar spinal motion. *Spine*; **13**: 50–53

Graham GP, Johnson S, Dent CM, Fairclough JA (1991) Comparison of clinical tests and the KT1000 in the diagnosis of anterior cruciate ligament rupture. *Br. J. Sports Med.*; **25**: 96–97

Greene WB, Heckman JD (eds) (1994) *The Clinical Measurement of Joint Motion.* American Academy of Orthopaedic Surgeons. Rosemont.

Hellebrandt FA, Duvall EN, Moore ML (1949) The measurement of joint motion: part III. Reliability of goniometry. *Phys. Ther. Rev.*; **29**: 302–307

Hoaglund FT, Yau AC, Wong WL (1973) Osteoarthritis of the hip and other joints in Southern Chinese in Hong Kong. *J. Bone Jt. Surg.*; **55A**: 547–557

LeStayo PC, Wheeler DL (1994) Reliability of passive wrist flexion and extension goniometric measurements: a multicenter study. *Phys. Ther.*; **74**: 162–176

Loebl WY (1967) Measurement of spinal posture and range of spinal movement. *Ann. Phys. Med.*; **9**: 103–110

Low J (1976) Reliability of joint measurements. *Physiotherapy*; **62**: 227–229

Mallon WJ, Brown HR, Nunley JA (1991) Digital ranges of motion: normal values in young adults. *J. Hand Surg.*; **16A**: 882–888

Mayer T, Brady S, Bovasso E, Pope P, Gatchel G (1993) Non-invasive measurement of cervical tri-planar motion in normal subjects. *Spine*; **18**: 2191–2195

Mellin GP (1986) Accuracy of measuring lateral flexion of the spine with a tape. *Clin. Biomech.*; **1**: 85–89

Moll JMH, Wright V (1971) Normal range of spinal mobility: an objective clinical study. *Ann. Rheum. Dis.*; **30**: 381–386

Nigg BM, Fisher V, Allinger TL, Ronsky JR, Engsberg JR (1992) Range of motion of the foot as a function of age. *Foot Ankle*; **13**: 336–343

Parker JW, Harrell PB, Alarcon GS (1988) The value of the Joint Alignment and Motion Scale in rheumatoid arthritis. *J. Rheumatol.*; **15**: 1212–1215

Reid DC, Burnham RS, Saboe LA, Kushner SF (1987) Lower extremity flexibility patterns in classical ballet dancers and their correlation to lateral hip and knee injuries. *Am. J. Sports Med.*; **15**: 347–352

Roach KE, Miles TP (1991) Normal hip and knee active range of motion: the relationship to age. *Phys. Ther.*; **71**: 656–665

Roass A, Anderson GBJ (1982) Normal range of motion of the hip, knee and ankle joints in male subjects, 30–40 years of age. *Acta Orthop. Scand.*; **53**: 205–208

Rothstein JM, Miller PJ, Roettger RF (1983) Goniometric reliability in a clinical setting: elbow and knee measurements. *Phys. Ther.*; **63**: 1611–1615

Rowley DI, Norris SH, Duckworth T (1986) A prospective trial comparing operative and manipulative treatment of ankle fractures. *J. Bone Jt. Surg.*; **68B**: 610–613

Stratford P, Agostino V, Brazeau C, Gowitzke BA (1984) Reliability of joint angle measurement: a discussion of methodology issues. *Physiother. Canada*; **36**: 5–9

Svenningsen S, Terjsen T, Auflem M, Berg V (1989) Hip motion related to age and sex. *Acta Orthop. Scand.*; **60**: 97–100

Wei S-H, McQuade KJ, Smidt GL (1993) Three-dimensional joint range of motion measurements from skeletal coordinate data. *JOSPT*; **18**: 687–691

Whittle M (1991) *Gait Analysis: an Introduction.* Oxford: Butterworth-Heinemann

Williams R, Binkley J, Bloch R, Goldsmith CH, Minuk T (1993) Reliability of modified-modified Schober and double inclinometer methods for measuring lumbar flexion and extension. *Phys. Ther.*; **73**: 26–37

Wynne-Davies R (1971) Familial joint laxity. *Proc. R. Soc. Med.*; **64**: 689–690

Youdas JW, Carey JR, Garrett TR (1991) Reliability of measurements of cervical spine range of motion – comparison of three methods. *Phys. Ther.*; **71**: 98–104

Chapter 10

Anthropometry

RG Burwell

Science is rooted in creative interpretation. Numbers suggest, constrain, and refute....

(Gould, 1992)

Introduction

Anthropometry is the measurement of the human body. It is that branch of physical anthropology which deals with human morphometry, biometry or metrology. Scientists measure the body and its segments with respect to lengths, widths, diameters, circumferences (girths) and areas. They calculate ratios and proportions based on two or more of these measurements, identify shapes, sizes and topography.

Orthopaedic surgeons in their daily practice use a variety of anthropometric techniques. Because the musculo-skeletal system of humans is so readily available for measurement by surface and radiological techniques, *morphometry* is widely and increasingly used in orthopaedic science.

Historical

The Egyptians of 40 centuries ago measured the world about them by the use of anatomical units. They based their domestic metrology on the *width of the hand* and its multiples (Rabey, 1968, 1979). In the size relationships of its various parts the human body exhibits very remarkable proportions which are known collectively as the canon. The ancient Greeks established the human figure as 7-*heads* in length some 2400 years ago and we regard as beautiful those individuals and models in whom these proportions are embodied as in classical statues. This canon of proportion of the human figure is equivalent to the foot-rule in measurement, the axiom in geometry and the Pole star in navigation (Hogarth, 1965).

According to Tanner (1981), anthropometry was born, not of medicine or science, but of the arts impregnated by the spirit of Pythagorean philosophy (Figure 10.1). Painters and sculptors needed instructions about the relative proportions of legs and trunk, shoulders and hips, eyes and forehead, so that they could more easily go about what we might nowadays consider the mundane occupation of making life-like images. However, the practice of measuring people emerged because of military requirements – tall soldiers were regarded as preferable to short ones. The first longitudinal growth study was made by Count de Montbeillard upon his son in the years 1759–77. In 1833 the introduction of the Normal Curve by Quatelet, who in many ways was the founder of modern

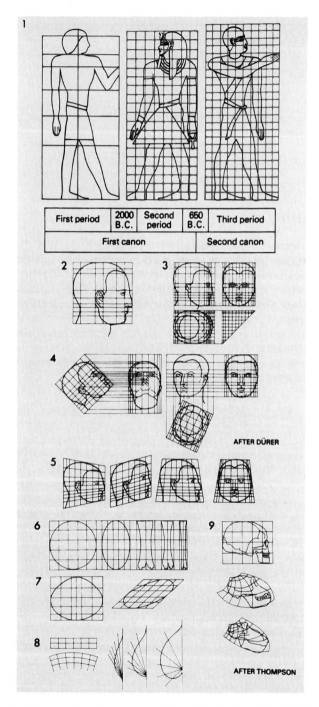

Figure 10.1 Synthetic co-ordinates in human morphology introduced by: 1 Ancient Egyptian artists, 2–5 Dürer, 6–9 D'Arcy Thompson. (Reproduced by kind permission of Dr G Rabey and MT Press Ltd)

statistics, provided a mathematical foundation for the study of human growth (Boyd, 1980; Tanner, 1981). Galton (1822–1911), a pioneer of modern statistics, believed that with sufficient labour and ingenuity anything might be measured and that measurement is the primary creation of a scientific study (Gould, 1992).

Definition

Anthropometry

Winter (1990) writes:

> Anthropometry is the major branch of anthropology that studies the physical measurements of the human body to determine differences in individuals and groups. A wide variety of physical measurements are required to describe and differentiate the characteristics of race, sex, age and body type. In the past the major emphasis of these studies has been evolutionary and historical. More recently a major impetus has come from the needs of technological development especially man-machine interfaces, work-space design, cockpits, pressure suits, armor and so on. Most of these needs are satisfied by basic linear, area and volume measurements. However, human movement analysis requires kinetic measures as well: masses, moments of inertia, and their locations. There exists also a moderate body of knowledge regarding joint centres of rotation, the origin and insertion of muscles, the angle and pull of tendons and the length and cross-sectional area of muscles.
>
> (Boyd, 1980; Tanner, 1981)

Classification

Anthropometry covers a wide field and is useful to consider it under several headings as follows.

Classical anthropometry

The word *anthropometry* was first used in relation to the measurement of anatomical components on the surface of the human body which can be termed '*classical anthropometry*' (Weiner and Lourie, 1969, 1981; Roebuck *et al.,* 1975; Cameron, 1984). The common measurements made include (Figure 10.2a,b,c,d):

- General body – stature, supine length, weight.
- Trunk – length, sitting height, crown–rump length.
- Widths – biacromial, bi-iliac and lateral chest.
- Sagittal – AP chest diameter.
- Limbs:
    - lengths: total leg length, tibial length, foot length and their asymmetries.
    - circumferences: thigh, subgluteal and calf and their asymmetries
- Fat folds – subscapular, triceps.
- Head – circumference, length and breadth.

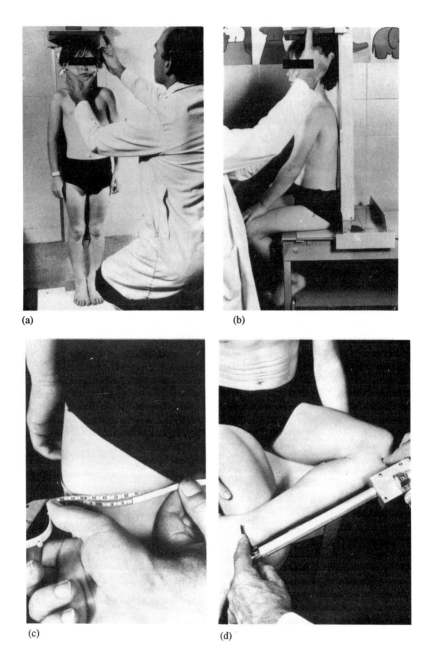

(a)   (b)

(c)   (d)

Figure 10.2 Some techniques in anthropometry: (a) Standing height using the Harpenden stadiometer; (b) Sitting height using the Harpenden sitting height table; (c) Subgluteal thigh circumference with a steel tape at the level of the gluteal fold – a useful measurement in hip disorders; (d) Tibial length using the Harpenden anthropometer

In analysing these data, anthropologists use a variety of derivatives including centiles, standard deviation scores, and ratios expressed as indices (Figures 10.3 and 10.4) (Burwell *et al.,* 1980; Falkner and Tanner, 1986; Winter, 1990). Many linear measurements of the body are distributed normally (Gaussian), but weight and skin folds are each skewed. In longitudinal studies of children's growth the velocity of growth in stature is plotted. The word *auxology* is used to refer to growth research (Pelto *et al.,* 1989).

Nutritional anthropometry is used particularly in developing countries where malnutrition is widespread. Body weight is by far the most frequently used

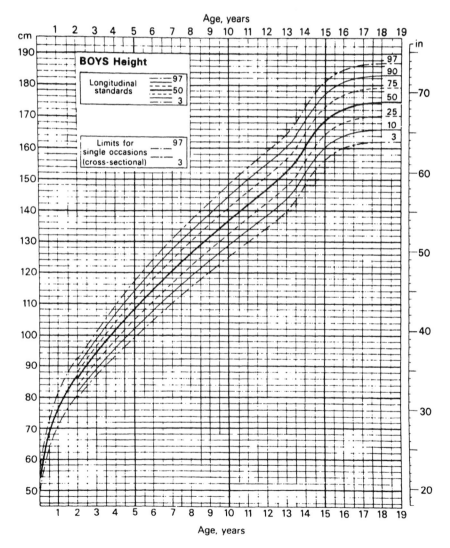

Figure 10.3 Standing height centile chart for boys. (Reproduced by permission of Castlemead Publications Ltd, Chart No GDB11A)

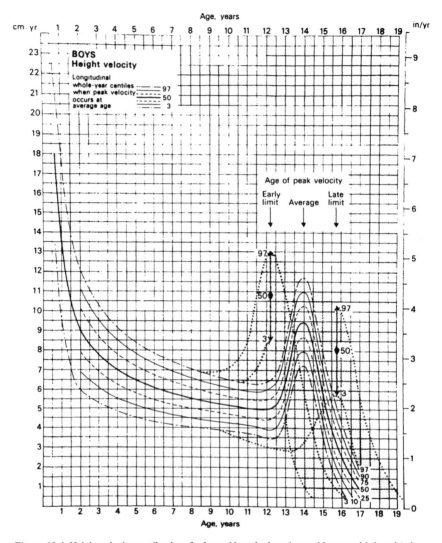

Figure 10.4 Height velocity centile chart for boys. Note the long interval between birth and 'take-off' into the adolescent growth spurt; the mid-growth spurt is not evident in this chart. (Reproduced by permission of Castlemead Publications Ltd, Chart No LVH V2A)

criterion to assess nutritional status of population groups (Vijayraghavan and Sastry, 1976).

Anthropometry of the head and face

Craniometry and the measurement of brain size were rigorously pursued in the nineteenth century (see Gould, 1992). Recently, the availability of MRI has reactivated the debate on brain size, gender and intelligence (Harvey and Krebs, 1990; Ankney, 1992; Rushton, 1992).

Maxillofacial surgeons and scientists have made outstanding contributions to anthropometry (Herron, 1974; Burke and Healy, 1993; Farkas, 1994). *Audiograms and speech spectrograms* can be viewed as anthropometric methods. *Stereotaxic surgery* of the brain uses anthropometry. *Forensic medicine* utilises measurements from skeletal remains, particularly the skull to identify an individual (Iscan and Helmer, 1993).

Radiological anthropometry

X-radiation of the human body provides images of bones and soft tissues which when measured is *radiological anthropometry* such as *pelvimetry*. The more recent use of CT, MRI and ultrasound, by providing images which can be measured, is contributing to the field of anthropometry. Radionuclide scintigraphy (Galasko and Weber, 1984) can provide quantitative data which is a *radionuclide anthropometry*. Anthropometric measurements are widely used in radiotherapy. Medical ultrasound is now being used in the orthopaedic metrology of lower limb bone torsions (Moulton *et al.*, 1993, 1994, 1995a,b).

Cadaveric, pathological and histological anthropometry

Measurements made on cadavers is *cadaveric anthropometry*. Most recently, thin sections of an entire human male cadaver have been digitised to create three-dimensional (3-D) images of the various parts of the human body ('Adam'). Similar thin sections of an entire female cadaver are currently being digitised for similar usage ('Eve').

Cartesian co-ordinates and deformations

Dürer (1471–1528) connected anatomical points to form a lattice which Descartes (1596–1650) developed as *the method of co-ordinates* as a generalisation from the proportional diagrams of the artist and the architect (Figure 10.1) (Rabey, 1979). D'Arcy Thompson (1942) showed that shape alteration, or deformations can result from geometrical co-ordinate transformations. The inherent geometrical information captured by Cartesian co-ordinates allows a much more efficient mechanism for identifying local shape differences than does traditional morphometrics relying on Euclidean distances between the landmarks. This capacity to localise shape differences is currently providing for a comprehensive description of the shape variation associated with each of developmental and physiological variables (Walker, 1994).

Biostereometrics

Biostereometrics is the spatial and spatio-temporal analysis of form and function based on principles of analytical geometry (Figure 10.5) (Herron, 1974; Burwell, 1978; Rabey, 1979). The science of biostereometrics deals not only with 3-D measurements of biological subjects in space but also with any variation of the measurements with time such as movement and growth. The potential of stereometric measurement of the human body was demonstrated over 500 years ago in Florence by Alberti.

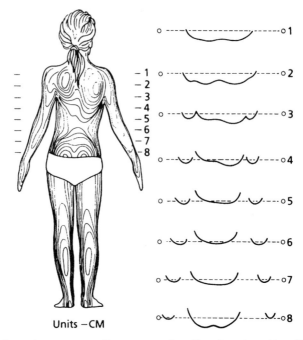

Units – CM

Figure 10.5 Stereophotogrammetry. Contour map and profiles of a patient with scoliosis in the standard standing position. (Reproduced by kind permissiom of Mr Hugg and the American Society of Photogrammetry, Burwell, 1978)

In basic terms, spatial and spatio-temporal measurements of the human body involves using the following systems (Figure 10.6): orientation, reference, recording, interface and analysis systems, also systems for expressing the data. The increasing power of computer hardware and software has made it possible to analyse and reconstruct 3-D structures but the problem of how to visualise three dimensions is inherent in all imaging systems, whether they are using coherent or incoherent light, stereo X-rays, CT and MRI scans or ultrasound. 3-D anthropometric data are being used in computer-aided design (CAD) for textile manufacturing (Jones *et al.*, 1989).

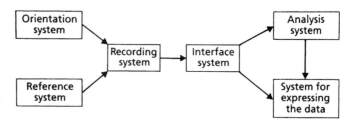

Figure 10.6 A flow diagram to show the relations of the systems used in biostereometrics

Kinanthropometry and kinesiology

Kinanthropometry, a branch of biostereometrics, is a relatively new scientific discipline that focuses solely on the measurement of size, shape, proportion, composition, maturation and gross function as related to such concerns as growth, exercise, performance and nutrition (Adrian and Cooper, 1995). The International Working Group in Kinanthropometry was founded in 1978 by the International Council of Sport Science and Physical Education, under the auspices of UNESCO. The International Society for the Advancement of Kinanthropometry was founded in 1986 (Malina, 1984). It is part of the wider field of kinesiology (Steindler, 1955; Soderberg, 1986).

Muscle anthropometry

Fundamental to the study of kinesiology and pathological motion are the terms and associated units used to describe motion and the forces producing or resulting from motion. Also essential are the factors which influence motion hence, relating these factors to movement is essential to understanding normal and abnormal movement (Soderberg, 1986). In calculating the forces produced by individual muscles during normal movement, some dimensions from the muscles themselves are needed. The functional or physiological cross-sectional area of a muscle is a measure of the number of sarcomeres in parallel with the angle of pull of the muscle. This is *muscle anthropometry* (Winter, 1990).

Anthropometric models – mechanical, mathematical and virtual reality

Mechanical models of parts of the human body based on anthropometric measurements have long been used. Computer-generated 3-D reconstructions provide the opportunity for measurement (Sutherland, 1986). Computer-aided simulation (Murphy *et al.,* 1986) and other mathematical models are employed, especially *finite element analysis* (Figure 10.7) (Huiskes and Chao, 1983; Choo *et al.,* 1989; Huiskes, 1992).

   Virtual reality can be defined as human interaction in an environment that is simulated by a computer. Currently the potential medical applications of this new technology are being explored in minimally invasive surgery, neurosurgery and 'tele-presence surgery' (Annotation, 1994). In this new technology 50–70 sensors are placed on the surface of the body and multiple cameras used to capture the images and movements for storage on a computer. The 3-D image is then placed on digital sets and motion algorithms are used to drive the movements. Software that enables shoppers to become models on a 'virtual' catwalk on their own television sets, is being used in a trial of 'interactive TV', in one commercial application. The model on the television screen accepts the shopper's 'vital statistics' and the system allows users to try on 'virtual' clothes in the comfort of their homes (Gray, 1992, 1994).

Anthropometry, growth theory and evolution

Historically, most disciplines begin with the descriptive phase. Bogin (1988) comments that one sign of a maturing discipline is when it begins to develop

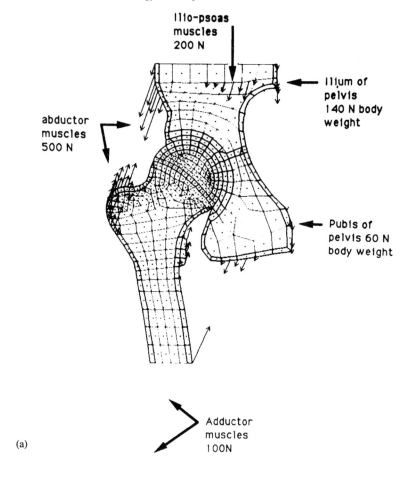

Illo-psoas
muscles
200 N

Illum of
pelvis
140 N body
weight

abductor
muscles
500 N

Publs of
pelvis 60 N
body weight

(a)

Adductor
muscles
100N

hypotheses to examine the nature of the processes that account for the descriptive data. Moreover, mature sciences are noted for their ability to simplify several hypotheses that have been independently verified into comprehensive theories that explain the known data and, in turn, indicate the kind of observations that should be made in further research. Human growth research is now entering the hypothesis testing stage, but a number of purely descriptive studies are still being produced. As Gould (1991) writes, 'Science is.... not a mechanized, robotlike accumulation of objective information, leading by laws of logic to inescapable interpretation'. 'Creative thought, in science as much as in the arts, is the motor of changing opinion'.

Despite the anatomical and biochemical evidence for the evolutionary origins of the human growth pattern, most works on human growth give little consideration to the evolution of man (Aiello and Dean, 1990).

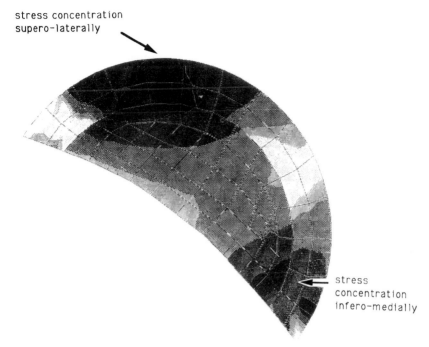

stress concentration
supero-laterally

stress
concentration
infero-medially

Figure 10.7 (a) Finite element model of a normal child's hip. (b) Typical distribution of maximal compressive stress in the 'normal' femoral head. (Reproduced from Choo *et al.*, 1989 by kind permission of the Editor of *The Structural Engineer*)

Some human skeletal and locomotor characteristics

Nothing in biology makes sense except in the light of evolution
(Dobzhansky, 1973)

The most decisive event in human evolution was bipedalism which started about 3–4 million years ago. It allowed the forelimbs to be freed for other purposes, such as manipulation, carrying things and making and using tools. The mouth too was freed from its arduous function of food consumption, paving the way for speech. The next event was increasing brain size, perhaps influenced by the interaction (positive feedback) between cultural and biological changes.

Skeletal growth and growth spurts (see also Chapter 11)

The human pattern of skeletal growth differs from other primates in at least two ways: addition of the juvenile period (between infancy and adolescence) and the markedly increased potential for statural growth at adolescence; these are features particular to the human growth curve (Bogin, 1988). The long period of human skeletal growth, almost 30% of the lifespan, serves to increase the height attained at skeletal maturity. Bone ageing in human evolutionary terms involves a delay of bone development (concept of neoteny[1]) (Gould, 1991) during the quiescent hormonal period lasting from 2–7 years of age.

The prolonged period of infancy and childhood in humans appears to be an evolutionary step taken by primates, and particularly man, to provide the opportunity for learning, brain growth and maturation (Lovejoy, 1981). From birth until the age of 4 or 5 years the rate of skeletal growth declines rapidly (Figure 10.4, *infantile growth spurt*). A slight increase in velocity peaking at about 7 years as a *mid-growth spurt* occurs before the onset of the *adolescent growth spurt* about 11 years in the 'typical' girl and 13 years in the 'typical' boy (Tanner and Cameron, 1980; Gasser *et al.,* 1985). There is a wide individual variation in the age at which an adolescent reaches *peak height velocity* (PHV). Menarcheal age is closely associated with adult body size and fatness (Lindgren, 1978; Tanner, 1992).

Skeletal size – height attained

Adult humans are among the largest animals on earth; more than 99% of animal species are smaller than man (Romer, 1954). Gould (1991) has argued that human skills and behaviour are finely tuned to the size of the body. He writes, '....I have been struck by how rarely our large size has been recognised as a controlling factor of our evolutionary progress'. A doubling of stature would have involved an eight-fold increase in weight, more than the legs could support. In humans the surface area is small relative to size so that we are ruled by gravitational forces acting upon our weight.

Skeletal shape – proportions and allometry

Age changes and allometry

The skeletal proportions change with increasing age from birth to 25 years (Figure 10.8). The proportions of the human body and their changes during growth show that profound internal laws of harmony regulate the formation of the human body. Genetic as well as environmental factors – such as climate, nutrition and trace elements, and the internal environment – control and change these proportions. Differential rates of growth of parts of the body relative to that of the body as a whole when expressed in mathematical terms is termed *allometry* (Huxley, 1932) which is the rule in primate development. Both positive and negative allometry take place in human development (e.g. leg *versus* trunk growth and foot *versus* tibial growth, respectively). *Allometry* brings about functional differences between the adult and child both in physical appearance and performance (Gould, 1966; Alexander, 1971; Bogin, 1988); it has adapted the physique of ethnic groups to climate (Ruff, 1993, 1994); and it is evident in the limbs of children with Perthes' disease (Burwell *et al.,* 1978; Harrison and Burwell, 1981).

Sexual dimorphism in skeletal size and shape

The term *sexual dimorphism* means morphological differences between the sexes which in the human includes size and shape (Glucksmann, 1978; Ghesquière

---

[1] Neoteny – the retention of the juvenile body form or particular features of it, in a mature animal. *Oxford Science Dictionary.*

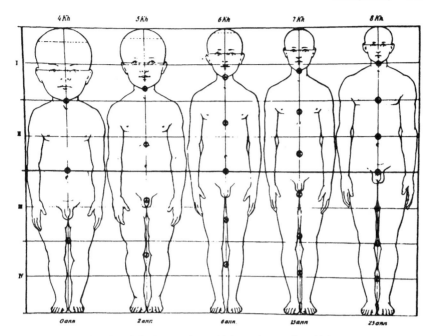

Figure 10.8 The changing skeletal proportions with increasing age from birth to 25 years. (Reproduced by kind permission of Professor VA McKusick and CV Mosby Ltd)

et al., 1985). The shape of the body is modelled in the first place by four of its constituent parts: bones, muscles, subcutaneous fat and skin. Sex differences in these components, individually and in combination, account for the differences in appearance. Gender is pervasive in its effects on skeletal size and shape so that anthropometric data from the sexes should only rarely be combined for statistical analysis.

Skeletal symmetry and asymmetry

Non-random asymmetry in long bones of the limbs
During evolution from the quadrupedal to the bipedal state the nervous system has become more *asymmetrical.* Handedness is *functional* rather than *structural* and is fundamentally a manifestation of cerebral rather than bodily asymmetry (Corballis, 1991). Most bilateral characteristics show some degree of asymmetry, i.e. a difference between the right and left sides. Studies of adult dried limb bones have shown that mild bilateral asymmetry in length is a feature of the appendicular skeleton which differs in amount between upper and lower limb bones as well as between individuals, the sexes and ethnic groups (Schultz, 1937; Malina and Buschang, 1984). *Upper limb bones* show asymmetry due to longer bones usually on the right, especially in females and less so in blacks. *Lower limb bones* show less asymmetry and when present the bones are usually longer on the left. The left clavicles are usually the longer (61%). Skeletal asymmetries which develop during growth are determined by genetic and environmental factors (Vagenas and Hoshizaki, 1991).

Non-random asymmetry in bones of the trunk

The normal *human trunk* frequently shows mild bilateral asymmetry evident as a hump on one side of the back and a small lateral spinal curve (Burwell *et al.*, 1983). The trunk shows marked *asymmetry* between its front and back. Abnormalities of this normal pattern of *bilateral (right–left) symmetry* and *antero–posterior asymmetry* are well recognised, the former as scoliosis, which is usually a 3-D deformity, and the latter as the kyphosis of Scheuermann's disease and ankylosing spondylitis.

Non-random asymmetry of limb malformations

Unilateral malformations of paired structures show a propensity to affect a particular side which is non-random: the right side in radial and fibular aplasia and hemihypertrophy; and the left side in post-axial polydactyly and hemiatrophy (Schnall and Smith, 1974).

Random (fluctuating) asymmetry (FA) is defined as the random difference between each side of certain measureable quantitative traits in an individual; the values are normally distributed around a mean of zero within the population (Livshits and Kobyliansky, 1989). In the limbs, FA may be evident as asymmetry in width at each of the elbow, wrist, knee, ankle and foot. FA is generally considered to be caused by developmental 'instability'.

Pelvis and lower limbs

The lower portion of the human body has evolved first, to facilitate the load-bearing and balance the requirements of walking upright and secondly, in females, to permit the birth of large-headed infants (Aiello and Dean, 1990). Crucial elements of these adaptations are in the form of the pelvis and the femorotibial angle at the knee. After the second year of life in normal humans, the femur and leg proper are at a valgus angle which enables both feet to be under the centre of gravity of the body when walking upright (Salenius and Vankka, 1975; Whitfield, 1993).

During walking, with every step and hundreds of times a day, each *heelstrike* sends shock waves through the body to the head causing accelerations of over three times that of gravity during walking (Voloshin and Wosk, 1982) to as high as 15 times gravity during running (Nigg, 1986). Such dynamic impulse loading under physiological conditions provides an important stimulus for bone growth and remodelling (Lanyon and Rubin, 1984).

Femorotibial angle – valgus and varus at the knee joint

The *femorotibial angle* (FTA) in the frontal plane is formed by the intersection at the knee joint of the long axes of the femur and tibia, represented by appropriate lines drawn on the radiograph (Insall, 1993).

Torsion in limb bones

During pre- and post-natal human development there are torsional changes in the femur, tibia and humerus which are determined multifactorially by factors including heredity, intra-uterine position and mechanical forces (Guidera *et al.*, 1994).

After birth in healthy children *femoral anteversion* decreases, and *lateral tibial torsion* increases, with age (Harris, 1983; Campos and Maiques, 1990). Clinical opinion asserts that as the femur detorts medially, the tibia torts laterally, but the statistical association between femoral anteversion and tibial torsion is weak or absent (Kobyliansky *et al.*, 1979; Takai *et al.*, 1985; Reikeras, 1991; Moulton *et al.*, 1993; Kirby *et al.*, 1994). Recent work has shown that lateral tibial torsion starts in the foetal period and continues after birth (Badelon *et al.*, 1989).

In the upper limbs, *humeral torsion* exists at birth and increases more during growth. Humeral head retroversion is decreased in non-traumatic anterior dislocation of the shoulder on the dominant and non-dominant sides (Kronberg and Broström, 1990).

Some anthropometric methods

The simplest measurements on the framework of the human body, such as the length of a long bone, are made in one dimension (1-D, Figure 10.2d). Less commonly are two-dimensional (2-D) measurements made, such as the length and width of a bone. In recent years 3-D measurements are increasingly being used to assess body size and shape and particularly of limb bones, the spine, trunk and face; and 4-D measurements to evaluate movement and growth.

The development of computer-aided design (CAD) and computer-aided manufacture (CAM) makes it possible to create 3-D models of different parts of the human skeleton for use in clinical practice and science.

Static techniques

Some static techniques of anthropometry used in measuring the musculo-skeletal system can be *classified* as follows:

- Surface – mechanical
  - optical
  - electrical
- Intracorporeal – non-invasive – X-radiation, including tomograms and CT scans.
  - magnetic resonance imaging
  - ultrasound
  - invasive – radio-opaque dyes
  - radio-active isotopes
  - intra-operative
- Models
  - mechanical
  - mathematical, including finite element analysis
  - virtual reality

Discussion here will be restricted to surface techniques.

Classical surface techniques

Classical anthropometry
This requires the use of special instruments which have gradually been developed in several countries of the world during the nineteenth and twentieth

centuries (Figure 10.2) (Weiner and Lourie, 1969, 1981; Roebuck *et al.*, 1975). A full range of modern instruments employing dial reading and digital reading counters has been designed by Professor Tanner and his colleagues at the Institute of Child Health, London, England. This Holtain–Harpenden range of anthropometric instruments is available commercially from Holtain Ltd (Crosswell, near Crymych, Dyfed, SA41 3UF, UK; in the USA, Pfister Import-Export Inc, 450 Barrell Avenue, Carlstadt, New Jersey 070072). *In using such instruments it is essential that the measurer (or anthropometrist) is trained not only to use the equipment correctly but also to employ, as far as possible, standard techniques of measurement* (Tanner *et al.*, 1969; Marshall, 1977; Lohman *et al.*, 1988; Tanner, 1992). Traditional techniques for measuring stature in untrained hands are generally considered to have an accuracy of often little better than ±1 cm. Eklund and Corlett (1984) developed an apparatus to measure stature more accurately.

Stature, sitting height, sub-ischial height and weight
In measuring the body as a whole, standing height (Figure 10.2a) and weight are generally recorded. If the sitting height (Figure 10.2b) is also measured, then subtracting the sitting height from the standing height gives an assessment of leg length below the ischial tuberosities termed the *sub-ischial height* (Figure 10.9). Up to the age of 2 years stature is measured as *supine length*; after that age it is customary to measure standing height. In subjects with true leg length discrepancy the pelvis should be levelled with wooden blocks under the appropriate foot.

Body widths
Widths of the trunk are measured as biacromial diameter, bi-iliac diameter, and lateral chest diameter using a Harpenden anthropometer (Figure 10.2d). Limb widths can be measured at the elbow, wrist, knee, ankle and foot using a bicondylar vernier (see Burwell *et al.*, 1980).

Knemometry
Valk *et al.* (1983) introduced the method of *knemometry*, which measures the exact distance between the heel and the knee in a sitting position. By this technique, changes in growth velocity, which occur within 3–4 days, can be made visible. The technique has shown that 'mini-growth-spurts' occur quite regularly every 3–8 weeks lasting for several days and alternating with periods of decreased growth velocity. During the spurt the growth velocity rose up to more than 200% of the mean individual growth velocity (Wales and Milner 1987; Hermanussen *et al.*, 1988a,b; Ahmed *et al.*, 1995).

Circumferences
Circumference asymmetry of a limb is conventionally used above the knee using a nylon tape and usefully at the hip and calf using a steel tape (Figure 10.2c). Chest circumference is used in the diagnosis of ankylosing spondylitis. The ratio of waist/thigh circumference is the 'best' index of centralised fat in children and adults (Mueller *et al.*, 1989).

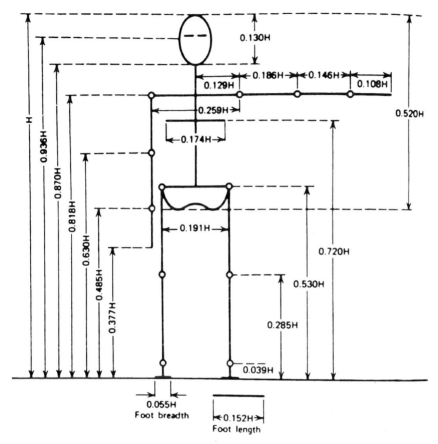

Figure 10.9 Body segment lengths expressed as a fraction of body height. (Reproduced by kind permission of Dr D A Winter and John Wiley & Sons Inc.)

Subcutaneous skin and fat folds

Triceps, subscapular and iliac skin and fat folds are rarely measured in orthopaedic practice. They are used to assess the nutritional state of a child, but *body weight* remains the most frequently used criterion (Vijayraghavan and Sastry, 1976). Subcutaneous fatness has also been measured using soft-tissue radiographs and ultrasound (Haymes *et al.,* 1976).

Body mass index

The body mass index, weight (W) divided by height (H) squared, also know as Quetelet's Index, is used widely as an index of overweight and obesity. It correlates highly with the percentage of the body weight as fat (percentage fat) and lowly with height. More recently, it has been proposed that BMI should be used as a measure of underweight individuals and populations (Norgan, 1994).

Surface area

A nomogram involving stature and weight is commonly employed to calculate the surface area of a child. For older children and adults, an approximate method of assessing surface area percentage involvement in the skin lesion such as burns, using the 'rule of 9's' (Buckler, 1979).

Growth measurements, cross-sectional and longitudinal studies
Most population studies of human development have been *cross-sectional*, i.e. individuals were each measured once and mean values deduced for various age groups. To provide information on the rate of change, or the velocity of growth, *longitudinal studies* must be used in which each individual is measured repeatedly at several ages over a period of time as in the National Child Development Study (Rona and Altman, 1977; Karlberg *et al.*, 1993).

Limb length symmetry and asymmetry
It is traditional in classical anthropometry to measure either the right or the left limbs because, for most subjects the bone asymmetry in length is mild and of little consequence. In the UK, left limbs are measured (Cameron, 1984). In anthropometric studies of congenital and idiopathic scoliosis, asymmetry of upper limb length was revealed which led to a re-evaluation of limb length asymmetry in healthy children (Burwell *et al.*, 1977, 1981, 1984; Taylor and Slinger, 1980), and to a review of growth and asymmetry (Dangerfield, 1994). In the feet asymmetry of ± 0.5 cm is common without any laterality; there is asymmetry of foot lengthening in moving from a non-weight-bearing to a weight-bearing position (Burwell *et al.*, 1996).

Joint laxity
Carter and Wilkinson (1964) described a clinical method for the diagnosis of *generalised joint laxity* which involves tests of laxity at each of the thumbs, fingers, elbows, knees and ankles. Each of these tests is *all or none*. The normal subjects were schoolboys and schoolgirls age 6–11 years and in them the prevalence of generalised joint laxity was 7% (Sutherland *et al.*, 1988; Cheng *et al.*, 1991). Burwell *et al.* (1981) assessed the thumb-to-forearm angle on a *continuous scale* using a trigonometric method which involves calculating the angle to which the thumb could be moved by manual pressure towards the radial border of the forearm. In 1274 normal Caucasian subjects aged 5–16 years (boys 628, girls 646), the thumb-to-forearm angle was related to age, sex and side. Fairbank *et al.* (1984a) evaluated six measurements of joint mobility in 446 normal adolescents. They found that each joint has a normal distribution of mobility and they concluded that joint laxity is the extreme of the normal spectrum of joint mobility. These workers found that 115 people aged 13–17 years, with a history of low back pain, tended to have decreased lower limb joint mobility (Fairbank *et al.*, 1984b).

Observer error, reliability and validity
It is generally recognised among anthropologists that measurements made on the surface of the living human body marking landmarks are reliable to within 5 mm, and this is the standard to which beginners are trained (Hoe *et al.*, 1994). More accurate measurements can be made upon radiographs, e.g. of limb bones using a scanogram or on images obtained by CT or MRI.

Studies of measurement error are usually organised in one of two ways: either with a single observer or with multiple observers. These situations give rise to two aspects of *reliability*. The first investigates the reliability of a single observer and is known as '*replicability*' (within observer or intra-observer reliability) and the second investigates multiple observers and is known as '*comparability*' (between observer or inter-observer reliability) (Burwell *et al.,* 1980; Cameron, 1984; Ulijaszek and Lourie, 1994). An additional concept is that of '*validity*' which is the extent to which a technique measures what it purports to measure. The assessment of validity needs an independent standard of reference which can be accepted as trustworthy.

Statistical techniques are needed in assessing reliability which include standard deviation, coefficient of variation, correlation coefficient, coefficient of reliability, simple and multiple regression analysis, and analysis of variance.

3-D surface techniques

Some methods for the *3-D measurement* of the human body are reviewed by Burwell (1978) and for spinal deformities by Burwell and Dangerfield (1992). Such techniques include the following: vector stereography (Morris and Harris, 1976; Pynsent *et al.,* 1983); moiré photography (Willner, 1979); integrated shape investigation system (ISIS) (Turner-Smith *et al.,* 1988); stereophotogrammetry (Figure 10.5) (Herron 1974; and for its radiological application, Saraste and Östman, 1986); raster stereography (Frobin and Hierholzer, 1990); AUSCAN (Assente *et al.,* 1987); optronic torsograph (Dawson *et al.,* 1989); Loughborough anthropometric shadow scanner (LASS) (Jones *et al.,* 1989); phase measuring profilometry (PMP) (Halioua *et al.,* 1980); Liverpool stereographic method (Dangerfield *et al.,* 1990); three-linear array back-scanning with airborne ultrasound (ATLAS) (Mauritzson *et al.,* 1986); ultrasonic topometry (Schumpe and Messler, 1987).

3-D scanning by LASS provides a new method for determining size and shape in body composition studies (Smith *et al.*, 1990; Brooke-Wavell *et al.,* 1994).

Movement techniques

Static (see also Chapter 9)

Goniometers

The simplest way of measuring joint movement is to use a commercial goniometer which measures the angle between the limb segments. Standard techniques for measuring and recording joint motion were published by the American Academy of Orthopaedic Surgeons (1965). An updated version of this information is now available (American Academy of Orthopaedic Surgeons, 1994). Greene and Heckman (1994) write:

> Although joint motion can be visually estimated, a goniometer enhances accuracy of measurement and is preferred at the elbow, wrist, finger, knee, ankle and hallux. These joints allow palpation of bony landmarks and reasonably consistent alignment of the goniometer. A goniometer may also be used for measuring hip and shoulder motion. The overlying soft tissue, however, does not allow the same degree of repeatability when aligning the goniometer in these areas (see also Lea and Gerhardt, 1995).

The starting, or zero position (Neutral Zero Position) (Cave and Roberts, 1936) is the extended 'anatomical position' of the extremity and to avoid confusion this position is described as 0° rather than 180°.

Dynamic (kinanthropometry) (see also Chapter 8)
Early papers relating to the human gait are those of Weber and Weber (1836) and
Braune and Fischer (1895–1904).

Movement description
To describe motion adequately a reference frame is required (Figure 10.6). A
concept of degrees of freedom is by definition the number of independent co-
ordinates in a system that are necessary to specify accurately the position of an
object in space, e.g. a pure hinge joint would have 1° of freedom because only
one co-ordinate exists around which motion will take place. To describe the
movement pattern (or 3-D trajectory) of any rigid body six parameters are
needed namely, three orientation parameters (involving *rotation* about each of *x*,
y and *z* axes), and three position parameters involving *translation* parallel to each
of *x*, *y* and *z* axes (Stokes *et al.*, 1989). The common combination of *rotation* and
translation is termed *general motion* (Adrian and Cooper, 1995).

Kinematic measurements may be made in either two dimensions or three. The
simplest kinematic measurements are made using a single camera in an
uncalibrated system. To achieve reasonable accuracy in kinematic measurement
it is necessary to use a 3-D system which involves making measurements from
more than one viewpoint, and the use of some form of calibration (Sutherland *et
al.*, 1988; Whittle, 1991; Rose and Gamble, 1994). Video-tape digitisers and
television-computer systems are now utilised. Using a force platform with a
kinematic system it is possible to perform calculations in which the limb is
treated as a mechanical system (combined kinetic-kinematic system).

Mechanical methods
Dvir (1995) reviews isokinetic *dynamometry* which is concerned with the
provision of a resistance and the measurement of the moment exerted by a
muscle against that resistance at each point in the range of motion. The CYBEX
II system is a dynamometer which has been widely used to record joint
movements and torque, in clinical testing and in rehabilitation (Lumex Inc., 2100
Smithtown Avenue, Ronkonkoma, NY 11779, USA). Another system is the
MedX lumbar extension testing and rehabilitation exercise machine (MedX
Corporation, Ocala, Fl 32670, USA). The B-200 Lumbar Dynamometer is a
commercially available instrument for testing range of motion, isometric
strength, velocity endurance and consistency of effort in low back pain patients
and normal subjects (Isotechnologies Carrboro, North Carolina, USA) (Gomez
et al., 1991).

Optical methods
These methods for surface measurement use reflective markers (e.g. CODA,
Charnwood Dynamics, Loughborough, UK; VICON, Oxford Metrics Ltd, Unit
8 Westway, Oxford, OX2 0JB, UK; MacReflex motion analysis system, Ögärdes
Vägen 2 433 30 Partille, Sweden), or light emitting diodes (e.g. Spinoscope®,
Gracovetsky, 1988). SPINETRAK is a 2-D spinal motion analysis system that
uses retro-reflective markers applied to specific body line marks to analyse
active spinal range of motion and velocity (Motion Analysis Corporation, Santa
Rosa, California, USA).

Electrogoniometers
These have been devised to measure the position of joints or parts of the body. A commercial electrogoniometer, *The Bird*™, uses an onboard 16-bit CPU to compute the position and orientation in space of its tiny receiver, creating an output of x, y and z co-ordinates (Ascension Technology Corporation, PO Box 527, Burlington, VT 05402, USA). The 3 SPACE ISOTRAK is an electromagnetic device for the measurement of the position orientation of a sensor in space (Hindle *et al.,* 1990; Pearcy, 1993). Another device for measuring angular position and motion is the Waterloo Spatial Motion and Recording Technique (WATSMART™, Northern Digital Inc., Waterloo, Ontario, Canada) (Cummings *et al.,* 1993). The Lumbar Motion Monitor (LMM) is a tri-axial electrogoniometer capable of assessing the instantaneous position of the thoraco-lumbar spine in three dimensions. It was designed, in essence, to be an exoskeleton of the spine, which tracks position, velocity and acceleration of the trunk as a function of time in the sagittal, frontal and transverse planes of the body (Marrass *et al.,* 1993; Chattanooga Group, Inc., 4717 Adams Road, PO Box 489, Hixson, TM 37343-0489, USA). Dopf *et al.* (1994) report an analysis of spine motion variability using a computerised goniometer (CA-6000 Spine Motion Analyser, Orthopedic Systems Inc., Hayward, California, USA).

Other instrumentation systems for assessing movement include electro-myography, force platforms and force plates (see Adrian and Cooper, 1995).

Orthopaedic anthropometry:stature and lower limbs

Every natural phenomenon ......is really composite, and every visible action and effect is a summation of countless subordinate actions
(D'Arcy Thompson, 1942)

Consideration here will be restricted to some anthropometric findings relating to *stature* and *lower limbs.* The anthropometry of the trunk with respect to spinal deformities is considered elsewhere (Burwell and Dangerfield, 1992). Morphometrically, healthy people differ with respect to age, sex, physique, social class, and ethnic factors.

Stature

The accurate measurement of stature requires the use of a stadiometer by a trained observer (Figure 10.2a).

Single readings
A single reading of the stature of a child in an orthopaedic clinic is a common practice. The reading may be plotted on the centile chart for sex and the 'normality' is assessed. In Britain, growth and development charts have been prepared by Tanner (1992) and his colleagues for certain body components which are commonly measured in paediatric practice (Buckler, 1979; Hensinger, 1986). In these charts the distribution for a given measurement of a normal population is provided as centiles (3rd–97th) about the 50th centile (Figures 10.3

and 10.4) (Cole TJ, 1989). The British Orthopaedic Association has charts for the growth record of children (Ref 91 & 92, Castlemead Publications, 4A Crane Mead, Ware, Herts, SG12 9PY, UK). National height standards for the USA and the Netherlands are available (Cole TJ, 1989).

Many factors influence the size of a child including genetics, nutrition, socio-economic status, psychosocial stress, ethnic factors and disease. In the UK there is variance in height between social classes (Mascie-Taylor and Boldsen, 1985; Rosenbaum et al., 1985).

Diurnal variation of stature

It is known that young subjects lose about 5 mm in height during the school day (Burwell et al., 1980). Using a special stadiometer designed to measure stature very accurately, several workers have evaluated the circadian variation in stature and the effects in spinal loading, the working day in nurses and a disease – ankylosing spondylitis (Tyrrell et al., 1985; Foreman and Troup, 1987; Hindle et al., 1987). Foreman and Troup (1987) used this apparatus to show that in nurses the loss of stature was greater during the 8-h working shift than during a 12-h period on their days off. There were significant correlations between loss of stature in both the total duration of lean/stoop postures and the total duration of lifting. Krag et al. (1990) in 10 healthy adult men and women showed that 26% of the 8-h loss occurred in the first hour upright and 41% of the 4-h recovery occurred in the first hour recumbent (Hoe et al., 1994).

Multiple readings

Linear growth velocity, measured as stature, is a very sensitive indicator of the basic health of a child. Variations can be quickly detected by accurate recording and charting of growth measurements at frequent intervals (Tanner 1992; Gasser et al., 1985, 1993). Data may be plotted on the height velocity chart for sex; and can be analysed either *longitudinally* or as a *'mixed' longitudinal study* (Goldstein, 1986; Chandler and Bock, 1991).

Abnormalities of stature – size

It is usually advised that investigation of the cause of *short stature* is required in all children whose standing height falls below the 3rd centile (= standard deviation score of –1.88, see below). *Very short stature* is defined as a measurement three standard deviations below the mean for the chronological age of the child. *Tall stature* above the 97th centile is less common (Tanner, 1992). Patients with tall stature should be examined for additional signs of Marfan's syndrome or other hereditary disorders of connective tissue (Nelle et al., 1994). To estimate the abnormality of stature, or of any other skeletal component, it is usual to use a *standard deviation score (SDS)* which corrects for age and sex. The SDS of stature for a child is obtained from the formula:

$$\text{SDS of stature} = \frac{\text{(stature of child)} - \text{(mean stature at given age)}}{\text{standard deviation at a given age}}$$

By convention, 'normal' is defined as within ±2 standard deviations from the mean for a given age and sex. Hence, 'abnormality', outside the 3rd and 97th centiles, will include a few 'normal' subjects.

Abnormalities of stature – proportions

Abnormalities of skeletal proportions are found in *short-trunk, short stature and short-leg short stature* (Wynne-Davies *et al.*, 1985) and in Perthes' disease (Burwell *et al.*, 1978; Harrison and Burwell, 1981; Burwell, 1988; Hall *et al.*, 1988).

Essentially there are two ways to decide whether a child (or adult) is proportionate or disproportionate in his/her skeletal growth (Tanner, 1953); by inspection (anthroposcopy); or by measurements made on the surface of the subject and/or on radiographs (anthropometry). Whether one uses *anthroposcopy* or needs *anthropometry* in the clinical assessment of a patient depends upon the degree of skeletal abnormality. The abnormality may be obvious, but in some individuals disproportionate growth can be revealed only after careful measurement and appropriate analysis. If anthropometry is used, the recordings may be analysed by the following methods:

1. Plotting on centile charts.
2. Calculating standard deviation scores (Hall *et al.*, 1988; Moulton *et al.*, 1995b).
3. Calculating ratios of two body regions and comparing the results with normal subjects.
4. Using 'relationship lines' between two body regions and comparing the results with normal subjects (Hiernaux, 1968; Eveleth, 1978; Burwell *et al.*, 1978, 1981).

Prediction of stature

The change of span relative to stature with increasing age is well-known from Quatelet's data (Boyd, 1980; Tanner 1981). *Span* has been used to give an indication of relative stature in patients with Marfan's syndrome and homocystinuria (Brenton *et al.*, 1972), but as a measure of upper limb length it has little to recommend it; it is hard to measure accurately and it combines both arm length and chest breadth. Alternatives to span as predictors of stature include *demi-span* (Bassey 1986; Smith *et al.*, 1995), and *tibial length* (Figure 10.2) (Zorab *et al.*, 1964; Dangerfield *et al.*, 1994).

The *prediction* of a child's adult height is commonly needed in practice and three methods are available (Bailey and Pinneau, 1952; Roche *et al.*, 1975; Tanner *et al.*, 1983).

In *scoliosis*, the loss of height due to the lateral spinal curvature can be corrected by one of three methods (Bjure and Nachemson, 1973; Hodgett *et al.*, 1986; Carr *et al.*, 1989).

Stature of adults

Several investigators have shown that both men and women decline in stature during normal ageing. For those of a Northern European background the decline between peak height and the age of 80 is 6 cm in men and 6.6 cm in women. Factors involved in these changes are posture, intervertebral discs and osteoporosis (Chandler and Bock, 1991). A survey of heights and weights of adults in Great Britain in 1980 is given by Rosenbaum *et al.* (1985). Secular height increases are still occurring in the stature of young adults living in Northern Europe.

Lower limbs

Anthropologists use a variety of methods to measure the *lengths* of the lower limbs (and their components) and these include:

- Standing height minus sitting height (= sub-ischial height).
- Symphyseal height (lower segment).
- Cristal height (iliac crest to floor).
- Ilio–spinal height (anterior–superior spine to floor).
- Total leg length.
- Trochanteric height.
- Tibial height.
- Lower leg (tibial) length (Figure 10.3d).
- Foot length.

In *orthopaedic practice* the *classical anthropometry* of the lower limbs relates to deformity, range of movement of joints, length of limbs and of limb segments, limb circumferences (Figure 10.2c,d) and skeletal growth. Deformity in the lower limbs is principally at the joints and is best analysed into deformity in 3-D: *frontal plane* (valgus/varus); *sagittal plane* (flexion contractures at the hip, knee, ankle and foot); and *transverse plane,* namely anteversion/retroversion of the femur and torsion of the tibia.

Clinical leg length and circumference measurements
Total leg length is generally measured with a nylon tape and with care, in a subject who is not obese, leg length inequality of 1 cm or more can usually be detected. The accuracy of measuring leg length inequality clinically was examined by Nichols and Bailey (1955) and more recently by Friberg *et al.* (1988), the latter validating their clinical techniques with radiological measurements. They found that more than half (53%) of the observations were erroneous when the criterion of leg length inequality was 5 mm; discrepancies occurred even when the radiological reading gave a leg length inequality of as much as 2.5 cm. A difficulty with their methods is that the upper datum line for the clinical method was the anterior–superior iliac spine and for the radiological measurement was the hip joint. Friberg *et al.* found that the *indirect* measurement of leg length inequality made by estimating the lateral pelvic tilt by manual palpation of the iliac crest for levelness (by placing wooden boards of known thickness under the perceived shorter limb until the iliac crests were thought to be level), was no more accurate than the *direct* method of using a tape measure.

Tibial length is best measured with a Harpenden anthropometer which is an accurate method when the subject is not obese (Figure 10.2d) (Burwell *et al.,* 1980). The circumference of the thigh is generally measured at a distance above either the patella (10 cm) or the lateral tibial plateau (17 cm) (Hughston, 1993). Useful *circumference measurements* for assessing asymmetries are subgluteal (for hip abnormalities) and calf, for both of which a steel tape is essential (Figure 10.2c).

Radiological leg length measurement
Radiological measurement provides the most accurate method of assessing leg length inequality (Giles and Taylor, 1981). Maresh (1970) published standards for the length of the femur, tibia and fibula for American white children. In view

of the errors of *teleroentgenography* used for her data, and the importance in orthopaedics of having accurate measurements of long bones of the lower limbs throughout growth, *orthoroentgenography* was subsequently used. Standards for such data have been published for the femur and tibia of normal American white boys and girls from 1–18 years (Anderson *et al.,* 1964). The means and standard deviations for each bone length are provided for each age, enabling standard deviations scores (see above) of bone lengths to be calculated in children suspected of having disproportionate skeletal growth in segments of the lower limbs. In a series of papers, Green and Anderson reviewed several earlier methods and reported a classical approach to this problem based on the principle of utilising a fixed year of incremental growth and skeletal age (Anderson *et al.,* 1963). Tupman (1962) using the method of Kunkle and Carpenter (1954) studied the growth of the femur and tibia in British children and published formulae from which at any skeletal age the remaining femoral and tibial growth can be calculated. Moseley (1977) using the *scanogram* method of Bell and Thompson (1950) reported a straight-line graph for leg length discrepancies. Altongy *et al.* (1987) report the use of *micro-dose digital radiographs* (which require 1% of the radiation needed to produce conventional images) for the measurement of leg length inequality. Aaron *et al.* (1992) found that *computed tomography* is more accurate than orthoroentgenography for the measurement of limb-length discrepancy in patients who have a flexion deformity of the knee.

Clinical significance of leg length inequality
A difference of 5 mm in the length of the lower limbs has been found to be present in about 40% of the adult population (Rush and Steiner, 1946) and 1 cm or more in 7% of the adult population (Taylor and Slinger, 1980); and there is evidence that the lower limbs may differ by as much as 2.2 cm without falling outside the limits of the normal distribution (Ingelmark and Lindström, 1963). The clinical significance of leg length inequality less than 2.5 cm and compensatory postural pelvic scolioses is uncertain and is frequently the subject of debate. Some authors believe the detriment caused by leg length inequality is cosmetic, whereas others contend that such asymmetry contributes to or causes pelvic tilt scoliosis (Ingelmark and Lindström, 1963; Farinet *et al.,* 1982; Giles and Taylor, 1982), low back pain, hip pain and unilateral overuse symptoms in the lower extremities (e.g. long-leg arthropathy), and even mechanical loosening of the prosthetic components after total hip arthroplasty (see Friberg, 1983; Friberg *et al.,* 1988). Some workers consider that leg length inequality predisposes an individual to acute and chronic injury of the sacro-iliac joint. In this connection Cummings *et al.* (1993) examined the effect of varying degrees of imposed leg length inequality on the symmetry of the hip (pelvic) bones in healthy adult women with relatively equal leg lengths. Using a Waterloo Spatial Motion and Recording Technique they found that the hip bone rotates posteriorly on the side of the lengthened limb and anteriorly on the shorter limb.

Femorotibial angle – valgus and varus at the knee joint
A clinical examination is used initially to assess valgus and varus at the knee. Upper *tibia vara* is commonly associated with lateral tibial torsion and increased femoral anteversion. When such a patient stands with the feet together, medial rotation at the hips cause the patella to squint with an apparent genu varum.

Many advocate that the femorotibial angle (FTA) and the mechanical axis of the lower limb should be calculated using standing radiographs of the hip, knee and ankle. The FTA has been used particularly in relation to osteoarthritis of the knee and tibial osteotomy (Jackson and Waugh, 1984; Insall, 1993).

The *quadriceps (Q) angle* was used by Insall reporting on chondromalacia patellae who considered that a Q angle of over 20° is definitely abnormal (Insall, 1979). Hvid and Andersen (1982) found the Q angle is larger in women than men with a median figure of 20° for women and 12° for men. This difference has been linked to the wider hips of women. There is a correlation between Q angle and hip medial rotation favouring the hypothesis that excess femoral neck anteversion leads to compensatory lateral tibial torsion and a high Q angle (Hvid and Andersen, 1982). Patellar height, higher in women than in men, is unrelated to the Q angle (Carson *et al.,* 1984). The vector stereograph has been used to measure the Q angle (Fairbank *et al.,* 1984c). The Q angle can also be assessed with the knee flexed at 90° (90° *tubercle–sulcus angle*) (Kelly and Insall, 1993).

Aglietti *et al.* (1993) *intraoperatively* measured the angle between the anterior–superior iliac spine (S), the deepest point of the sulcus femoralis (S), and the top of the tibial tuberosity (T) half way between the medial and lateral margins of the patellar tendon *(SST angle)*. This measure was obtained at surgery using a goniometer. The SST angle represents a measure of the valgus vector of the extensor apparatus and is not affected by the patella position as the surface Q angle.

Goutallier *et al.* (1978) measures the valgus at the knee using *CT images* and superimposed a cut through the tibial tuberosity upon a cut through the upper part of the femoral sulcus. The lateral displacement at the tip of the tuberosity from the deepest part of the sulcus is measured and termed, in the English vernacular, the *TT–SF distance*. Distances greater than 20 mm are said to be definitely abnormal.

Torsion of the femur and tibia

Femoral anteversion in clinical practice is estimated by laying the patient prone and measuring the amount of medial rotation at the hip. We have found that femoral anteversion accounts for only 25% of the medial rotation measured (Cole AA, 1989). Ruwe *et al.* (1992) reported an apparent improvement on this method, but again we have found this method to be of limited value (Cavdar *et al.,* 1995). Femoral anteversion, of course, is only one factor which determines the structural stability of the hip: *acetabular anteversion* is more difficult to measure but attempts have been made by some workers (Dechambre and Teinturier, 1966; Wientroub *et al.,* 1981).

In the 1950s, several X-ray techniques were developed to measure femoral anteversion in children with hip problems and some data were obtained from the 'normal' hips of children with other orthopaedic conditions (biplanar roent-genography, stereophotogrammetry, axial roentgenography and fluoroscopy) (Dunlap *et al.,* 1953; Kirby *et al.,* 1993). In the 1970s, new imaging techniques became available and were applied to problems associated with torsional abnormalities in the femur which assisted in the selection of patients for, and the pre-operative planning of, derotational osteotomy of the femur. These techniques include *computer tomography* (CT), *magnetic resonance imaging* (MRI) (Galbraith *et al.,* 1987) and *ultrasound* (Moulton and Upadhyay, 1982; Clarac *et al.,* 1985; Kirby *et al.,* 1993). Virtual reality technology has also been applied to assess femoral anteversion (Gosling *et al.,* 1993).

Tibial torsion has been measured using surface techniques, X-ray techniques including CT (Takai *et al.,* 1985; Eckhoff and Johnson, 1994) and most recently by ultrasound (Burwell *et al.,* 1994; Kirby *et al.,* 1994, 1996). Medial tibial torsion, a feature of the new-born and young children with toeing-in gait, persists in 8–9% of adolescent schoolchildren and 3–5% of adults, and more in women (Hutter and Scott, 1949; Ritter *et al.,* 1976; Staheli *et al.,* 1985). Ultrasound findings obtained by measuring the femoral anteversion and tibial torsion suggest firstly, that the *summated rotational alignment* of each lower limb predicts *toeing-in and toeing-out* (Fabry *et al.,* 1994; Moulton *et al.,* 1994); secondly, that *patellofemoral pain* in adolescents and young adults is associated with abnormalities of tibial torsion and femoral anteversion (Eckhoff *et al.,* 1994; Moulton *et al.,* 1995a,b). In patients with *medial-type osteoarthritis* of the knee, lateral tibial torsion is significantly lower than in normal adults (Yagi, 1994).

Radiological anthropometry of the knee joint

Radiographic examination of the knee includes antero-posterior (AP) and lateral views. Lateral radiographs enable the patellofemoral joint to be assessed for patella alta and patella baja (Carson *et al.,* 1984; Deutsch *et al.,* 1993). Two other projections may be included in routine knee examinations – a tunnel view and a patellofemoral view (Pavlov, 1993). In assessing patients with patellofemoral disorders tangential views have been described by several workers and used to calculate sulcus angle, congruence angle, lateral patellofemoral angle, and patellofemoral index. CT and MRI are now supplementing such conventional radiography (Deutsch *et al.,* 1993).

Conclusion

From its narrow origin in the arts and the military, anthropometry has developed through growth studies to include measurements of the human body traditionally in the gross and not the microscopic. Measurement provides the evidence to describe deformity, movement and the effects of treatment. Statistical methods enable clinical findings to be compared with data from normal subjects, including means (or medians) and standard deviations. To obtain the latter type of data anthropometric techniques are needed which can be applied ethically to healthy subjects; such techniques include surface topography, ultrasound and MRI – the safety of which has to be continually assessed (CMO, 1994).

In the last 20 years, there have been two major developments of anthropometric methods: firstly, 3-D and 4-D measurements, the latter involving movements and less commonly growth; and secondly, computer-generated anthropomorphic images.

The problems to be tested by anthropometry are legion, and the techniques ever increasing. Beyond the descriptive phase, hypotheses need to be developed to examine the nature of the processes that account for the descriptive data. In medicine, the ultimate goal is the *prevention* of disease.

Acknowledgements

The writer is indebted to Action Research (1972–1993) and subsequently AO/ASIF and the Arthritis and Rheumatism Council for funding, Professor TM Mayhew for some facilities, Dr AA Cole for reading the text and Mrs EP Sykes for the typescript.

References

Aaron A, Weinstein D, Thickman D, Eilert R (1992) Comparison of orthoroentgenography and computed tomography in the measurement of limb-length discrepancy. *J. Bone Jt Surg.*; **74A**: 897–902

Adrian MJ, Cooper JM (1995) Fundamental biomechanical concepts, Chapter 1, pp. 3–20. In *Biomechanics of Human Movement*, 2nd edition. Maddison: Brown & Benchmark

Aglietti P, Buzzi R, Insall JN (1993) Disorders of the patellofemoral joint, Chapter 12, pp. 241–385. In: Insall JN (ed.) *Surgery of the Knee,* volume 1, 2nd edition. New York: Churchill Livingstone

Ahmed SF, Wallace WHB, Kelnar CJH (1995) Knemometry in childhood: a study to compare the precision of two different techniques. *Ann. Hum. Biol.*; **22**: 247–252

Aiello L, Dean C (1990) *An Introduction to Human Evolutionary Anatomy.* London: Academic Press

Alexander RM (1971) *Size and Shape.* Institute of Biology's studies in biology No 29. London: Edward Arnold

Altongy JF, Harcke HT, Bowen JR (1987) Measurement of leg length inequalities by micro-dose digital radiographs. *J. Pediatr. Orthop.*; **7**: 311–316

American Academy of Orthopaedic Surgeons (1966) *Joint Motion: Method of Measuring and Recording.* London: British Orthopaedic Association

American Academy of Orthopaedic Surgeons (1994) In: Greene WB, Heckman JD (eds) *The Clinical Measurement of Joint Motion.* Rosemont Illinois: American Academy of Orthopaedic Surgeons

Anderson MM, Green WT, Messner MB (1963) Growth and predictions of growth in the lower extremities. *J. Bone Jt Surg.*; **45A**: 1–14

Anderson M, Messner MB, Green WT (1964) Distribution of lengths of the normal femur and tibia in children from one to eighteen years of age. *J. Bone Jt Surg.*; **46A**: 1197–1202

Ankney CD (1992) The brain size/IQ debate. *Nature*; **360**: 292

Annotation (1994) Applications of virtual reality to surgery. *B. M. J.*; **308**: 1054–1055

Assente R, Ferrigno G, Santambrogio GC, Vigano R (1987) Application of AUSCAN system for evaluation of postural changes induced by a brace, pp. 97–104. In: Stokes IAF, Pekelsky JR, Moreland MS (eds) *Surface Topography and Spinal Deformity.* Proceedings of the Fourth International Symposium, 29–30 September 1986, Mont Sainte Marie Québec. Stuttgart: Gustav Fischer

Badelon O, Bensahel H, Folinais D, Lassale B (1989) Tibiofibular torsion from the fetal period until birth. *J. Pediatr. Orthop.*; **9**: 169–173

Bailey N, Pinneau SB (1952) Tables for predicting adult height from skeletal age: revised for use with Greulich-Pyle hand standards. *J. Pediatr.*; **40**: 423–441

Bassey EJ (1986) Demi-span as a measure of skeletal size. *Ann. Hum. Biol.*; **13**: 499–502

Bell JS, Thompson WAL (1950) Modified spot scanography. *Am. J. Roentgenol.*; **63**: 915–916

Bjure J, Nachemson A (1973) Non-treated scoliosis. *Clin. Orthop. Rel. Res.*; **93**: 44–52

Bogin B (1988) *Patterns of Human Growth.* Cambridge: Cambridge University Press

Boyd E, (1980) *Origins of the Study of Human Growth.* University of Oregon Health Sciences Center

Braune W, Fischer O (1895–1904) *The Human Gait.* Maquet P, Furlong, R (translators). Berlin: Springer-Verlag 1987

Brenton DP, Dow CJ, James JIP, Hay RL, Wynne-Davies R (1972) Homocystinuria and Marfan's syndrome: a comparison. *J. Bone Jt Surg.*; **54B**: 277–298

Brooke-Wavell K, Jones PRM, West GM (1994) Reliability and repeatability of 3-D body scanner (LASS) measurements compared to anthropometry. *Ann. Hum. Biol.*; **21**: 571–577

Buckler JMH (1979) *A Reference Manual of Growth and Development.* Oxford: Blackwell Scientific Publications

Burke PH, Healy MJR (1993) A serial study of normal facial asymmetry in monozygotic twins. *Ann. Hum. Biol.*; **20**: 527–534

Burwell RG (1978) Biostereometrics, shape replication and orthopaedics, pp. 51–85. In: Harris D, Copeland K (eds) *Orthopaedic Engineering.* Oxford: Orthopaedic Engineering Centre and Biological Engineering Society

Burwell RG (1988) Perthes' disease: growth and aetiology. *Arch. Dis. Child.*; **63**: 1408–1412

Burwell RG, Dangerfield PH, Vernon CL (1977) Anthropometry and scoliosis, pp. 123–163. In: *Scoliosis*, Proceedings of a Fifth Symposium, 21–26 September 1976. London: Academic Press

Burwell RG, Dangerfield PH, Hall DJ, Vernon CL, Harrison MHM (1978) Perthes' disease. An anthropometric study revealing impaired and disproportionate growth. *J. Bone Jt Surg.*; **60B**: 461–477

Burwell RG, Vernon CL, Dangerfield PH (1980) Skeletal measurement, Chapter 38, pp. 317–329. In: Owen R, Goodfellow J, Bullough P (eds) *Scientific Foundations of Orthopaedics and Traumatology.* London: William Heinemann

Burwell RG, Dangerfield PH, Vernon CL (1981) Bone asymmetry and joint laxity in the upper limbs of children with adolescent idiopathic scoliosis. *Ann. R. Coll. Surg. Engl.*; **63**: 209–210

Burwell RG, James NJ, Johnson F, Webb JK, Wilson YG (1983) Standardised trunk asymmetry scores – a study of back contour in healthy children. *J. Bone Jt Surg.*; **65B**: 452–462

Burwell RG, Dangerfield PH, James NJ, Johnson F, Webb JK (1984) Anthropometric studies of normal and scoliotic children. Axial and appendicular asymmetry, sexual dimorphisms and age-related changes, pp. 27–44. In: Jacobs RR (ed.) *Pathogenesis of Idiopathic Scoliosis.* Proceedings of an International Conference. Chicago: Scoliosis Research Society

Burwell RG, Dangerfield PH (1992) Anthropometry, Chapter 9, pp. 191–227. In: Findlay G, Owen R (eds) *Spine, A combined orthopaedic and neurosurgical approach.* Oxford: Blackwell Scientific Publications

Burwell RG, Kirby AS, Aujla RK, Moulton A, Wallace WA (1994) Laterality and sexual dimorphism in the prediction of torsional asymmetry in the femora and tibiae of young adolescents: a nervous system interpretation. *Clin. Anat.*; **7**: 54–55

Burwell RG, Cole AA, Moulton A (1996) Asymmetry of foot lengthening in moving from a non-weight-bearing to a weight-bearing position. *Clin. Anat.* In press

Cameron N (1984) *The Measurement of Human Growth.* London: Croom Helm

Campos FF, Maiques JAT (1990) The development of tibiofibular torsion. *Surg. Radiol. Anat.*; **12**: 109–112

Carr AJ, Jefferson RJ, Weisz I, Turner-Smith AR (1989) Correction of body height in scoliosis patients using ISIS scanning. *Spine*; **14**: 220–222

Carson WG Jr, James SL, Larson RL, Singer KM, Winternitz WW (1984) Patellofemoral disorders: physical and radiographic evaluation. Part II Radiographic examination. *Clin. Orthop. Rel. Res.*; **185**: 178–186

Carter C, Wilkinson J (1964) Persistent joint laxity and congenital dislocation at the hip. *J. Bone Jt Surg.*; **46B**: 40–45

Cavdar S, Burwell RG, Cole AA, Kirby AS, Moulton A, Webb JK (1995) The relation between femoral anteversion, tibial torsion and back shape in children with adolescent idiopathic scoliosis (AIS). *Clinical Anatomy*; **8**: 367

Cave F, Roberts SM (1936) A method for measuring and recording joint function. *J. Bone Jt Surg.*; **18**: 455–465

Chandler PJ, Bock RD (1991) Age changes in adult stature: trend estimation from mixed longitudinal data. *Ann. Hum. Biol.*; **18**: 433–440

Cheng JCY, Chan PS, Hui PW (1991) Joint laxity in children. *J. Pediatr. Orthop.*; **11**: 752–756

Choo BS, Hogg ADC, Burwell RG, Moulton A, Worthington DS (1989) A study of stress factors in Perthes' disease of the hip, using the finite element method. *The Structural Engineer*; **67**: 92–94

Clarac J-P, Pries P, Laine M, Richer J-P, Freychet H, Goubalt F, Barret D, Hurmic A, Vandermarque P, Drouineau J (1985) Mesure de l'antétorsion du col fémoral par échographie. Comparison avec la tomodensitométrie. *Rev. Chir. Orthop.*; **71**: 365–368

CMO (1994) Safe use of diagnostic ultrasound. In: *CMO's Update 4 Department of Health*

Cole AA (1989) A study of pelvic dynamics in gait and hip rotation whilst standing in relation to the spine in health and deformity. Thesis: Department of Human Morphology, University of Nottingham

Cole TJ (1989) Using the LMS method to measure skewness in the NCHS and Dutch National height standards. *Ann. Hum. Biol.*; **16**: 407–419

Corballis MC (1991) *The Lopsided Ape: Evolution of the Generative Mind.* Oxford: Oxford University Press

Cummings G, Scholz JP, Barnes K (1993) The effect of imposed leg length difference on pelvic bone symmetry. *Spine*; **18**: 368–373

Dangerfield PH (1994) Asymmetry and growth, Chapter 2, pp. 7–29. In: Ulijaszek SJ, Mascie-Taylor CGN (eds) *Cambridge studies in biological anthropology 14, Anthropometry: The individual and the population.* Cambridge: Cambridge University Press

Dangerfield PH, Groves D, Pearson J (1990) Advanced computer analysis of moiré contour images and the assessment of ribcage deformity in scoliosis. *J. Bone Jt Surg.*; **72B**: 338

Dangerfield PH, Griffiths RD, Edwards RHT (1994) A new chart for height elongation in cases of Duchenne muscular dystrophy. *Clin. Anat.*; **7**: 54

Dawson EG, Kropf MA, Purcell GA, Kanin LEA, Kabo JM, Burt CM (1989) *Optoelectronic Evaluation of Trunk Deformity in Scoliosis.* In combined meeting of Scoliosis Research Society and European Spinal Deformity Society, Amsterdam, 17–22 September 1989

Dechambre H, Teinturier P (1966) Étude radiographique de l'antéversion du cotyle. *J. Radiol. d'Electrologie*; **47**: 207–212

Deutsch AL, Shellock FG, Mink JH (1993) Imaging of the patellofemoral joint: emphasis on advanced techniques, Chapter 5, pp. 75–103. In: Fox JM, Del Pizzo W (eds) *The patellofemoral joint.* New York: McGraw-Hill, Inc.

Dobzhansky T (1973) Nothing in biology makes sense except in the light of evolution. *Am. Biol. Teacher*; **35**: 125–129

Dopf CA, Mandel SS, Geiger DF, Mayer PJ (1994) Analysis of spine motion variability using a computerized goniometer compared to physical examination. A prospective clinical study. *Spine*; **19**: 586–595

Dunlap K, Shands AR Jr, Hollister LC Jr, Gaul JS Jr, Streit HA (1953) A new method for determination of torsion of the femur. *J. Bone Jt Surg.*; **35A**: 289–311

Dvir Z (1995) *Isokinetics. Muscle Testing, Interpretation and Clinical Applications.* London: Churchill Livingstone

Eckhoff DG, Johnson KK (1994) Three-dimensional computed tomography reconstruction of tibial torsion. *Clin. Orthop. Rel. Res.*; **302**: 42–46

Eckhoff DG, Montgomery WK, Kilcoyne RF, Stamm ER (1994) Femoral morphometry and anterior knee pain. *Clin. Orthop. Rel. Res.*; **302**: 64–68

Eklund J, Corlett E (1984) Shrinkage as a measure of the effect of the load on the spine. *Spine*; **9**: 189–194

Eveleth PB (1978) Differences between populations in body shape of children and adolescents. *Am. J. Phys. Anthropol.*; **49**: 373–381

Fabry G, Cheng LX, Molenaers G (1994) Normal and abnormal torsional development in children. *Clin. Orthop. Rel. Res.*; **302**: 22–26

Fairbank JCT, Pynsent PB, Phillips H (1984a) Quantitative measurements of joint mobility in adolescents. *Ann. Rheum. Dis.*; **43**: 288–294

Fairbank JCT, Pynsent PB, van Poortvliet JA, Phillips H (1984b) Influence of anthropometric factors and joint laxity in the incidence of adolescent back pain. *Spine*; **9**: 461–464

Fairbank JCT, Pynsent PB, van Poortvliet JA, Phillips H (1984c) Mechanical factors in the incidence of knee pain in adolescents and young adults. *J. Bone Jt Surg.*; **66B**: 685–693

Falkner F, Tanner JM (1986) Human Growth, 2nd edition. Vol I Developmental biology, Vol II Postnatal growth, neurobiology, Vol III Methodology, ecological, genetic and nutritional effects on growth. London: Plenum Press

Farinet G, Piasco D, Boffa W (1982) Studio radiologico con teleradiografia panoramica della dismetria degli arti nella scoliosi. *La Radiologica Medica*; **68**: 903–906

Farkas LG (1994) *Anthropometry of the Head and Face*, 2nd edition. Raven

Foreman TK, Troup JDG (1987) Diurnal variations in spinal loading and the effects on stature: a preliminary study of nursing activities. *Clin. Biomech.*; **2**: 48–54

Friberg O (1983) Clinical symptoms and biomechanics of lumbar spine and hip joint in leg length inequality. *Spine*; **8**: 643–651

Friberg O, Nurminen M, Korhonen K, Sorninen E, Mänttari ET (1988) Accuracy and precision of clinical estimation of leg length inequality and lumbar scoliosis: comparison of clinical and radiological measurements. *International Disability Studies*; **10**: 49–53

Frobin W, Hierholzer E (1990) *Video Raster Stereography, a Method for On-line Surface Measurements,* pp. 155–157. In: Neugebauer H, Windischbauer G (eds) Surface topography and body deformity. Proceedings of the Fifth International Symposium, 29 September–1 October 1988, Vienna, Austria. Stuttgart: Gustav Fischer

Galasko CSB, Weber DA (1984) *Radionuclide Scintigraphy in Orthopaedics.* Edinburgh: Churchill Livingstone

Galbraith RT, Gelberman RH, Hagek PC, Baker LA, Sartoris DJ, Rab GT, Cohen MS, Griffin PP (1987) Obesity and decreased femoral anteversion in adolescents. *J. Orthop. Res.*; **5**: 523–526

Gasser T, Müller H-G, Köhler W, Prader A, Largo R, Molinari L (1985) An analysis of the mid-growth and adolescent spurts of height based on acceleration. *Ann. Hum. Biol.*; **12**: 129–148

Gasser T, Ziegler P, Kneip A, Prader A, Molinari L, Largo R (1993) The dynamics of growth of weight, circumferences and skinfolds in distance, velocity and acceleration. *Ann. Hum. Biol.*; **20**: 239–259

Ghesquière J, Martin RD, Newcombe F (1985) *Human Sexual Dimorphism.* Symposia of the Society for the Study of Human Biology. London: Taylor and Francis

Giles LGF, Taylor JR (1981) Low-back pain associated with leg length inequality. *Spine*; **6**: 510–521.

Giles LGF, Taylor JR (1982) Lumbar spine structural changes associated with leg length inequality. *Spine*; **7**: 159–162

Glucksmann A (1978) *The Sex Determination and Sexual Dimorphism in Mammals.* London: Wykeham Publications Ltd

Goldstein H (1986) Efficient statistical modelling of longitudinal data. *Annals of Human Biology*; **13**: 129–141

Gomez T, Beach G, Cooke C, Hrudey W, Goyert P (1991) Normative database for trunk range of motion, strength, velocity, and endurance with the Isostation with the B-200. *Spine*; **16**: 15–21

Gosling JP, Lomas DJ, Prager RW, Berman LH (1993) *Virtual Reality Technology in the Assessment of Femoral Anteversion.* In 79th Scientific Assembly and Annual Meeting of RSNA Chicago, paper 1378

Gould SJ (1966) Allometry and size in ontogeny and phylogeny. *Biol. Rev.*; **41**: 587–640

Gould SJ (1991) *Ever since Darwin: Reflections in Natural History,* pp. 63–69, pp. 161–162, pp. 179–185. London: Penguin Books

Gould SJ (1992) *Measuring Heads,* Chapter 3, pp. 73–112. *The Mismeasure of Man.* London: Penguin Books

Goutallier D, Bernageau J, Lecudonnec B (1978) Mesure de l'écart tubérosité tibiale antérieure-gorge de le trochlée (TA-GT): technique résultats intérêt. *Rev. Chir. Orthop.*; **64**: 423

Gracovetsky S (1988) Appendix 2: *The Spinoscope,* pp. 447–462. In The Spinal Engine. Vienna: Springer-Verlag

Gray S (1992) Computer catwalk puts world of fashion into focus. *The Times* December 2, London, England

Gray S (1994) Try on a new dress on your TV screen. *The Sunday Times* November 27, London, England

Greene WB, Heckman JD (1994) *The Clinical Measurement of Joint Motion.* Rosemont, Illinois: American Academy of Orthopaedic Surgeons

Guidera KJ, Ganey TM, Keneally CR, Ogden JA (1994) The embryology of lower extremity torsion. *Clin. Orthop. Rel. Res.*; **302**: 17–21

Halioua M, Liu H-C, Chin A, Bowings TS (1990) Automated topography of the human forms by phase-measuring profilometry and model analysis, pp. 91–100. In: Neugebauer H, Windischbauer G (eds) Surface topography and body deformity. Proceedings of the Fifth International Symposium, 29 September–1 October 1988, Vienna, Austria. Stuttgart: Gustav Fischer

Hall AJ, Barker DJP, Dangerfield PH, Osmond C, Taylor JF (1988) Small feet and Perthes' disease. *J. Bone Jt Surg.*; **70B**: 611–613

Harris NH (1983) Torsional deformities of the lower extremities, Chapter 9, pp. 220–238. In: Harris NH (ed.) *Postgraduate Textbook of Clinical Orthopaedics.* London: Wright PSG

Harrison MHM, Burwell RG (1981) Perthes' disease: a concept of pathogenesis. *Clin. Orthop. Rel. Res.*; **156**: 115–127

Harvey PH, Krebs, JR (1990) Comparing brains. *Science*; **249**: 140–146

Haymes EM, Lundegren HM, Loomis JL, Buskirk ER (1976) Validity of the ultrasonic technique as a method of measuring subcutaneous adipose tissue. *Ann. Hum. Biol.*; **3**: 245–251

Hensinger RJ (1986) *Standards in pediatric orthopedics.* New York: Raven Press

Hermanussen M, Geiger-Benoit K, Burmeister J, Sippell WG (1988a) Knemometry in childhood: accuracy and standardisation of a new technique of lower leg length measurement. *Ann. Hum. Biol.*; **15**: 1–16

Hermanussen M, Geiger-Benoit K, Burmeister J, Sippell WG (1988b) Periodical changes of short term growth velocity (mini-growth-spurts) in human growth. *Ann. Hum. Biol.*; **15**: 103–109

Herron RE (1974) *Biostereometrics 74- an epilogue,* p. 635. In: *'Biostereometrics 74'* Proceedings of the Symposium of Commission V. International Society of Photogrammetry on Biomedical and Bioengineering Applications of Photogrammetry. Washington, DC, 10–13 September 1974. Virginia, USA: American Society of Photogrammetry

Hiernaux J (1968) Bodily shape differentiation of ethnic groups and of the sexes through growth. *Hum. Biol.*; **40**: 44–62

Hindle RJ, Murray-Leslie C, Atha J (1987) Diurnal stature variation in ankylosing spondylitis. *Clin. Biomech.*; **2**: 152–157

Hindle RJ, Pearcy MJ, Cross AT, Miller DHT (1990) Three-dimensional kinematics of the human back. *Clin. Biomech.*; **5**: 218–228

Hodgett SG, Burwell RG, Webb JK (1986) *Trunk height loss in idiopathic scoliosis in AP and oblique spinal radiographs,* p. 92. In: Proceedings of the European Spinal Deformity Society First Congress, 16–19 April 1986 (see Burwell and Dangerfield, 1992)

Hoe A, Atha J, Murray-Leslie C (1994) Stature loss from sustained gentle body loading. *Ann. Hum. Biol.*; **21**: 171–178

Hogarth B (1965) *Proportions and Measurements, Observations on Changing Proportions,* Chapter IV, pp. 67–72. In: Dynamic Anatomy. New York: Watson-Guptill Publication

Hughston JC (1993) *Extensor Mechanism Examination,* Chapter 4, pp. 63–74. Section II, Clinical. In: Fox JM, Del Pizzo W (eds) The patellofemoral joint. New York: McGraw-Hill Inc.

Huiskes R (1992) Mathematical modelling of the knee, Chapter 21, pp. 419–439. In: *Biology and Biomechanics of the traumatized synovial joint: the knee as a model.* Rosemont: American Academy of Orthopaedic Surgeons

Huiskes R, Chao EYS (1983) A survey of finite element analysis in orthopaedic biomechanics: the first decade. *J. Biomech.*; **16**: 385–409

Hutter CG, Scott W (1949) Tibial torsion. *J. Bone Jt Surg.*; **31A**: 511–518

Huxley JS (1932) *Problems of Relative Growth,* 2nd edition. London: Methuen.

Hvid I, Andersen LI (1982) The quadriceps angle and its relation to femoral torsion. *Acta Orthop. Scand.*; **53**: 577–579

Ingelmark BO, Lindström J (1963) Asymmetries of the lower extemities and pelvis and their relations to lumbar scoliosis. A radiographic study. *Acta Morphol. Neerl. Scand.*; **5**: 221–334

Insall J (1979) 'Chondromalacia patellae': patella malalignment syndrome. *Orthop. Clin. N. Am.*; **10**: 117–127

Insall JN (1993) Osteotomy, Chapter 22, pp. 633–676. In: Insall JN (ed.) *Surgery of the knee,* Volume 2, 2nd edition. New York: Churchill Livingstone

Iscan MY, Helmer RP (1993) *Forensic Analysis of the Skull.* New York: Wiley-Liss

Jackson JP, Waugh W (1984) Osteoarthritis of the knee, Chapter 13, pp. 279–320. In: Jackson JP, Waugh W (eds) *Surgery of the Knee Joint.* London: Chapman and Hall

Jones PRM, West GM, Harris DH, Read JB (1989) The Loughborough anthropometric shadow scanner (LASS). *Endeavour, New Series*; **13**: 162–168

Karlberg J, Gelander L, Albertsson-Wikland K (1993) Distinctions between short- and long-term human growth studies. *Acta Paediatr. Scand.*; **82**: 631–634

Kelly MA, Insall JN (1993) *Clinical Examination*, Chapter 4, pp. 63–82. In: Insall JN (ed.) Surgery of the knee, Volume 1, 2nd edition. New York: Churchill Livingstone

Kirby AS, Aujila RK, Burwell RG, Cole AA, Moulton A (1996) A cross-sectional ultrasound study of femoral anteversion and tibial torsion in healthy children aged 5–17 years. *Clin. Anat.* In press

Kirby AS, Burwell RG, Aujla RK, Moulton A, Wallace WA (1994) A new ultrasound method for measuring tibial torsion (TT angles) and findings in young adolescents. *Clin. Anat.*; **7**: 55–56

Kirby AS, Wallace WA, Moulton A, Burwell RG (1993) Comparison of four methods of measuring femoral anteversion. *Clin. Anat.*; **6**: 280–288

Kobyliansky E, Weissman SL, Nathan H (1979) Femoral and tibial torsion. A correlation in dry bones. *Int. Orthop. (SICOT)*; **3**: 145–147

Krag MH, Cohen MC, Haugh LD, Pope MH (1990) Body height change during upright and recumbent posture. *Spine*; **15**: 202–207

Kronberg M, Broström L-Å (1990) Humeral head retroversion in patients with unstable humero-scapular joints. *Clin. Orthop. Rel. Res.*; **260**: 207–211

Kunkle HM, Carpenter EB (1954) A simple technique for X-ray measurement of limb-length discrepancies. *J. Bone Jt Surg.*; **36A**: 152–154

Lanyon LE, Rubin CT (1984) Static vs dynamic loads as an influence on bone remodelling. *J. Biomech.*; **17**: 897–905

Lea RD, Gerhardt JJ (1995) Current concepts review: Range-of-motion measurements. *J. Bone Jt Surg.*; **77A**: 784–798

Lindgren G (1978) Growth of school children with early, average and late ages of peak height velocity. *Ann. Hum. Biol.*; **5**: 253–267

Livshits G, Kobyliansky E (1989) Study of genetic variants in the fluctuating asymmetry of anthropometrical traits. *Ann. Hum. Biol.*; **16**: 121–129

Lohman TG, Slaughter MH, Swlinger A, Boileau RA (1978) Relationship of body composition to somatotype in college men. *Ann. Hum. Biol.*; **5**: 147–157

Lohman TG, Roche AF, Marterell R (1988) *Anthropometric Standardisation Reference Manual*. Champaign, Illinois: Human Kinetic Books

Lovejoy OC (1981) The origin of man. *Science*; **221**: 341–350

Malina RM (1980) *Kinanthropometric Research in Human Auxology*, pp. 437–451 In: Borms J, Hauspie R, Sand A, Susanne C, Hebbelinck M (eds) Human growth and development. New York: Plenum Press

Malina RM, Buschang PH (1984) Anthropometric asymmetry in normal and mentally retarded males. *Ann. Hum. Biol.*; **11**: 515–531

Maresh MM (1970) In: McCammon RW (ed.) *Human Growth and Development*, pp. 157–200. Springfield, Illinois: Chas. C Thomas

Marrass WS, Lavender SA, Leurgans SE, Rajulu SL, Allread WG, Fathallah FA, Ferguson SA (1993) The role of dynamic three-dimensional trunk motion in occupationally-related low back disorders. The effect of workplace factors, trunk position, and trunk motion characteristics on risk of injury. *Spine*; **18**: 617–628

Marshall WA (1977) *Human Growth and its Disorders*. London: Academic Press

Mascie-Taylor CGN, Boldsen JL (1985) Regional and social analysis of height variation in contemporary British sample. *Ann. Hum. Biol.*; **4**: 315–324

Mauritzon L, Benoni G, Ilver J, Lindstrom K, Willner S (1986) *Three-linear Array Back Scanning with Airborne Ultrasound*, pp. 47–51. In: Harris JD, Turner-Smith (eds) Surface topography and spinal deformity. Proceedings of the Third International Symposium 27–28 September 1984 Oxford, England. Stuttgart: Gustav Fischer

Morris JRW, Harris JD (1976) Three-dimensional shapes. *Lancet*; **1**: 1189–1190

Moseley CF (1977) A straight-line graph for leg-length discrepancies. *J. Bone Jt Surg.*; **59A**: 174–179

Moulton A, Upadhyay SS (1982) A direct method of measuring femoral anteversion using ultrasound. *J. Bone Jt Surg.*; **64B**: 469–472

Moulton A, Burwell RG, Wallace WA, Aujla RK, Kirby AS (1993) The development and application of ultrasound methods for measuring femoral anteversion: relevance to clinical practice. *J. Bone Jt Surg.*; **75B**: Orthopaedic Proceedings Supplement II, 163

Moulton A, Burwell RG, Cole AA, Kirby AS, McKim Thomas H (1994) A new ultrasound appraisal of rotational alignment in the lower limbs between the hip and ankle: application to toeing-in and toeing-out. *Clin. Anat.*; **7**: 164

Moulton A, Burwell RG, Cole AA, Kirby AS (1995a) Anterior knee pain in young subjects; rotational alignment in the lower limbs measured by ultrasound. *Clin. Anat.*; **8**: 151

Moulton A, Burwell RG, Mayhew TM (1995b) Anterior knee pain in children and young adults evaluated by ultrasound measurement of femoral anterversion (FAV), tibial torsion (TT), femoro-tibial rotation (FTR) and summated rotational alignment of the lower limbs (RA). *Scientific reports: The Arthritis and Rheumatism Council for Research*

Mueller WH, Marbella A, Harrist RB, Kaplowitz HJ, Grunbaum JA, Labarthe DR (1989) Body circumferences as alternatives to skinfold measures of body fat distribution in children. *Ann. Hum. Biol.*; **16**: 495–506

Murphy SB, Kijewski PK, Simon SR *et al.* (1986) Computer-aided simulation, analysis and design in orthopedic surgery. *Orthop. Clin. N. Am.*; **17**: 637–649

Nelle M, Tröger J, Rupprath G, Bettendorf M (1994) Metacarpal index in Marfan's syndrome and in constitutional tall stature. *Arch. Dis. Child.*; **70**: 149–150

Nichols PJR, Bailey NTJ (1955) The accuracy of measuring leg-length differences. An 'observer error' experiment. *B. M. J.*; Nov 19: 1247–1248

Nigg BM (1986) Quoted by Salathé EP Jr *et al.* (1990) The foot as a shock absorber. *J. Biomech.*; **23**: 655–659

Norgan NG (1994) Relative sitting height and interpretation of the body mass index. *Ann. Hum. Biol.*; **21**: 79–82

Pavlov H (1993) Radiographic examination, Chapter 5, pp. 83–110. In: Insall JN (ed.) *Surgery of the Knee*, Vol 1, 2nd edition. New York: Churchill Livingstone

Pearcy MJ (1993) Twisting mobility of the human back in flexed postures. *Spine*; **18**: 114–119

Pelto GH, Pelto PJ, Messer E (1989) *Research Methods in Nutritional Anthropology.* Tokyo: the United Nations University

Pynsent PB, Fairbank JC, Clack FJ, Phillips H (1983) The computer recording of anatomical points in 3-dimensional space. *J. Biomed. Eng.*; **5**: 137–140

Rabey G (1968) *Morphanalysis.* London: Hatch Pinner & Co.

Rabey G (1979) *Analytic Medicine.* Vol 1: Conventions. Lancaster: MTP Press Ltd.

Reikeras O (1991) Is there a relationship between femoral anteversion and leg torsion? *Skeletal Radiol.*; **20**: 409–411

Ritter MA, DeRosa GP, Babcock JL (1976) Tibial torsion. *Clin. Orthop. Rel. Res.*; **120**: 159–163

Roche AF, Wainer H, Thissen D (1975) *Skeletal Maturity: the Knee Joint as a Biological Indicator.* New York and London: Blenheim Medical Book Company

Roebuck Jr JA, Kromer KHE, Thomsom WG (1975) *Engineering Anthropometry Methods.* New York: John Wiley and Sons, Inc.

Romer AS (1954) The human body: skin, nervous system, Chapter 17, pp. 280–313. In: Man and the vertebrates, Vol 2. London: Penguin Books

Rona RJ, Altman DG (1976) National study of health and growth: standards of attained height, weight and triceps skin fold in English children 5–11 years old. *Ann. Hum. Biol.*; **4**: 501–523

Rose J, Gamble JG (1994) *Human Walking*, 2nd edition. Rose J, Gamble JG (eds). Baltimore: Williams and Wilkins

Rosenbaum S, Skinner RK, Knight IB, Garrow JS (1985) A survey of heights and weights of adults in Great Britain, 1980. *Ann. Hum. Biol.*; **12**: 115–127

Ruff CB (1993) Climatic adaptation and hominid evolution: the thermoregulatory imperative. *Evolution. Anthropol.*; **2**: 53–60

Ruff CB (1994) Morphological adaptation to climate in modern and fossil hominids. *Yearbook of Physical Anthropology*; **37**: 65–107

Rush WA, Steiner HA (1946) A study of lower extremity length inequality. *Am. J. Roentgenol.*; **56**: 616–623

Rushton JP (1992) The brain size/IQ debate. *Nature*; **360**: 292

Ruwe PA, Gage JR, Ozonoff MB, DeLuca PA (1992) Clinical determination of femoral anteversion: comparison with established techniques. *J. Bone Jt Surg.*; **74A**: 820–830

Salenius P, Vankka E (1975) The development of the tibiofemoral angle in children. *J. Bone Jt Surg.*; **57A**: 259–261

Saraste H, Östman A (1986) Stereophotogrammetry in the evaluation of the treatment of scoliosis. *Int. Orthop.* (SICOT); **10**: 63–67

Schnall BS, Smith DW (1974) Nonrandom laterality of malformations in paired structures. *J. Pediatr.*; **85**: 509–511

Schultz AH (1937) Proportions, variability and asymmetries of the long bones of the limbs and clavicles in man and apes. *Hum. Biol.*; **9**: 281–328

Schumpe G, Messler H (1987) *Comparison of Parameters Used for the Measurement of Spinal Deformity by Means of Optrimetric, Ultrasonic and Radiographic Technique*, pp. 203–212. In: Stokes IAF, Pekelsky JR, Moreland MS (eds) Surface topography and spinal deformity. Proceedings of the Fourth International Symposium, 29–30 September 1986, Mont Sainte Marie, Québec. Stuttgart: Gustav Fischer

Smith SH, Jones PRM, West GM (1990) Three-dimensional scanning: a new tool in the study of human body composition. *Ann. Hum. Biol.*; **17**: 340

Smith WDF, Cunningham DA, Paterson DH, Koval JJ (1995) Body mass indices and skeletal size in 394 Canadians aged 55–86 years. *Ann. Hum. Biol.*; **22**: 305–314

Soderberg GL (1986) *Kinesiology, Application to Pathological Motion.* Baltimore: Williams and Wilkins

Staheli LT, Corbett M, Wiss C, King H (1985) Lower-extremity rotational problems in children. Normal values to guide management. *J. Bone Jt Surg.*; **67A**: 39–47

Steindler A (1955) *Kinesiology of the Human Body Under Normal and Pathological Conditions.* Springfield: Chas C Thomas

Stokes VP, Andersson C, Forssberg H (1989) Rotational and translational movement features of the pelvis and thorax during adult human locomotion. *J. Biomech.*; **22**: 43–50

Sutherland CJ (1986) Practical application of computer-generated three-dimensional reconstructions in orthopedic surgery. *Orthop. Clin. N. Am.*; **17**: 651–656

Sutherland DH, Olshen RA, Biden EN, Wyatt MP (1988) *The Development of Mature Walking.* Clinics in Developmental Medicine No 104. Oxford: Blackwell Scientific Publications Ltd.

Takai S, Sakakida K, Yamashita F, Suzu F, Izuta F (1985) Rotational alignment of the lower limb in osteoarthritis of the knee. *Int. Orthop. (SICOT)*; **9**: 209–216

Tanner JM (1953) *Growth and Constitution.* In: Kroeber AL (ed.) Anthropology Today. An encyclopaedic inventory. Chicago: University of Chicago Press

Tanner JM (1981) *A History of the Study of Human Growth.* Cambridge: Cambridge University Press

Tanner JM (1992) *Physical Growth Development and Puberty,* Chapter 8, pp. 389–445. In: Campbell AGM, McIntosh N, (eds) Forfar and Arneil's Textbook of Paediatrics, 4th edition. London: Churchill Livingstone

Tanner JM, Cameron N (1980) Investigation of the mid-growth spurt in height, weight and limb circumferences in single-year velocity data from the London 1966-67 growth survey. *Ann. Hum. Biol.*; **7**: 565–577

Tanner JM, Hiernaux J, Jarman S (1969) *Growth and Physique Studies,* pp. 1–71. In IBP Handbook No 9 Human Biology. A guide to field methods compiled by JS Weiner and JA Lourie. Oxford: Blackwell Scientific Publications

Tanner JM, Whitehouse RH, Cameron N, Marshall WA, Healy MJR, Goldstein H (1983) *Assessment of Skeletal Maturity and Prediction of Adult Height (TW2 Method).* London: Academic Press

Taylor JR, Slinger BS (1980) Scoliosis screening and growth in Western Australian students. *Med. J. Aust.*; **1**: 475–478

Thompson D'Arcy W (1942) *On Growth and Form.* An abridged edition by JT Bonner (ed.). Cambridge: Cambridge University Press, 1992

Tupman GS (1962) A study of bone growth in normal children and its relationship to skeletal maturation. *J. Bone Jt Surg.*; **44B**: 42–67

Turner-Smith AR, Harris JD, Houghton GR, Jefferson RJ (1988) A method for analysis of back shape in scoliosis. *J. Biomech.*; **21**: 497–509

Tyrrell A, Reilly T, Troup J (1985) Circadian variation in stature and the effects of spinal loading. *Spine*; **10**: 161–164

Ulijaszek SJ, Lourie JA (1994) Intra- and inter-observer error in anthropometric measurement, Chapter 3, pp. 30–55. In: Ulijaszek SJ, Mascie-Taylor CGN (eds) *Cambridge Studies in Biological Anthropology 14. Anthropometry: the Individual and the Population.* Cambridge: Cambridge University Press

Vagenas G, Hoshizaki B (1991) Functional asymmetries and lateral dominance in the lower limbs of distance runners. *Int. J. Sport Biomech.*; **7**: 311–329

Valk IM, Chabloz AMEL, Smals AGH, Kloppenborg PWC, Cassorla FG, Schutte EAST (1983) Accurate measurement of the lower leg length and the ulnar length and its application in short term growth measurement. *Growth*; **47**: 53–66

Vijayraghavan K, Sastry JG (1976) The efficacy of arm circumference as a substitute for weight in assessment of protein-calorie malnutrition. *Ann. Hum. Biol.*; **3**: 229–233

Voloshin A, Wosk J (1982) An *in vivo* study of low back pain and shock absorption in the human locomotor system. *J. Biomech.*; **15**: 21–27

Wales JKH, Milner RDG (1987) Knemometry in assessment of linear growth. *Arch. Dis. Child.*; **62**: 166–171

Walker J (1994) A new morphometrics? *Evolution. Anthropol.*; **3**: 37

Weber W, Weber E (1836) *Mechanics of the Human Walking Apparatus.* Translated by P Maquet and R Furlong. Berlin: Springer-Verlag, 1992

Weiner JS, Lourie JA (1969) *Human Biology, a Guide to Field Methods.* IBP Handbook No. 9. Oxford: Blackwell Scientific Publications

Weiner JS, Lourie JA (1981) *Practical Human Biology.* London: Academic Press

Whitfield P (1993) The natural history of evolution. Life and change. Introduction; p. 44: London

Wientroub S, Boyde A, Chrispin AR, Lloyd-Roberts GC (1981) The use of stereophotogrammetry to measure acetabular and femoral anteversion. *J. Bone Jt Surg.*; **63B**: 209–213

Whittle MW (1991) *Gait Analysis: An Introduction.* Oxford: Butterworth-Heinemann

Willner S (1979) Moiré topography for the diagnosis and documentation of scoliosis. *Acta Orthop. Scand.*; **50**: 295–302

Winter DA (1990) *Biomechanics and the Motor Control of Human Movement,* 2nd edition. New York: John Wiley and Sons, Inc.

Wynne-Davies R (1975) Infantile idiopathic scoliosis. Causative factors, particularly in the first six months of life. *J. Bone Jt Surg.*; **57B**: 138–141

Wynne-Davies R, Hall CM, Apley AG (1985) *Atlas of Skeletal Dysplasias. Section Seven, Short Limbs and Trunk,* pp. 239–308. Edinburgh: Churchill Livingstone

Yagi T (1994) Tibial torsion in patients with medial-type osteoarthrotic knees. *Clin. Orthop. Rel. Res.*; **302**: 52–56

Zorab PA, Harrison A, Harrison WJ (1964) Estimation of height from tibial length. *Lancet*; **2**: 1063

Chapter 11

Growth and bone age

MA Preece and LA Cox

Introduction

The phenomenon of growth, more than any other, distinguishes the child from the adult. Throughout the first 2 decades of life the child continually changes size and matures, both in size and function. This process has considerable implications to paediatrics in both anatomical and physiological considerations. In this chapter we will consider the more general aspects of growth leaving the more specific to other authors.

The height growth curve (see also Chapter 10)

Distance curve

The data shown in Figure 11.1 is from the oldest published study of growth of a child (Tanner, 1962). The upper panel (11.1a) demonstrates the height growth curve for a single boy from birth to 18 years. This type of growth curve is usually referred to as the height-attained or distance curve of growth. It is the most commonly used representation and the most closely associated with height as observed in everyday life. It contains all the information about growth in height of the individual child.

Velocity curve

In Figure 11.1(b) the measurements are represented in a different way. Here, the distance data is converted into height velocity in centimetres per year. This is calculated from the distance data by dividing the difference between two height measurements, as near to one year apart as possible, by the exact time elapsed between them. The calculated velocity is plotted at the mid-point of the time interval over which it was measured to give the velocity curve. This representation of growth is particularly useful as it shows more detail of the growth process and is a more sensitive chronicle of events that have occurred in any one year than is the height distance measurement at the same time. The latter subsumes measurements of all previous heights before. Thus the more sensitive velocity curve may show rather dramatic changes in growth during disease, where the simpler distance curve would obscure them.

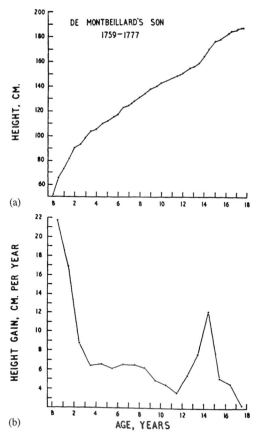

Figure 11.1 Growth in height of the son of the Count de Montbeillard from birth to 18 years. (a) (above) shows the height attained or distance curve and (b) (below) shows the height velocity curve. From Tanner (1962) with permission

In general, there are three epochs of growth: early, rather fast growth before the age of 2; a relatively unchanging pattern of growth during the preschool and primary school years and then the adolescent growth spurt.

During the first year of life the infant has an average height velocity of about 25 cm per year (Tanner *et al.*, 1966a,b). However this is a time when the velocity is changing dramatically and shorter time periods should be considered. The average velocity during the first 3 months is 40 cm per year in boys and 36 cm per year in girls, falling to 15 cm per year and 16 cm per year, respectively, by the last 3 months of that year. During the next 3 years there is a further deceleration to achieve a rather constant velocity of about 5–6 cm per year. This continues with gentle slowing until puberty. Figure 11.1 shows clearly the simple changes described above but also illustrates a phenomenon which is less constant. A slight increase in growth velocity is seen in this curve between the ages of about 6 and 8 years which is sometimes referred to as the juvenile or mid-growth spurt (Molinari *et al.*, 1980). This is a rather inconstant feature and in many individual children cannot be seen. Its physiological significance remains obscure but it is worth noting that unlike the adolescent growth spurt, the mid-growth spurt is of equal intensity and comparable timing in both sexes.

An almost universal event in children's height growth is the adolescent growth spurt. At about 10 years in girls and 12 years in boys the rate of growth increases dramatically, reaching a peak on average 2 years later. This period will be discussed in more detail later when considering the differences between the sexes. At this point it suffices to note that the mean peak growth velocity of boys is about 10 cm per year and of girls about 8 cm per year.

The deceleration in growth velocity that is seen from birth onwards is the continuation of a process that started long before birth. The true time of peak growth velocity is at about 32 weeks of gestation for growth in length and at about 25 weeks of gestation for weight gain (Davies, 1981).

Growth of other body parts

Figure 11.2 shows schematically the four major growth patterns seen in different body parts (Tanner, 1962). In all cases the vertical axis shows the percentage of mature size at any one age represented on the horizontal axis. The heavy horizontal line at 100% represents mature size. It can be seen that there are quite striking differences between the general pattern of growth of the brain and head, the reproductive organs, the lymphatic tissues and the overall general pattern which mostly refers to skeletal but also some other tissues. The pattern described

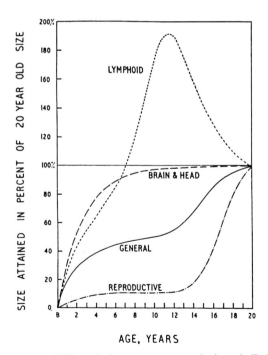

Figure 11.2 Growth curves of different body systems represented schematically. From Tanner (1962) with permission

as general can be seen to be essentially similar to that for growth in height and largely this is true for most other skeletal measures. The major exception is the cranium which follows the brain closely in its growth. In this case it can be seen that there is considerable growth in the first 4–5 years of life; about 80% of mature size is achieved in cranial growth by the age of 4. There is a small adolescent growth spurt but on the scale of this figure it is not discernible. It is important to note, however, that this pattern reflects the growth of the cranium but not the facial bones. The growth patterns of the face are very complex but they seem to have, if anything, more similarity to the growth of the long bones.

The reproductive organs grow little in the first years of life and it is not until the onset of puberty that there is a dramatic change in size. This applies to the testes, ovaries, epididymus, prostate, seminal vesicles, fallopian tubes and uterus.

Finally, the pattern of growth of lymphatic tissues should be noted. This is unique in that there is a period of overgrowth in the later school years when there is a period of 'excessive' size which may have been at least in part responsible for earlier fashions for tonsillectomy, often inappropriately.

Sexual dimorphism in skeletal growth

Figure 11.3(a) shows the height growth curves of a typical boy and a typical girl from birth to 19 years of age (Tanner *et al.*, 1966a). Figure 11.3(b) shows the equivalent velocity curves. Here we can discuss some of the differences between the sexes; much of the sexual dimorphism in skeletal shape is accounted for by changes at puberty rather than before.

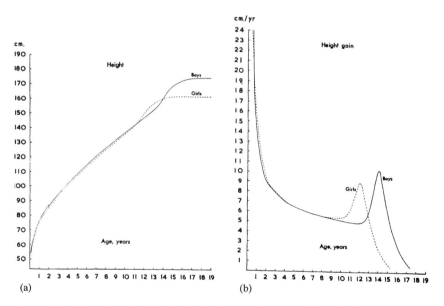

Figure 11.3. Height (a) and height velocity (b) of a typical boy and girl from birth to maturity. From Tanner (1966a) with permission

There is little difference between boys and girls before 10 years of age. Then the typical girl starts her adolescent growth spurt and for a few years is taller than the same-aged boy. Some 2 years later the boy starts his spurt and by the age of 14 is the taller. The major difference in mature height between men and women (14.0 cm in the UK (Freeman *et al.*, 1990)) is established at puberty. About 12 cm comes from the extra 2 years of prepubertal growth of boys and the remainder from their more intense growth spurt. There is, further, a notable difference between the sexes in the intensity of the segmental growth spurts. In boys the sitting height growth spurt is more intense than in girls although the leg spurts are about equal (Preece *et al.*, 1992). This is explained by the fact that growth of the spine, in boys at least, is largely testosterone-dependent and secretion of this hormone is rapidly increasing at this time. There are also considerable changes in other skeletal dimensions that appear now. While only a little of the difference between men and women's leg length is achieved during puberty (about 10%) around 50% of the difference between men and women's sitting height and biacromial diameter is achieved during pubertal growth. In contrast, bi-iliac diameter, reflecting pelvic breadth, is one of the few measurements where girls have a more prolonged and more intense adolescent growth spurt than boys and some 40% of mature size difference between the sexes is achieved during puberty (Preece *et al.*, 1992).

Tissue components

Body fat is usually estimated using skinfold calipers to measure the subcutaneous fat thickness. X-rays of limbs can be used to estimate fat, muscle and bone diameters. Subcutaneous fat measurements by skinfold calipers are very prone to error. Nevertheless, clearly defined patterns of subcutaneous fat growth have been reported and standards are available for use. Clinically, they are the most practical method for measurement of fat.

The X-ray method is limited in its usefulness today because of the recognition that X-rays can be harmful, particularly in longitudinal studies. However, longitudinal growth curves obtained at an earlier time, demonstrate patterns of normal growth of these tissues (Figure 11.4) (Tanner *et al.*, 1981).

Bone diameters

The distance curves for the mean humerus and tibia widths from the age of 3 onwards are shown in Figure 11.4(a). The humerus width in boys is, on average, slightly greater than the girls' until the female adolescent growth spurt starts. For about 2 years the means are then equal after which the boys' greater growth spurt commences. In tibia width there is no sex difference before the onset of puberty but by maturity both bones show a 13% greater width in the male than in the female.

Limb muscle

In Figure 11.4(b) calf and arm muscle widths are illustrated. Before puberty the curves are very similar to those for bone although the sex difference in the arm muscle is somewhat greater. At puberty there is marked growth spurt in both

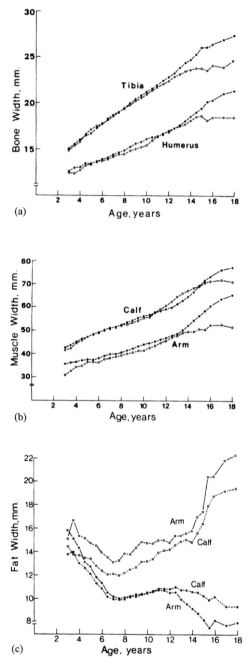

Figure 11.4 Mean widths of various limb components for boys (*filled circles*) and girls (*open circles*). (a) Humerus and tibia; (b) arm and calf muscle; and (c) arm and calf fat. From Tanner *et al.* (1981) with permission

limbs in boys; in girls the arm muscle increases only slightly while calf muscle exceeds that of boys between the ages of 11 and 15. By full maturity the male preponderance is much greater in the arm (about 20%) than in the calf (10%).

Limb fat

Figure 11.4(c) shows the fat layer widths for arm and calf. Boys have less fat than girls at both sites from age 4 onwards. The difference is increased during childhood and particularly so at puberty. In both sexes fat width falls from age 3 to about 7 and then starts to rise. In boys the rise is replaced from about 12 to 18 by a further loss which is greater in the arm than in the calf. In girls fat accumulates fairly continuously excepting a period during puberty (10–12 years of age) when arm fat remains fairly constant. Fat changes as measured by skinfold calipers show a similar pattern when the triceps skinfold is used as a measure of limb fat. The changes are less dramatic but reflect the same events.

Growth gradients

Not all parts of the body grow at the same tempo. By this we mean that different body segments, such as trunk and limbs or subsections of limbs, reach particular proportions of mature size at different ages (Cameron et al., 1982). In general there is a peripheral to central gradient in the limbs such that the more distal segments, such as the hand or foot, are the earliest to reach mature size and have their adolescent peak growth velocity at earlier ages. Thus in any given child the foot or hand is the more likely to finish growing before the more proximal body parts such as the upper leg or spine. Although not a universal rule, this pattern occurs in the majority of children. As far as the trunk and lower limb relationships are concerned, in 65% of children the sequence is one of sub-ischial leg length preceding total height which in turn precedes sitting height.

Normal variation

Every measured variable has a range of normal variation in a population. It would be impracticable to go through every measurement in turn in a chapter such as the present and therefore attention will only be given to height as an example.

Height standards

Figure 11.5 shows recently published British standard curves for height for boys (Freeman et al., 1990). These data are based on large, nationally representative samples of children studied in a cross-sectional manner. This is important as longitudinal data is nearly always collected from a selected population of children which could lead to an underestimate of population variance. They may also contain selection biases. The centiles shown follow ideas recently discussed by Cole (1994) where nine centile lines are displayed (0.4th, 2nd, 9th, 25th, 50th, 75th, 91st, 98th and 99.6th centiles) which are evenly spaced 0.67 SDs apart.

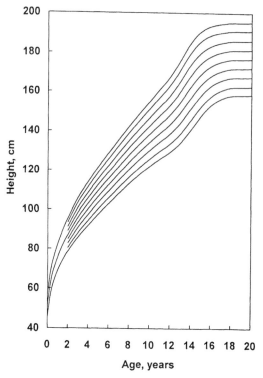

Figure 11.5 Contemporary cross-sectional growth curves for British boys. The growth curves represent (from bottom to top) the 0.4th, 2nd, 9th, 25th, 50th, 75th, 91st, 98th and 99.6th centiles. From Freeman *et al.* (1995) with permission and see also Cole (1994)

It is conventional for children to be measured lying down until the age of two years and standing thereafter. However, in cross-sectional analyses if proper measurement technique is used so that postural effects are minimised, no difference is discernible between supine and standing measurements (Lindgren and Hauspie, 1989; Freeman *et al.*, 1990).

Correction for family height

The above standards derive from population surveys; they can be made more accurate for a given child if the heights of the parents are taken into account. The easiest way of doing this is to plot the parents' centiles at the right-hand edge of the chart; age 20 for these standards. This is quickly done by plotting first the actual height of the like-sexed parent and, secondly the father's height, minus 14 cm or the mother's height plus 14 cm, for the unlike-sexed parent. The 14 cm is the mean difference between adult men and women in the UK (Freeman *et al.*, 1990). This should be adjusted appropriately in other countries according to local data.

The above technique also goes some way towards making allowances for racial differences. An ideal would be race-specific standards for large multi-racial societies but these are seldom available.

Puberty

Some of the skeletal changes that occur during puberty have already been discussed. Many of these events are important in the development of differences in shape between the adult male and female but these are, of course, compounded by other changes in growth that are occurring in the soft tissues. Here we will restrict ourselves to discussing the changes of the classical puberty stages which are an essential part of evaluation of a child's progression through puberty.

The systems in current use depend on the criteria formalised by Tanner (1962). These depend upon rating breast and pubic hair development on a five point scale and axillary hair on a three point scale for girls and external genitalia, pubic and axillary hair on similar scales for boys.

The breast stages are illustrated in Figure 11.6 and are defined as follows:

Stage 1. Pre-adolescent: elevation of the papilla only.
Stage 2: Breast bud stage: elevation of breast and papilla as a small mound. Enlargement of areolar diameter.
Stage 3. Further enlargement and elevation of breast and areola, with no separation of their contours.
Stage 4. Projection of areola and papilla to form a secondary mound above the level of the breast.
Stage 5. Mature stage: projection of papilla only, due to recession of the areola to the general contour of the breast.

The stage 4 development of the areolar mound does not occur in all girls; in a quarter it is absent and in a further quarter relatively slight.

Genitalia stages for boys are shown in Figure 11.7.

Stage 1. Pre-adolescent: testes, scrotum and penis are of about same size and proportions as in early childhood.
Stage 2. Enlargement of scrotum and of testes. The skin of the scrotum reddens and changes in texture. Little or no enlargement of penis at this stage.
Stage 3. Enlargement of penis, which occurs at first mainly in length. Further growth of testes and scrotum.
Stage 4. Increased size of penis with growth in breadth and development of glands. Further enlargement of testes and scrotum; increasing darkening of scrotal skin.
Stage 5. Genitalia adult in size and shape.

Pubic hair distributions for both sexes are illustrated in Figure 11.8.

Stage 1. Pre-adolescent stage: the vellus over the pubes is not further developed than over the abdominal wall.
Stage 2. Sparse growth of long, slightly pigmented downy hair, straight or only slightly curled, appearing chiefly at base of the penis or along the labia.
Stage 3. Considerably darker, coarser and more curled. The hair spreads sparsely over the junction of the pubes.
Stage 4. Hair now resembles adult in type but the area covered by it is still considerably smaller than in the adult. No spread to the medial surface of the thighs.

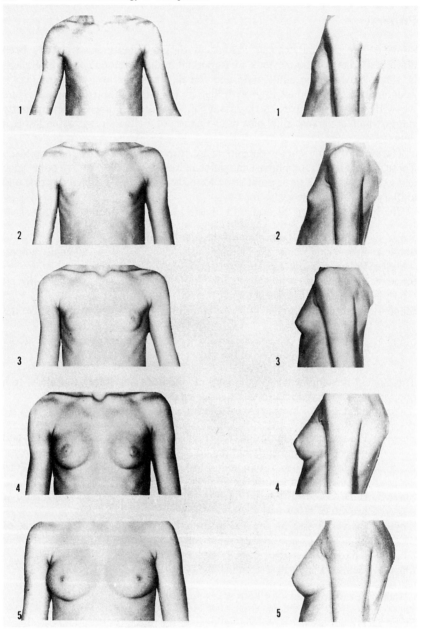

Figure 11.6 Breast stages. From Tanner (1962) with permission

Stage 5. Adult in quantity and type with distribution of the horizontal (or classically 'feminine' pattern). Spread to the medial surface of thighs but not up linea alba or elsewhere above the base of the inverse triangle.

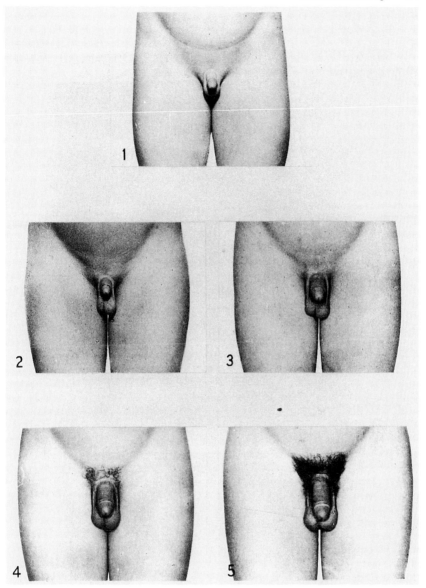

Figure 11.7 Genitalia stages. From Tanner (1962) with permission

Axillary hair in both sexes has only three stages: stage 1 shows no hair; stage 2 a small amount and stage 3 normal adult distribution of hair.

In much the same way as we discussed variation in height for age, we should also discuss variation in attainment of different pubertal stages. Standards for achievement of puberty stages are available for British adolescents (Tanner and Whitehouse, 1976).

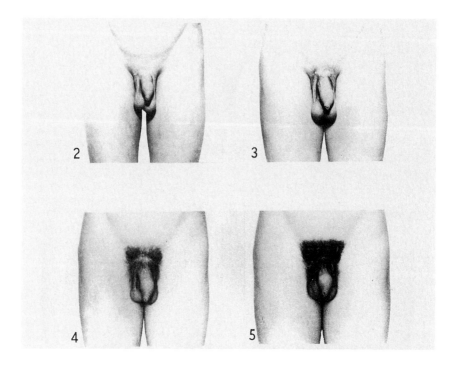

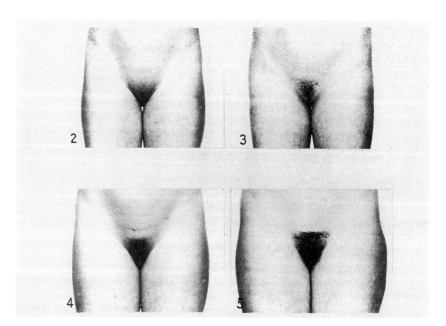

Figure 11.8 Pubic hair stages. From Tanner (1962) with permission

Indices of maturation

Chronological age is a poor measure of maturity. The average maturing boy completes his growth at 18 years of age, whereas an early developer may do so at 15 or 16 years; a later developer may still be growing at 20 years of age. With girls the same is true except that the whole process occurs some 2 years earlier. The growth of an early developer is advanced for the entire period of growth including puberty unless the advance is due to a late-acquired factor such as disease. Precocious puberty is an instance when growth rate is accelerated but time of growth is shortened. The opposite applies in the case of a process such as malnutrition which leads to growth delay. In both of these cases final height may be reduced. Because these differences in the pattern of maturation are not accounted for by chronological age, other measures are needed to categorize a child as advanced or delayed in maturation. The variable pattern of an individual's maturation rate can be conveniently referred to as 'tempo'. Several measures of physiological maturity have been advocated, all depending on defining a sequence of events that occur in an invariant order and which always occur in every individual that reaches maturity. Implicitly each individual must reach the same final event at maturity.

The puberty stages described in the previous section are indices of maturity and are very appropriate ones in the peripubertal age group. They are, however, inappropriate in the younger child and also in those children who have already successfully completed puberty but are not necessarily fully grown. For this reason other methods of maturational assessment have been developed of which skeletal age is by far the most important.

An additional but very valuable pubertal indicator in females is menarche, the attainment of the first menstrual period. This is rather strongly related to the timing of the adolescent growth spurt; in the great majority of girls menarche occurs after peak height velocity has been passed. In one study, 16% of girls attained menarche in the same year as the peak height velocity, a further 55% in the following year and the remainder by 3 years after peak height velocity (Hagg and Taranger, 1979). It can, therefore, be said that if a girl has attained menarche, she is probably in the slowing-down phase of the growth spurt.

Skeletal age

There have been several methods developed to assess the skeletal maturity of growing children. The first attempt at producing an atlas as a means of assessing skeletal maturity was made by Todd (1937). The children used in this study were referred to the research group by paediatricians and were therefore above average socio-economic and educational status. Radiographs were taken of the left shoulder, elbow, hand, knee, and foot. This group of children, with additions over the years became known as the Brush Foundation Study and it was this group that were used to expand the ideas of Todd to produce atlas type standards for the hand and wrist (Greulich and Pyle, 1959), the knee (Pyle and Hoerr, 1955) and the ankle and foot (Hoerr et al., 1952).

Discussion continues as to which area of the skeleton best indicates the maturity and growth potential of an individual. The major criterion has to be that the area chosen can be X-rayed with minimal radiation, and with as few views as possible. The hand and wrist remains the most popular as historically it was the first to be used, it only needs one view, and there are many bones in a small area.

The most commonly used system is that of Greulich and Pyle (1959), which used fewer standards than Todd's original with a larger sample of children and incorporated the Bailey Pinneau prediction of adult height in the second edition (Bayley and Pinneau, 1952). The standard chosen to represent a particular age was the one that best expressed the mode of a ranked series of one hundred radiographs that showed the entire span of maturity seen in the age group concerned.

The atlas method of producing standards has several disadvantages. The assessor is supposed to pick the standard that most closely matches the film being investigated, if no exact match is found then each bone is checked against individual standards and a mean bone age calculated. In practice, the overall standard most closely resembling the film in question is chosen and that becomes the bone age. The assessor tends to concentrate on only a few bones leading to a biased reading. It is not uncommon for a single radiograph to yield bone ages that are several years apart when assessed by different observers. Another difficulty is that the standards, by virtue of the sample they were drawn from were relatively advanced compared with other American children and even more when compared to European children. At present, the secular trend for earlier maturation has almost removed the social bias with modern Americans, but Europeans are still, on average, 6–9 months delayed (Preece, 1988).

Methods that use a bone-specific scoring system are preferred. These use criteria for set stages in maturation employing written descriptions together with illustrations and considerably reduce subjectivity. Several systems have evolved for both the knee (Roche et al., 1975a) and the hand and wrist (Roche et al., 1975b; Tanner et al., 1983a). The most frequently used system is the TW2 method, which also incorporates a methodology for predicting adult height (Tanner et al., 1983a), the equations for which have been extended (Tanner et al., 1983b).

Each of 20 bones in the left hand and wrist can be rated by this system: the radius; ulna; digits 1, 3 and 5; and the carpals. Because the pattern of maturation is similar in boys and girls only one set of criteria were produced and the sex differences taken into account when the individual ratings are converted into a weighted numerical score. Summation of these scores gives the possibility of three maturity scores, the total 20-bone score (TW20), the radius, ulna, and short bone score (RUS) and the carpal score (carpal). In practice, the RUS score is the most useful, as the carpus is very variable in the way it matures and extremely difficult to rate, because the criteria are not easy to define. Also in most normal children the carpus is mature at an early age (a mean of 11 years for girls and 13 years for boys). It is also the RUS score that is used in the prediction of adult height. Standards for maturity scores for British children have been produced but are rarely used as the scores are usually converted to a bone 'age' which clinicians generally find more convenient. The method can be used for any population, but if bone age standards are to be used then specific standards for each country should be developed by applying the method to radiographs of local normal children.

Reliability

Beunen and Cameron (1995) showed that the same assessor gave the same stage rating on two occasions in 90% of instances and that different assessors gave the same rating in 75–85% of instances; a self taught rater using only the instructions from the book could become as reliable as an experienced assessor. The 96% confidence limits for a single RUS bone age is ±0.5 'years'. Reliability varies over the age span as later in maturity some individual ratings on a single bone can alter the bone age by as much as 0.5 'years'.

One of the authors (LAC) on a blind test–retest series had a standard error of measurement of 0.1 'years'. This rater compared a series of many hundreds of radiographs that had been rated by one of the originators of the system and the inter-observer error was a mean difference of 0.35 'years'.

Digitisation of radiographs and increasingly accessible computer technology would appear to offer ways of increasing objectivity and reducing errors. Two computer-based systems have been described (Hill and Pynsent, 1994; Tanner and Gibbons, 1994) but these still require considerable validation before they will be ready for adoption in routine clinical use.

Height age

The concept of height age has permeated much literature about growth disorders since the 1950s. Unfortunately it incorporates a basic misunderstanding of the requirements for defining developmental age. An implicit assumption of developmental age is that all individuals reach the same endpoint at maturity which is clearly not so for stature. A child may have a delayed height age for two reasons: delayed maturation, absolute short stature or both. A child has a delayed skeletal age for only one reason: delayed maturation.

Height age is assigned by noting the age at which the average child of the same sex has the same height as the patient. It does not recognise that the child's family might be unusually short (or tall) and that therefore the population average is not relevant. Further, it takes no note of the normal variation within a family which is not dependent on maturity and is about 17 cm at adult size. The only valid way to use height as a measure of maturity would be to compare an individual's height as a proportion of their own mature height – clearly a retrospective exercise and of little clinical value. Certainly height age has no place in modern auxological thinking.

It is important to consider how each maturity indicator correlates with others. It is quite striking that there is poor correlation between any one system once chronological age (which simply measures the passage of time) has been allowed for (Preece and Cox, 1986). This is less surprising if we stop thinking of the maturity indicators as direct measures of maturity, but rather as indirect measures of an inner biological clock, all using slightly different criteria. They show the same general pattern but the details are distorted and may differ considerably.

References

Bayley N, Pinneau S (1952) Tables for predicting adult height from skeletal age. *J. Pediatr.*; **40**: 423–441

Beunen G, Cameron N (1995) The reproducibility of TW2 skeletal age assessments by a self-taught assessor. *Ann. Hum. Biol.*; **7**: 155–162

Cameron N, Tanner JM, Whitehouse RH (1982) A longitudinal analysis of the growth of limb segments in adolescence. *Ann. Hum. Biol.*; **9**: 211–220

Cole TJ (1994) Do growth chart centiles need a face lift? *B. M. J.*; **308**: 641–642

Davies DP (1981) Physical growth from fetus to early childhood. In: Davis JA, Dobbing J (eds) *Paediatrics*. London: Heineman, pp. 303–339

Freeman JV, Cole TJ, Chinn S, Jones PRM, White EM, Preece MA (1995) Cross-sectional stature and weight reference curves for the UK, 1990. *Arch. Dis. Child.*; **73**: 17–24

Greulich WW, Pyle SI (1959) *Radiographic Atlas of Skeletal Development of the Hand and Wrist.* Stanford: Stanford University Press

Hagg U, Taranger J (1979) Menarche and voice change as indicators of the pubertal growth spurt. *Acta Odontol. Scand.*; **38**: 179–186

Hill K, Pynsent PB (1994) A fully automated bone-ageing system. *Acta Paediatr. Scand. [Suppl.].*; **406**: 81–83

Hoerr NL, Pyle SI, Francis CC (1969) *Radiographic Atlas of Skeletal Development of the Foot and Ankle*. Springfield, Illinois: Charles C. Thomas

Lindgren GW, Hauspie RC (1989) Heights and weights of Swedish school children born in 1955 and 1967. *Ann. Hum. Biol.*; **16**: 397–406

Molinari L, Largo RH, Prader A (1980) Analysis of the growth spurt at age seven (mid-growth spurt). *Helv. Paediatr. Acta.*; **35**: 325–334

Preece M, Cox L (1986) Estimation of biological maturity in the older child. In: Bittles A, Collins KJ (eds) *The Biology of Human Ageing*. Cambridge: Cambridge University Press, pp. 67–80

Preece MA, Pan H, Ratcliffe SG (1992) Auxological aspects of male and female puberty. *Acta Paediatr. Scand. [Suppl.]*; **383**: 11–13

Preece MA (1988) Prediction of adult height: methods and problems. *Acta Paediatr. Scand. [Suppl.]*; **347**: 4–10

Pyle SI, Hoerr NL (1955) *Radiographic Atlas of Skeletal Development of the Knee*. Springfield, Illinois: Charles C. Thomas

Roche AF, Wainer H, Thissen D (1975a) *Skeletal Maturity. The Knee Joint as a Biological Indicator*. New York: Plenum

Roche AF, Wainer H, Thissen D (1975b) *Predicting Adult Stature for Individuals*. Basel: S Karger AG

Tanner JM (1962) *Growth at Adolescence*. Oxford: Blackwell

Tanner JM, Gibbons RD (1994) Automatic bone age measurement using computerized image analysis. *J. Pediatr. Endocrinol.*; **7**: 141–145

Tanner JM, Whitehouse RH (1976) Clinical Longitudinal Standards for height, weight, height velocity, weight velocity, and the stages of puberty. *Arch. Dis. Child.*; **51**: 170–179

Tanner JM, Whitehouse RH, Takaishi M (1966a) Standards from birth to maturity for height, weight, height velocity, and weight velocity: British children, 1965 – I. *Arch. Dis. Child.*; **41**: 454–471

Tanner JM, Whitehouse RH, Takaishi M (1966b) Standards from birth to maturity for height, weight, height velocity, and weight velocity: British children, 1965 – II. *Arch. Dis. Child.*; **41**: 613–635

Tanner JM, Hughes PCR, Whitehouse RH (1981) Radiographically determined widths of bone muscle and fat in the upper arm and calf from age 3–18 years. *Ann. Hum. Biol.*; **8**: 495–517

Tanner JM, Whitehouse RH, Cameron N, Marshall WA, Healy MJR, Goldstein H (1983a) *Assessment of Skeletal Maturity and Prediction of Adult Height (TW2 Method)*. London: Academic Press

Tanner JM, Landt KW, Cameron N, Carter BS, Patel J (1983b) Prediction of adult height from height and bone age in childhood: a new system of equations (TW Mark II) based on a sample including very tall and very short children. *Arch. Dis. Child.*; **58**: 767–776

Todd TW (1937) *Atlas of Skeletal Maturation (Hand)*. St Louis: C.V. Mosby

Chapter 12

Deformity and cosmesis of the lower limbs

M Saleh, M Burton, A Milne, M Sims and R Tattersall

Introduction

Limb deformity may be congenital in origin or acquired. Common aetiologies that present to our clinic include congenital limb deficiency, sequelae of poliomyelitis, osteomyelitis, septic arthritis and trauma. Deformity may be defined as a derangement of the integrity or axis of a bone and/or associated joints. At the point where the deformity is recognisable, there is likely to be an associated reduction in function. Scarring and other soft tissue defects may be described as disfigurement and these generally do not have the same functional connotations but do have a variety of subjective ones. Interestingly satisfaction with one's appearance may improve function through a sense of well-being (Saleh, 1995). In this chapter we will deal mainly with the lower limbs, since this is where the preponderance of surgery is performed and symmetrical limbs are an important prerequisite to function (the principles however may be usefully extrapolated to the upper limbs). We also aim to explore the subjective experiences of patients under the term 'cosmesis'.

Reconstructive surgical techniques (Table 12.1) are used to control pain, reverse functional loss, eradicate bone infection and control or reduce the risk of arthritis occurring which may be related to poor posture and an abnormal gait pattern. Since the area of limb reconstruction is a relatively new field, emphasis is placed on limb alignment and maximising the potential of joints to work in the correct plane and with the optimum available excursion or range. So little is known about the most appropriate correction that we use the axis of the contralateral limb as a model. If the other limb is deformed or damaged, an ideal model may be used (Paley and Tetsworth, 1992a,b). These reference systems must take into consideration the effects of secondary deformities and the limitations of available surgical techniques. If the deformity occurs in early

Table 12.1 Limb reconstructive surgery

Realignment osteotomy
Arthrodesis/arthroplasty
Limb equalisation
Osteosynthesis
Soft tissue distraction
Articulated distraction

childhood, subsequent growth may be influenced in such a way that correction may be limited, or even impossible (Saleh and Scott, 1992; Saleh and Goonatillake, 1995). In adult life the degree of corrigibility is directly related to the time for which the deformity has been present and the number of adaptive and compensatory mechanisms that are established. Improved cosmetic effect is generally considered by professionals to be a secondary gain and not justifiable as a sole indication for treatment, however, patients often take a very different view (Clark and Malchow, 1984; Saleh and Burton, 1991). When surgery is planned for angular and length correction there are often significant cosmetic benefits. One only has to see the smile on a patient's face following correction of a genu recurvatum deformity to recall the pleasure that cosmetic improvement gives. We know of one paper which considers length and 'form' and describes a number of bone widening procedures to improve the external contours of the limb (Ilizarov et al, 1979).

Planning of mechanical aspects of treatment is often exhaustive; however, there is little intentional regard to the assessment of appearance before, during or after treatment. The importance of preparing the patient to cope in terms of body image and self respect during what might be a long treatment period is slowly being recognised. As far as possible, patients are advised of postoperative scarring and other disfigurements although even this seemingly simple task is difficult with available resources.

The purpose of this chapter is to provoke discussion about and provide new insight into an old orthopaedic dilemma – the extent to which function and deformity guide surgery and whose definition and quantification to accept. We have chosen not to isolate these issues but to consider them equally using the concept of cosmesis. We will come to the definition of cosmesis later but first, why the need for such a concept?

There are two broad perspectives on surgery, namely that of the professionals and that of the patient. Within those perspectives many issues are raised; is the surgery technically possible? Is it justified? Why does the patient want it? What does the patient expect? What are the risks? Conventionally these issues are dealt with technically in terms of deformity and function. However, this division leaves a gap which, paradoxically, is the most important aspect of limb reconstruction surgery – what it 'means' to the patient. These two perspectives are often at odds (Amadio, 1993). The mismatch arises because the 'meaning' of surgery is necessarily subjective. Each surgeon, each patient and technical procedure are variables combining every time to produce a unique situation. Each case for limb reconstruction ideally involves a 'best fit' approach – best fit for the patient and surgeon alike. This must be the result of negotiation which at present is based on a narrow scope of existing measures of outcome focusing on function and deformity and is surgeon lead. There is no account taken of the meaning of the process to the patient and their life.

At this point we need to define cosmesis, since it provides a framework in which to broaden existing measures of outcome. Cosmesis comes from a Greek word meaning 'to adorn and arrange' (Shorter Oxford English Dictionary, 1973) and has entered modern usage both as the art of preserving beauty and function and as the surgical procedures which correct disfigurement (Butterworth's Medical Dictionary, 1978). It is this necessarily subjective slant which provides a more holistic approach to the assessment of limb reconstruction surgery. Information which is subjective and does not fit rigid scientific research criteria, for example photographic images and patient satisfaction measures combined with functional criteria, allows a 'best fit' approach to be used.

This approach has been summarised by the Outcomes Committee of the American Academy of Orthopaedic Surgeons; 'If orthopaedists do not know all that is important to their patients, and if they do not measure those things, they should not be surprised if their assessment of results and that of their patients are discordant.......Outcomes research certainly will not eliminate all such problems but it can help orthopaedists to understand them better and, at least, to try to address them' (Amadio, 1993).

Current assessment methods – in Sheffield

History

A careful and methodical interview technique is important. If the discrepancy is long standing, compliance in the use of orthoses and any previous surgical attempts at correction will provide useful information on the likelihood of secondary fixed deformities. Direct questioning should establish whether back, hip and other lower limb symptoms are present as well as any neurological compromise. A history of osteomyelitis, radiotherapy or other bone disease may militate against full reconstruction. A full medical history should be taken to establish anaesthetic and surgical risk factors for example, cardiopulmonary compromise. Psychosocial factors are important, since treatment may extend over many months or in some cases years. Assessment of the patient's and family's ability to cope with the stress of surgery as well as schooling/work, housing and financial needs must be undertaken as these are valid reasons for considering simpler treatment options. In this manner information is compiled towards a qualitative problem list which will become the basis of surgical planning and patient preparation. Most of the information obtained is unscored and probably unscoreable. However, attempts may be made to quantify entry criteria both for subsequent longitudinal study and exit analysis. In an attempt to address these two issues, we have scored major symptom complexes on a five point scale which is in current use but not as yet validated (Table 12.2).

Examination

The lower limbs should initially be examined with the patient standing to assess spinal posture and limb alignment. With corrective blocks placed under the foot leg length may be assessed as well as fixed spinal deformity. Lateral bending is particularly useful to exclude fixed spinal deformity (Figure 12.1 and 12.2). Scoliosis, hip deformity, genu valgus or varus, heel and forefoot posture should be noted.

Aligning the iliac crests with the patient standing on corrective blocks is the most accurate simple clinical test for length discrepancy if there is no pelvic hypoplasia. It is reliable, repeatable and compares favourably as a measurement technique with radiological methods (Eichler, 1972). Leg length may also be assessed by supine tape measurements from the anterior superior iliac spine to the medial malleolus or heel. These surface landmarks are often poorly defined leading to significant measurement errors. The site of the discrepancy may be

Table 12.2 Symptom complexes

PAIN
0   No pain
1   Mild
2   Discomfort
3   Distressing
4   Horrible
5   Excruciating

FUNCTION
0   I am able to perform all activities I want to.
1   I am able to perform all the activities I want to around the home but have some difficulties out of doors
2   I am able to perform all the activities I want to around the home and with my job/home duties but unable to participate at my usual level of leisure activities, e.g. sport, social outings.
3   I am able to perform all the activities I want to around the home but unable to carry on my chosen occupation or participate in sport or social outings. (If a housewife please consider if you have needed extra help or whether jobs are being neglected.)
4   I have difficulty and am slow at performing usual activities around the home and cannot go out without assistance, e.g. walking stick/crutch or another person
5   I need constant help around the home to perform daily activities and need assistance from another person to go out of doors.

DEFORMITY
0   I do not feel my leg is deformed.
1   I feel my leg is seen as a deformity but this does not upset or worry me.
2   I feel my leg is seen as a deformity and this upsets me slightly.
3   I feel my leg is seen as a deformity and this upsets me quite a lot.
4   I feel my leg is seen as a deformity and this upsets me severely.
5   I feel my leg is grossly deformed.

readily appreciated by flexing both hips and knees to between 70° and 90° and lining up the heels. Assessment of proximal femoral and foot shortening may be made by direct inspection. Laboratory based anthropometric measurements using specifically designed benches, rulers and callipers reduce these errors, particularly if a standardised technique is used.

Supine examination must evaluate scarring and establish or exclude any joint deformity or instability. The soft tissues are examined for scarring, sinuses and other deformities. The surface area involved in the scar may be measured and charted. Scar depth should also be assessed, since it produces unsightly appearances due to the way that shadows are cast by available light. A modified tyre depth gauge may be used. Deep tethering is not only unsightly but may pose problems in wound closure. A full neurovascular assessment including power in the hip, knee, ankle and foot should be performed. The extent and distribution of shoe wear should be noted.

The alignment and range of movements at all joints must be measured, since this is an important index of the type and amount of correction that is possible, for example a varus deformity of the tibia with a fixed valgus of the hind foot requires a double level correction and a 10° varus of the tibia should only be corrected if the subtalar joint can accommodate for the change in foot position. Range of movement (ROM) measurement is important in order to detect change and also to produce objective information about a specific problem, for example a reduced knee flexion. Visual estimation of ROM is considered to be unreliable

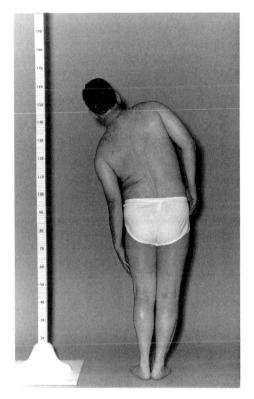 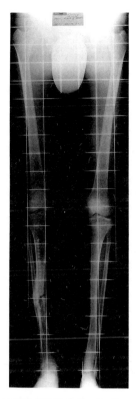

Figure 12.1 Lateral bending – examination to exclude fixed spinal deformity

Figure 12.2 Mechanical axis view (teleradiograph)

(Hellebrandt, 1949). Goniometry, although more accurate (Watkins, 1991), is not without problems (Goodwin *et al.,* 1992). Goniometric measurement of large 'simpler' joints is said to be valid and show a relatively high intra-observer agreement. However, techniques to measure movements of a more complex joint, such as the subtalar joint, are usually less precise and associated with higher intra-observer errors (Elveru *et al.,* 1988). Similar errors are associated with electrogoniometry which remains a popular technique in the clinical setting (Whittle, 1991). Therefore, a single observer using a standard goniometric technique is recommended. Given the problems of ROM data, little reliance should be placed on its scientific value. If detailed information is required, then plain radiographs are said to be the only reliable method (Backer *et al.,* 1989). Upper limb examination follows similar principles and will not be described further.

Radiography

Plain radiography is used to delineate the bony contribution of a deformity and this should be achieved with acceptable reproducibility and minimal radiation dosage. Various assessments are made, including the weight-bearing mechanical axis, limb length, joint alignment and contracture and bony integrity. Most methods of imaging limbs do have certain intrinsic problems with image distortion, and these must be taken into account. Accurate and reproducible positioning and exposures must be employed. Specialist training and specialisation within the X-ray department is vital for these methods to be used successfully.

In the normal skeleton, the lower limbs are of approximately equal length. The normal anatomical alignment is such that the weight-bearing mechanical axis of the limbs is aligned through the centre of the femoral head, the knee joint and the centre of the ankle joint (Moreland *et al.*, 1987). A standard mechanical axis X-ray may be taken against a 5 cm grid (Figure 12.2). The image produced demonstrates the weight-bearing axis of joints and quite good bony detail, but is inaccurate for the measurement of leg length because of magnification and the unpredictable effects of variations of the object film distance from one side to the other (Horsfield and Jones, 1986).

A standing parallel beam scanogram provides an image, with negligible distortion, of the lower limb joint planes and leg length (Saleh and Milne, 1994). Where a gross discrepancy in leg length is found clinically, wooden blocks can be positioned under the shorter of the limbs to allow more precise positioning of the legs prior to radiographic examination. Metal markers can be placed on the heels so that calcaneal height can be included in the measurement. Flexion deformity is still a problem. This can be solved by careful positioning, measuring knee flexion and object film distance, when positioning for the radiograph, and using simple geometry, in the final measurement, to compensate for parallax error.

Joint alignment and the axis of a single segment may be measured on anteroposterior and lateral supine films. These views must include the knee and ankle joints so that angular deformity may be measured. Rotational mal-alignment may be noted but for measurement ultrasound, CT scanning or MRI may be used. For more accurate measurement of angulation, parallax error may be excluded by taking spot films using a fluoroscopic table (Figure 12.3) or for interoperative alignment using an alignment grid (Saleh *et al.*, 1991). Knee and ankle joint contracture may be accurately assessed using lateral radiographs from mid-femur to mid-tibia with the knee fully extended and mid-tibia to toes in forced ankle dorsiflexion (or weight-bearing). Localised bony architecture, such as the detail of a non-union, may be visualised using coned radiographs and made comparative by fixing the position and exposure factors.

Radiographic images may be difficult to reproduce sequentially, due to

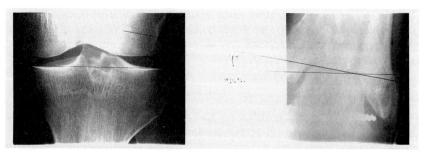

Figure 12.3 Spot films showing joint plane alignment

variables which are unpredictable over time. Recording the exposure factors used for each investigation can help with image density reproducibility. The limb being treated may suffer from disuse osteoporosis and, therefore, the objective contrast within the image zone may have to be reduced, even if all other variables are kept constant. Radiographic techniques are subject to operator variability. Centring points for a standard image can vary by several centimetres. This will introduce errors into longitudinal studies which are difficult to compensate for. The use of fluoroscopy can allow for reproducible positioning and centring of the X-ray beam but will increase radiation dose. The use of an automatic exposure aid such as an Iontomat will reduce image densitometry errors to a minimum in experienced hands. The scatter control grid will increase image contrast but will also increase radiation dose. Parallel beam radiography, CT scanning and MRI scanning allows for the minimisation of image distortion variability when measuring deformity directly from the resulting image. Closely collimated images, known as coned views, can both increase image contrast and reduce radiation dose, producing highly detailed images of specific bony sites.

Photography

Photography may be used to record the patient's appearance before and after surgery. Predefined views are taken (Figure 12.4) and may be enhanced by the use of a grid (Figure 12.5).

Although static, these views may also record functional limitations such as squatting or kneeling. Since we do not routinely measure rotational deformities using imaging techniques, we use photographs to monitor this aspect of deformity correction (Figure 12.6). Where leg length or overall height is altered, it is helpful to fix the object distance so that magnification effects are avoided in sequential comparative photographs. Close-up views may help to record the extent and depth of scarring, however, standard lighting techniques must be used to portray the indentation effects. Recent advances with digitisation techniques are used to measure surface area and contour mapping (Stacey *et al.,* 1991).

Functional testing

Although functional ability is assessed as part of most general outcome measures, the level of clinically useful information is limited and often does not translate across different patient groups. Since little has been written about the outcome following reconstructive surgery, we devised a simple subjective survey style questionnaire, asking patients to rate on a four-point scale, their ability to walk on even/uneven ground, run, jump, etc. This has given us baseline information about our patient population, and we are now in a position to progress to a more sensitive method of measurement. The TELER system is an emerging method of assessment which will allow the change in functional ability to be measured with greater specificity and sensitivity than has been previously documented (le Roux, 1993).

Detecting change and producing a unique score is, however, possible using physiological measures; i.e. timed walking tested. According to Wade, 'The timed walking test is remarkably simple, reliable, valid, sensitive, communicable, useful and relevant, almost the perfect measure!' (Wade, 1992).

Standard photographic views

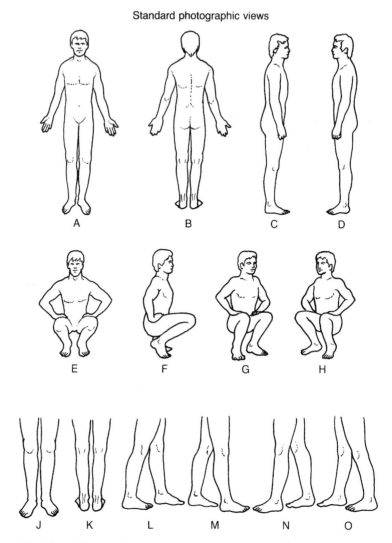

Figure 12.4 Standard photographic views

Although it is said that this type of test is not able to assess quality of walking, there is evidence to suggest that greater speed is associated with improved quality (Wade *et al.,* 1987). Taking timed walking tests a stage further is the Physiological Cost Index (PCI) developed by Butler. This allows the energy efficiency of gait to be measured (Butler *et al.,* 1984).

The evaluation of dynamic deformities, for example, during gait, may be made by visual observation; however, this has been shown to have significant errors compared with gait analysis (Saleh and Murdoch, 1985). Interactive video and gait analysis systems are already well established in the sports and leisure industries.

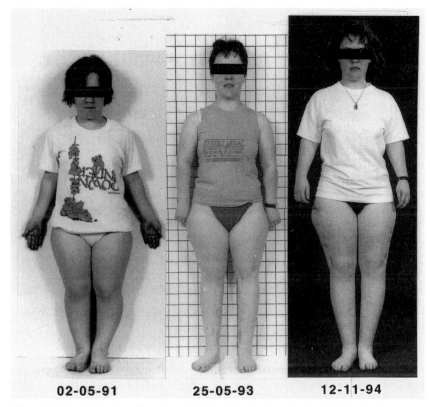

02-05-91   25-05-93   12-11-94

Figure 12.5 Standard views of a patient. (a) Before lengthening; (b) after tibial lengthening; (c) after tibial and femoral lengthening

General outcome measures

General outcome measures are considered to be of greater importance than traditional measures, such as range of motion and radiological parameters (Radford, 1993). There are a number of questionnaires/scales, some of which are disease specific, such as AIMS and others are for general use. The most commonly used in orthopaedics are:

The Sickness Impact Profile (Bergner *et al.*, 1981) (UK version – Functional Limitation Profile) which is well validated with high reliability, provides useful information but is lengthy (136 items) and is therefore impractical for regular use. In some areas of research the SIP is of great value. MacKenzie *et al.* (1993) used it to measure outcome following fractures of the lower limb. This provided useful information about ambulation, sleep and rest, emotional behaviour, home management, recreation and pastimes and work. This measure was rejected by our team as we intended to make repeated measurements.

The Nottingham Health Profile is wide ranging but looks only at the negative aspects of health and a score of nought does not indicate a lack of problems (Fallowfield, 1990). The validity and reliability is said to be satisfactory in

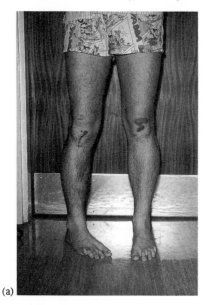 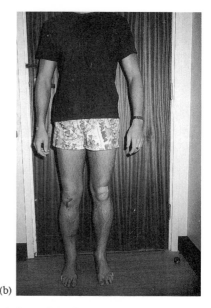

(a)   (b)

Figure 12.6 Tibial malunion in internal rotation (a) before and (b) after correction. Note value of photography

measuring perceived health status (Bowling, 1991). Although it is sensitive to gross change, it would appear that the subtle changes experienced by limb reconstruction patients would not be detected.

Arthritis Impact Measurement Scale (AIMS): although it was originally designed for patients with arthritis, AIMS has been used, in a modified form, for other orthopaedic conditions. Lerner *et al.* (1991) used AIMS in a modified form to measure functional ability of patients with post-traumatic non-union, chronic refractory osteomyelitis and lower limb amputation.

SF36 is very user friendly and is becoming more popular. It has face validity but only some of the areas have been tested for all aspects of validity and its reliability remains uncertain (Outcome Briefing, 1994). The physical activity section is insensitive to detect the more subtle changes experienced by patients undergoing limb reconstruction. It has proved useful when evaluating across groups (Ruta, 1994). Insensitivity is a criticism that can be levelled at most measures when dealing with the technical challenge and population of reconstruction candidates.

Psychological Adjustment to Illness Scale (PAIS) assesses the patient's adjustment to long-term illness/disability, it covers all the usual domains (physical, social, domestic, sexual, occupational and psychological) in 46 items and is self reporting. Although this scale is simple to complete, it has rather a complex scoring system. This allows it to be split into specific domains, allowing problem areas to be identified. It is a well developed tool employed in medical research and as a consequence T scores have been produced for a number of illnesses such as cardiac, renal and diabetes and we envisage that we will be able to produce such scores for various categories of limb reconstruction patients.

Cosmesis/body image

In order to enable patients to make an informed choice about surgery, it is necessary to include issues of body image. Ideally, we would like to evaluate the patient's perception of their body image prior to treatment and the importance they place on this before embarking on a prolonged treatment which will involve altered body image. It is important not just to consider how the patient will look at the end of surgery but also to inform them of the altered body image they will experience whilst undergoing the treatment, for example, the device to be used, use of wheelchairs and scarring.

Current English literature contains no specific orthopaedic outcome measures regarding body image either in terms of the expectations of patients or their requirements. Baird (1985) devised an assessment tool to diagnose altered body image in immobilised patients whilst in hospital. Drench (1994) discusses the responses to, and strategies for coping with, changes in body image. Wassner (1982) discusses the impact of mutilating surgery or trauma, whilst Seligson (1989) shows that feelings about body image during external fixation will affect the patient's prognosis. The remaining literature relates to other medical disciplines (Leppa, 1990; Sarver, 1993; Theologis *et al.,* 1993) and is not directly relevant to the limbs. PAIS was used in our outcome studies, but out of 46 questions, only one relates to body image.

Results

In order to complement standard reporting of results such as alignment, union and length, other outcome measures have been reviewed in our unit. Since November 1992, 165 limb reconstruction patients have entered a prospective study to monitor the functional, psychosocial, pain and ROM outcome at 3, 6, 12, 24 and 36 months following completion of treatment. Two validated scales have been used to measure psychosocial well-being, Psychosocial Adjustment to Illness Scale (PAIS) (Derogatis, 1983), and pain, the McGill Short Form Pain Questionnaire (Melzack, 1987).

Although PAIS produces a global measure of patient function we needed more detail about postoperative physical abilities. Such information is also required by patients preoperatively who are concerned regarding their possible subsequent functional level. Since little has been written about the outcome following reconstructive surgery, we devised a simple subjective survey style questionnaire asking patients to rate on a four-point scale their ability to walk on even/uneven ground, run, jump, etc. With this baseline information, we are now in a position to progress to a more sensitive method of measurement. In the future, modifications will be possible to increase the specificity and sensitivity using for example the TELER system.

The TELER (Treatment Evaluation by le Roux) (le Roux, 1993) allows small changes in patient's ability to be detected. This method can be used to compare outcome within groups and across groups, it can be as detailed or as gross as the assessor wishes. It is a very flexible system but is still in its infancy and requires further work to establish its usefulness within orthopaedics. The TELER is made up of a series of indicators which are '....an ordinal measuring scale for tracing change' (le Roux, 1993). The Indicators can be patient specific and negotiated or they can be generic. Each indicator has six reference points, 0 representing the least ability (either patient specific or general) and 5 being the patient or general goal. The progression from 0–5 is hierarchical in 'clinically significant' stages. This measure is under licence to A.A. le Roux.

The PAIS score for body image 38 patients in five categories of injury complexity were assessed and no relationship was found between severity of injury or perception of body image.

Measuring pain in isolation from other factors was considered to be necessary since for many of our patients pain was the primary complaint. The McGill Short Form Pain Questionnaire was chosen since it provides reliable and valid information on the quality and intensity of pain and has a present pain index. The inclusion of four 'affective' words make it possible to judge any psychogenic influence which may be present. Despite the pedigree of this scale, it is not without problem. Some of the descriptors are culturally adrift from our population, for example 'gnawing' was a word our patients did not understand nor could they find easy substitutes. Other descriptors are inappropriate for orthopaedic patients, for example 'tiring/exhausting' is classed as an 'affective item', however it often has a physiological cause.

Discussion

In Sheffield, as a result of our experience to date we use the following model as a process to start filling in the gaps between the surgeon's and patient's goals. At their first outpatient appointment, the patients are questioned about their perception of whether they feel their limb is deformed or not and to what degree the deformity bothers them (Table 12.2). The surgeon and patient state their individual goals of treatment, for example, promote union, correct deformity, pain control, improve function of the limb and appearance of the limb.

Standard view photographs are taken to provide a visual record (Figure 12.4). These are repeated during the treatment and at the end of the treatment period. Copies of photographs are frequently purchased by the patients so that they can remember what their limb looked like prior to surgery. For achondroplasic lengthening, the standard photographs can be manipulated using the appropriate software to simulate the postoperative appearances (Nicholls and Saleh, 1988; Nicholls, 1990). Such photographs may be used to select the appropriate operation (Figure 12.7) and motivate the patient during treatment.

Prior to surgery, the patients and their carers attend for an information day which allows them to discuss their expectations and enables the staff to discuss the physical and psychological implications of the treatment. A patient and carers support group is available and has particular value for patients who can see at first hand the functional and cosmetic results of surgery.

The amount of scarring occurring as a result of treatment is discussed with the patients and they are informed that pin site infections predispose to more pronounced scarring. Scarring may be disguised using cosmetic camouflage make-up. Silicone prostheses may be used to correct the contours of the soft tissues (Thomas, 1994). Scars and flaps may be successfully revised using plastic surgery techniques. External fixator pins which are drawn through the skin during lengthening leave particularly deep tethered scars but are generally amenable to massaging of scar tissue and revision surgery (Saleh and Howard,

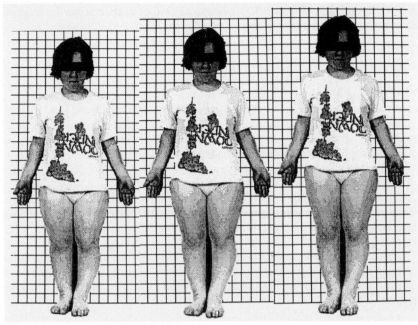

Figure 12.7 Composite simulation of the effects of lengthening. (a) Pre-operatively; (b) with 15 cm lengthening; (c) with 30 cm lengthening. Note effect in body proportions and arms (compare the effect of this simulation with the clinical result in same patient shown in Figure 12.5)

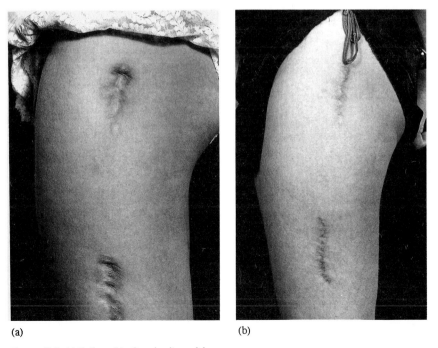

(a)   (b)

Figure 12.8 (a) Before, (b) after pin site revision

1994) (Figure 12.8). All these methods can be employed to improve the patient's satisfaction with their body image.

Conclusions

The outcome of lower limb surgery has routinely been reported using surgeon oriented measurement scales such as union (Saleh 1992; Ribbans *et al.*, 1992), eradication of infection, length and alignment (Saleh and Rees, 1995), joint ranges and occasionally limb function. The dichotomy persists between surgeon and patient's objectives, patients being more interested in function and cosmesis. We are in the process of developing a sensitive measure of functional ability for this category of patient. Broader perceptions of outcome, such as psychosocial evaluations and activity/functional levels, are well established. Reviewing our PAIS results, there are limitations in its specificity for limb reconstruction and we hope to address this in due course. Using PAIS there appears to be no relationship between the extent of a patient's injuries and their perception of body image. Therefore, totally independent assessments of cosmesis for each individual must be considered when proposing treatment. Despite these advances, however, it must be stated that patient satisfaction scales and evaluation of cosmesis remain primitive.

References

Amadio PC (1993) Outcomes measurements (editorial). *J. Bone Jt Surg.*; **75A**: 1583–1584

Backer M, Kofoed H (1989) Passive ankle mobility. Clinical measurement compared with radiography. *J. Bone Jt Surg.*; **71B**: 696–698

Baird SE (1985) Development of a nursing assessment tool to diagnose altered body image in immobilized patients. *Orthopaedic Nursing.*; **4**: 47–54

Bergner M, Bobbitt HR, Carter WB, Gatson BS (1981) The sickness impact profile: development and final revision of a health status measure. *Med. Care*; **XIX**: 787–805

Bowling A (1991) *Measuring Health. A Review of Quality of Life Measurement Scales.* Oxford: Oxford University Press

Butler P, Engelbrecht M, Major RE, Tait JH, Stallard J, Patrick JH (1984) Physiological cost index of walking for normal children and its use as an indicator of physical handicap. *Dev. Med. Child Neurol.*; **26**: 607–612

Butterworth's Medical Dictionary, 2nd edition (1978) Editor MacDonald Critchley, London

Clark JD, Malchow D (1984) How to avoid errors in limb salvage decisions. *Orthop. Rev.*; **XIII**: 197–205

Derogatis LR (1977) *The Psychosocial Adjustment to Illness Scale – Self Report Version.* Baltimore: Clinical Psychometric Research

Drench ME (1994) Changes in body image secondary to disease and injury. *Rehabilitation Nursing*; **19** (No 1): 31–36

Eichler J (1972) Methodological errors in documenting leg length and leg length discrepancies. *Der Orthopade*; **1**: 14–20

Elveru RA, Rothstein JM, Lamb RL (1988) Goniometric reliability in clinical setting. Subtalar and ankle joint measurements. *Phys. Ther.*; **68**: 672–677

Fallowfield L (1990) *The Quality of Life. The Missing Measurement in Health Care.* London: Souvenir Press

Goldberg D (1972) *Detection of Psychiatric Illness by Questionnaire.* Oxford: Oxford University Press

Goodwin J, Clark C, Deakes J, Burdon D, Lawrence C (1992) Clinical methods of goniometry: a comparative study. *Disability and Rehabilitation*; **14**: 10–15

Hellebrandt, FA, Duvall EN, Moore ML (1949) The measurement of joint motion. Part III, reliability of goniometry. *Phys. Ther. Rev.*; **29**: 302–307

Horsfield D, Jones SN (1986) Assessment of inequality in length of the lower limb. *Radiography*; **52**: 223–227

Ilizarov GA, Kaplunov VI, Shevtzov VG, Trokhova VG, Shatohin VD (1979) Methods of modelling of the leg and its elongation. *Orthop Traumatol Protez*; **11**: 28–32

Karlsson J, Peterson L (1991) Evaluation of ankle joint function: the use of a scoring scale. *Foot*; **1**: 15–19

Leppa CJ (1990) Cosmetic surgery and the motivation for health and beauty. *Nursing Forum*; **25**: 25–31

le Roux AA (1993) TELER: the concept. *Physiotherapy*; **79**: 755–758

Lerner RK, Esterhai JL, Polomono RC, Cheatle MC, Heppenstall RB, Brighton CT (1991) Psychosocial, functional and quality of life assessment of patients with post-traumatic fracture non-union, chronic refractory osteomyelitis and lower extremity amputation. *Arch. Phys. Med. Rehabil.*; **72**: 122–126

MacKenzie EJ, Cushing BM, Jurkovich GJ, Morris JA, Burgess AR, de Lateur BJ, McAndrew MP, Swiontkowski MF (1993) Physical impairment and functional outcomes six months after severe lower extremity fractures. *J. Trauma*; **34**(4): 528–538

Melzack R (1987) The Short Form McGill Pain Questionnaire. *Pain*; **30**: 191–197

Moreland J, Bassett L, Hanker G (1987) Radiographic analysis of the axial alignment of the lower extremity, *J. Bone Jt Surg.*; **69A**: 745–749

Nicholls M (1990) Computer aided manipulation of photographs for leg lengthening. *J. Audio Visual Media Medicine*; **13**: 13–16

Nicholls MJ, Saleh M (1988) Composite photographs in leg lengthening. *J. Audio Visual Media Medicine*; **11**: 96–99

Outcomes Briefing MOS SF36 Nuffield Institute for Health, August 1994 Issue 4, Leeds, England

Paley D, Tetsworth K (1992a) Mechanical axis deviation of the lower limbs: pre-operative planning of uniapical angular deformities of the tibia or femur. *Clin. Orthop. Rel. Res.*; **280**: 48–64

Paley D, Tetsworth K (1992b) Mechanical axis deviation of the lower limbs: pre-operative planning of multiapical frontal plane angular and bowing deformities of the tibia or femur. *Clin. Orthop. Rel. Res.*; **280**: 65-71

Radford PJ (1993) General outcome measures. In: Pynsent PB, Fairbank JCT, Carr AJ (eds) *Outcome Measures in Orthopaedics*. Oxford: Butterworth-Heinemann, pp. 59–80

Ribbans WJ, Stubbs D, Saleh M (1992) Non-union surgery part II: the Sheffield experience – one hundred consecutive cases: results and lessons. *Int. J. Orthop. Trauma*; **2**: 129–134

Ruta DA, Abdalla MI, Garratt AM, Coutts A, Russell IT (1994) SF36 health survey questionnaire I reliability in two patient based studies. *Quality in Health Care*; **3**: 180–185

Saleh M (1992) Non-union surgery part I – basic principles of management. *Int. J. Orthop. Trauma*; **2**: 2–14

Saleh M (1995) Personal communication

Saleh M, Burton M (1991) Patient selection and management in achondroplasia: leg lengthening. *Orthop. Clin. N. Am.*; **22**: 589–599

Saleh M, Goonatillake H (1995) The management of congenital leg length inequality. The value of early axis corrections. *J. Pediatr. Orthop.*; **Part B. 4**: 150–158

Saleh M, Howard AC (1994) Improving the appearance of pin-site scars. *J. Bone Jt Surg.*; **76B**: 906–908

Saleh M, Milne A (1994) Weight bearing parallel beam scanography for the measurement of leg length and joint plane alignment. *J. Bone Jt Surg.*; **76B**: 156–157

Saleh M, Murdoch G (1985) In defence of gait analysis: observation and measurement in gait assessment. *J. Bone Jt Surg.*; **67B**: 237–241

Saleh M, Rees AR (1995) Bifocal surgery for deformity and bone loss – bone and compression – distraction compared. *J. Bone Jt Surg.*; **77B**: 429–434

Saleh M, Scott B (1992) Pitfalls and complications in leg lengthening: the Sheffield experience. *Semin. Orthop.*; **7**: 207–222

Saleh M, Harriman P, Edwards DJ (1991) A radiological method for producing precise limb alignment. *J. Bone Jt Surg.*; **73B**: 515–516

Seligson D, Zinner K, Lusebrink V (1989) The patient's perception of the fixator in external fixation and functional bracing. Green S, Coombs R, Sarmiento A (eds). London: Orthotext

Shorter Oxford English Dictionary (1973). Oxford: Oxford University Press

Sarver DM, Johnston MW (1993) Orthognathic surgery and aesthetics: planning treatment to achieve functional and aesthetic goals. *Br. J. Orthodont.*; **20**: 93–100

Stacey MC, Burnand KG, Layer GT, Pattison M, Browse NL (1991) Measurement of the healing of venous ulcers. *Aust. N. Z. J. Surg.*; **61(II)**: 844–848

Theologis TN, Jefferson RJ, Simpson AHRW, Turner-Smith AR, Fairbank JCT (1993) Quantifying the cosmetic defect of adolescent idiopathic scoliosis. *Spine*; **18**: 909–912

Thomas KF (1994) *Partial Leg Prosthesis in Prosthetic Rehabilitation.* London: Quintessence Publishing Co. Ltd

Wade DT (1992) *Measurement in Neurological Rehabilitation.* Oxford: Oxford University Press

Wade DT, Wood VA, Heller A, Moggs J, Langton-Hewer R (1987) Walking after stroke: Measurement and recovery over first three months. *Scand. J. Rehab. Med.*; **19**: 25–30

Wassner A (1982) The impact of mutilating surgery or trauma on body-image. *Int. Nurs. Rev.*; **29**(3): 86–90

Watkins MA, Riddle DL, Lamb RL, Personius WJ (1991) Reliability of goniometric measurements and visual estimates of the knee range of motion obtained in a clinical setting. *Phys. Ther.*; **7**: 15–21

Whittle M (1991) *Gait Analysis: An Introduction.* Oxford: Butterworth-Heinemann

Chapter 13

Deformity and cosmesis of the spine

(*Methods and interpretation*)

TN Theologis and JCT Fairbank

Introduction

Alteration in body shape is a common presenting feature of spinal deformity, and this is undoubtedly a cosmetic problem (Aaro and Ohlund, 1984; Houghton, 1984; Webb, 1991). Measuring spinal deformity should therefore include measuring the shape of the back.

Spinal deformity and the resulting body surface deformity were recognised well before radiography was available. Adams (1865) was the first to give a detailed description of scoliosis as a three-dimensional deformity of the spine, based on clinical observation and cadaveric findings. The introduction of radiography opened new horizons in the study of spinal abnormalities. Numerous techniques and an impressive level of technology have evolved for the measurement and evaluation of spinal deformity.

From the scientific and surgical point of view, it is the skeletal deformity which is important, as it is the deformity of the underlying skeleton that produces the body surface deformity. For the patient, however, it is the surface deformity that matters. Patients are concerned about their body appearance and this is usually the reason why they attend clinics (Aaro and Ohlund, 1984; Houghton, 1984). Accordingly, various techniques have evolved for the study of body surface topography and the underlying skeletal deformity. It is important to understand that these two groups of techniques are addressing the problem of spinal deformity from different approaches and they are not necessarily directly comparable. Furthermore, both skeletal and body surface imaging and measurement are complimentary and one cannot replace the other.

It is clear that spinal deformity causes a significant psychological distress to patients, disturbs their body-image perception and has various psychosocial implications (Bengtsson *et al.,* 1974; Clayson, 1979; Edgar and Mehta, 1988). It is also clear that body appearance and the presence of a cosmetic defect are responsible for the psychological distress of these patients; it has been shown that the degree of deformity correlates positively to the severity of the psychological disturbance (Bengtsson *et al.,* 1974; Cochran *et al.,* 1983). The importance of cosmesis as a criterion in assessment of spinal deformity is apparent. What is not clear is which features of the deformity are responsible for the cosmetic defect and which measurements should be recorded.

An outline of the most known methods of measuring spinal deformity are presented below. Their value in providing information on the cosmetic defect of the patient is discussed.

Clinical appearance of spinal deformity

Definitions

There are three basic types of spinal deformity: scoliosis, kyphosis and lordosis. Scoliosis is a lateral rotatory curvature of the spine. Kyphosis and lordosis are curves of the spine in the sagittal plane, which exist normally but can increase to an abnormal degree. Spinal deformities can also be classified according to magnitude, location, direction and aetiology. The Scoliosis Research Society has established a complex classification model for spinal deformities and a glossary for the terminology associated with it (Moe, 1978). Every individual spinal deformity, therefore, can be described taking into consideration all the above mentioned parameters, as, for example 'a 60° left thoracic scoliosis due to cerebral palsy' or 'a 100° thoracolumbar congenital kyphosis'.

Clinical assessment

Obtaining the history of the disease and performing a complete and detailed clinical examination of the patient is the cornerstone of spinal deformity assessment. The onset of the deformity, its progression and any subsequent treatment should be recorded. History and examination may reveal an underlying disease causing the deformity. The patient's chronological and physiological age are important factors in prognosis. The patient's presenting complaint, apart from the cosmetic deficit, is also crucial in planning any treatment: pain, neurological deficit, cardiopulmonary problems and functional complications should be taken into account.

Observation and physical examination will reveal the effect of spinal deformity on body appearance and any subsequent complications affecting other areas of the body. In scoliosis patients, a unilateral rib prominence (hump), due to vertebral rotation should be noted. Any discrepancy in shoulder level or any pelvic tilt can be observed and measured. The balance of the thorax over the pelvis can be assessed with a plumb bob string held over the prominent spinous process of the seventh cervical vertebra. Any asymmetry of the scapulae and the waistline should be recorded. Unilateral skin creases at the waistline indicate trunk imbalance and subcostal skin folds indicate a shortened anterior abdominal wall. Any increase or decrease of the normal sagittal curves of the back and any anterior tilt or shift of the trunk may be observed from a side view of the patient. Finally, the anterior chest is examined to detect any existing pectus excavatum or carinatum or any unilateral anterior thoracic prominence, usually existing on the side opposite to the posterior prominence (rib hump).

The range of movement of the spine can also be assessed in flexion, extension, lateral flexion and rotation. The forward bending test will reveal any asymmetry in the two sides of the back and will provide the examiner with another impression of the size of the rib prominence. The asymmetry can be measured using simple instruments such as a spirit level (Moe *et al.,* 1978) or the scoliometer (Burwell *et al.,* 1990) and measurements should be recorded and monitored.

Clinical examination is essential in the initial assessment of the deformity, its aetiology and complications. From the point of view of the cosmetic impairment, the examiner will get a general impression of the body deformity and some simple measurements of some of the parameters of the deformity. The examiner, however, will only have a personal impression and opinion on the patient's cosmetic deformity. The examiner's impression of deformity will be based on personal previous experience and aesthetic criteria. Furthermore, opinion on cosmesis may differ substantially between the examiner and patient. In cases where cosmesis is an important criterion for treatment of spinal deformity, the surgeon involved does not have a measurable parameter on which to make the decisions with regard to treatment.

In conclusion, the clinical examination of the patient is an important and substantial part of the assessment but does not provide the examiner with an objective measurement of cosmesis.

Measuring spinal deformity

Measuring skeletal deformity

Plain radiographs

Radiographs are by far the most widespread method of imaging and measuring spinal deformity. Traditional standing postero–anterior and lateral views convert the three-dimensional anatomy of the spine into two biplanar images. Additional information may be provided with special projections such as the Ferguson view (Moe *et al.,* 1978), the derotated view (Stagnara, 1974) and side and forward flexion and extension views to evaluate flexibility.

Measurement of the scoliotic deformity in the coronal plane has been the established routine for many decades. Ferguson (1930) was the first to describe such a method, but the Cobb method (1948) was the one adopted by the Scoliosis Research Society in 1966 and has since been established as the standard measurement of the scoliotic deformity. The Cobb measurement quantifies the coronal plane angular deformity of the end vertebrae (Figure 13.1). The other most apparent deformities are all reflected to some extend in the coronal plane angular position of the end vertebrae.

The same principles of measuring spinal deformity have been applied to the sagittal plane, to measure kyphosis and lordosis. Again, the idea is to measure the angular deformity of the end vertebrae in this plane (Figure 13.2). The problem with using the equivalent of the Cobb angle in the sagittal plane is that the normal spine has physiological lordotic and kyphotic curves and the examiner has to be aware of the range of normality of these curves before diagnosing one as abnormal. Several studies on normal subjects provide the baseline for comparison (Stagnara *et al.,* 1982; Propst-Proctor and Bleck, 1983; Bernhardt and Bridwell, 1989).

There are certainly disadvantages in the use of the Cobb angle in scoliosis measurement. A single plane measurement is used for a three-dimensional deformity. The Cobb angle does not provide any information on the rotational element of the deformity. Several ways of measuring vertebral rotation have been suggested in order to overcome this problem (Nash and Moe, 1969; Mehta, 1972; Perdriolle, 1979). Even with this additional measurement, radiography is inadequate for outlining the overall body deformity. Thulbourne and Gillespie (1976) studied the relationships between rotation of the vertebral bodies, the degree of the lateral curvature of the spine and the rib–vertebra angle and found

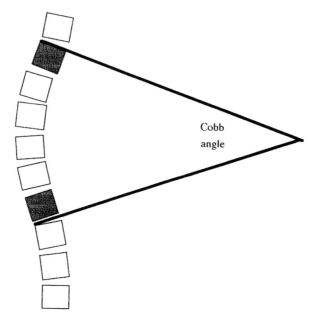

Figure 13.1 Measurement of the Cobb angle

no clear linear relationship between these three parameters. They concluded that the deformity of the spine in scoliosis does not necessarily correlate with the deformity of the back.

Another problem with the use of the Cobb angle is the reliability of its measurement. In recent studies (Carman *et al.,* 1990; Morrissy *et al.,* 1990) it was found that the error in measurement was close to 5°. This is also the change in Cobb angle that most authors define as progression of a scoliosis. It becomes apparent that the Cobb angle is unreliable for identifying a mild progression.

Three-dimensional radiographic methods

Bi-plane radiography has been suggested for better representation of the three-dimensional scoliotic deformity. The spine is measured from two radiographs taken in immediate succession from different angles (Brown *et al.,* 1976; Stokes *et al.,* 1987). The three-dimensional reconstruction is performed using a topographic technique called spatial triangulation. This method, however, is time-consuming and it involves extra radiation.

Computerised tomography (CT) and magnetic resonance imaging (MRI) have also been used for the study of scoliosis. CT has initially been used for the measurement of vertebral rotation and rib cage deformity (Aaro and Dahlborn, 1982). Both techniques have been used in three-dimensional imaging of the spine (Drerup, 1992). A disadvantage of the technique is that the patient is supine and not in the normal erect posture during imaging. CT demands a contiguous set of scans for a comprehensive 3-D reconstruction. However, the frequent application of the method is prohibited by the increased radiation dose. MRI is safe and 3-D investigations can be performed. The resolution of MRI is about 1 mm in each

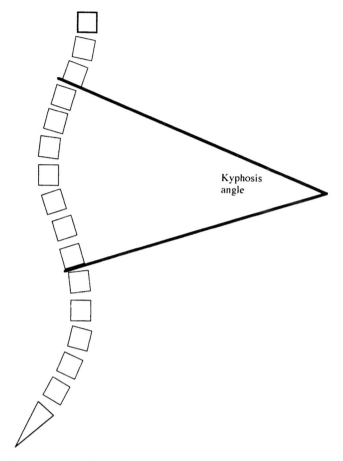

Kyphosis
angle

Figure 13.2 Measurement of kyphosis

direction. However, the MRI precision deteriorates substantially at the boundaries of the measurement volume (Drerup, 1992). Furthermore, frequent application of the technique is not practical for financial reasons.

Conclusions

The evolution of radiographic techniques over the last few decades and the introduction of computerised analysis of data have helped in the understanding of the three-dimensional structure of the deformed spine. They remain an irreplaceable tool in assessing the patient with spinal deformity. They often establish aetiological factors of spinal deformity, such as congenital or hereditary vertebral anomalies and they are important in assessing the skeletal age of the patient. Furthermore, they demonstrate any existing curve rigidity (flexion–extension and lateral flexion views) and underlying neurological conditions (MRI). The Cobb angle and vertebral rotation measurements have been used in clinical and research practice for many years and have stood the test of time despite the disadvantages mentioned above. For the vast majority of orthopaedic surgeons, decision-making on the treatment of spinal deformity patients is largely based on these measurements.

It has been shown, however, that imaging and measurement of skeletal deformity, no matter how detailed and precise, is not sufficient for the assessment of the body surface deformity (Thulbourne and Gillespie, 1976). Since cosmesis depends upon body appearance only, it cannot be represented by and measured on skeletal images. In conclusion, radiographs are important for the overall assessment and treatment of spinal deformity but are not sufficient for the assessment of cosmesis.

Measuring body surface

The first requirement in developing a method of assessing the cosmesis of the deformed human body is a suitable imaging technique. This should provide measurable parameters and should also be reliable and of clinical value. Ideally, the image and measurements made from it should be comprehensible both to the surgeon and to the patient.

Research and clinical trials on methods of imaging the back of patients with spinal deformities started in the early 1970s. The motive was to reduce the exposure of children and adolescent patients to X-rays. Conventional radiographic method of monitoring spinal curves increase the risks of breast cancer as young patients with spinal deformities are closely followed up at least until skeletal maturity is attained (Hoffman *et al.,* 1989; Dutkowsky *et al.,* 1990). Measurement and analysis of the surface of the back was therefore introduced as an alternative method of monitoring spinal deformity. It was hoped that surface, non-invasive measurements would be sufficiently reliably to detect the presence, progression and successful treatment of spinal deformities. Some of the best known of these techniques are presented in the following paragraphs.

Moiré technique

Moiré fringes occur when light is transmitted through two diffraction gratings superimposed on each other. This effect was first described by Lord Raleigh in the nineteenth century. In 1970, the Japanese scientist Hiroshi Takasaki demonstrated that these fringes represent lines of equal altitude, i.e. isohypses of an object. The Moiré technique made possible the presentation of a three-dimensional image on a two-dimensional photograph. This has been used to advantage for the representation of body deformities.

Moiré fringe topography has been developed over the past years. The main problem to be overcome is the lack of quantitative data from the contour maps for analysis and follow-up. Several methods of quantification have been suggested, based on the technique of digitising the Moiré pictures. However, the methods are still complicated and time-consuming. The technique also lacks reproducibility, since the picture depends on the position and posture of the patient. In addition to the expected variation in the stance of the patient between examinations, a significant alteration in posture, due to the spinal deformity, may be missed or misinterpreted. The interpretation of Moiré patterns, the standardisation of Moiré contouring equipment, patient positioning and error handling are still subjects of research.

Groves *et al.* (1990) presented an advanced computer analysis of Moiré images. According to the authors, the method enables the measurement of clinically accepted parameters of scoliosis deformity on Moiré images. They also suggest an algorithm based on their measurements, which represents a normalised measure of three-dimensional asymmetry around the spine. Similarly, Steinnocher *et al.* (1990) presented a method of automated evaluation of digitised Moiré images. The aim of the method was to recognise the asymmetry of the back, without the use of time-consuming complicated analysis.

Karras (1990) and Klein and Rooze (1990) studied the accuracy and reliability of Moiré method. They showed that lens distortion and film plane orientation can lead to a significant error. Moiré topography yields inferior results to stereophotogrammetry. Both the above studies show that errors can be decreased by the appropriate correction of the co-ordinates.

Windischbauer and Neugebauer (1990) presented a review of the evolution and progress of the Moiré technique through the years. The authors thought that Moiré figures were the most simple means of representing surface patterns in 'real time', that image acquisition and processing should be computerised, though this may be time-consuming and the data analysis could reveal rotational, lateral and angular deviations.

The Moiré technique has been accepted for routine clinical practice in a wide number of scoliosis centres around the world and is usually used in parallel with conventional radiography. It is routinely used in the assessment of back surface deformity and, particularly, the trunk asymmetry and the size of the rib hump (Suzuki *et al.*, 1992).

Rastersstereographic techniques

Rasterstereography is a modification of stereophotogrammetry, a common topographic technique. In stereophotogrammetry, an object is viewed by two or more cameras from different angles and its three-dimensional structure is studied. In rasterstereography, one of the cameras is replaced by projecting a grid onto the body. The shape of the body surface is recorded together with a control point system so that different measures of surface topography can be made.

Frobin and Hierzholzer (1984) improved the method by introducing a metric camera to the system, i.e. a camera with a fixed image co-ordinate system. This eliminated the need to calibrate the apparatus before each examination, and offered a substantial simplification and acceleration in automatic image processing time. The authors studied the accuracy of the system and found a standard deviation of 0.1% in the measurements. From the clinical viewpoint, the method is quick, reproducible and accurate but it does not provide any numerical data. Hierzholzer and Drerup (1990) used the same method in combination with a computerised system, in order to achieve a three-dimensional reconstruction of the spinal midline. The results were encouraging, since in more than 95% of the cases studied, the deviation of the results from the corresponding frontal radiographs was of the same order as the accuracy of radiographic measurements.

Frobin and Hierzholzer (1990) presented video rasterstereography as a method of back surface measurement. The apparatus consisted of a projector with raster slide and a video camera containing an image sensor. The video camera was directly connected to the image processing computer. The system enabled an accurate and operationally simple measurement and shape analysis of the back surface and the results were available in only a few minutes. Hierzholzer and Drerup (1992) evaluated the clinical use of the same system. They suggested that surface topography and plain radiography should not be directly compared and favoured comparison of their method with three-dimensional radiography. They concluded that surface topography was reliable and sufficient.

Ultrasound techniques

Ultrasound techniques have been suggested for three-dimensional imaging of spinal deformity, with the advantages of non-invasiveness and cheapness.

Mauritzson et al. (1984) presented work with airborne ultrasound. The principle is simple. A short sound pulse is transmitted from an ultrasound transducer directed towards the patient's back. The propagation time for the sound wave to travel from the transducer to the patient and back again is proportional to the distance. If a number of transducers are placed in a vertical linear array along the back, it is then possible to get multiple measuring points of the profile along this line. The method produces quantifiable data and is fairly fast. The authors do not comment on the reproducibility of the method or whether alterations in the positioning of the patient can produce a significant error. A similar method was developed in France and was used for surface reconstruction and also patient re-education treatment. The results were encouraging (Mouchref et al., 1992).

Another ultrasound technique was developed in Newcastle-upon-Tyne (Ions et al., 1984; Oates et al., 1990). Their technique, however, aimed at imaging the spine, did not provide any back surface data. Wojcik et al. (1990) used a standard static image B-mode ultrasound scanner to image the rib cage deformity and the spinal rotation with the patient in a prone position. They measured the angle between a line drawn parallel to the posterior elements (laminae) of a selected spinal segment and a line parallel to the posterior elements of the sacrum. They found that the measurement of spinal rotation was significantly correlated with the vertebral rotation measured on X-rays. However, the radiographic techniques are themselves unreliable (see above).

Optical scanners

Halioua et al. (1990) presented a technique called phase measuring profilometry. This is an optical sensing technique where a sinusoidal grating structure is projected onto the subject, detected by a solid state array camera and processed by a computer. The body surface is presented as a set of equally spaced horizontal cross sections and analysed in terms of relative and local parameters. This approach, combined with the ability to digitally introduce rigid body rotations and translations, makes the system insensitive to subject positioning. The authors showed that human forms are represented with error of <1 mm. The method permits the extraction of intrinsic shape information in an objective and repeatable fashion.

Another optical scanner was presented by Merolli and Tranquilli-Lealli in 1990. The system consisted of a light source (a dot-array projector) and an image processing system. The visual output of the system was a colour map in which the surface under examination was presented on a screen in small rectangles, each having a colour according to its distance from the light source, i.e. depending on its altitude. No numerical data were provided by the system and no reliability test has been performed.

The Integrated Shape Investigation System (ISIS, Oxford Metrics) is another optical scanner, designed and developed in Oxford since 1983. The basic

elements of the system are a light projector, a video camera and a microcomputer. The projector produces a horizontal plane of light, which the camera
views at an angle from below. The two-dimensional co-ordinates of the line, seen
as the light falls on a three-dimensional surface, are recorded directly by the
microcomputer. These co-ordinates, together with a full knowledge of the
geometry of the system, enable the three-dimensional shape of the illuminated
strip of surface to be computed. By swinging the projector unit about a horizontal
axis, the line of light moves down the back under examination and a complete
record of shape can be built up. The principle of this procedure is based on
photogrammetry. In its commercial version, the ISIS system can acquire over
7000 measurement points with a surface reconstruction accuracy of 1.5 mm
(standard error) to describe the surface and outline data (Turner-Smith, 1988).
The scanning lasts 1–2 s and the printed display is available in less than 10 min.

On the scan display, three views of the patient's back are shown, one in each
orthogonal plane (Figure 13.3). Several parameters are measured on each
display. Flexion, defined as the angle between the body and the true vertical and
rotation of the patient about a vertical axis are shown at the bottom of the scan.
Lateral asymmetry, the equivalent of the Cobb angle, derived from surface shape
data, is also displayed. In the transverse plane, the angle of inclination of the
back surface at several levels is measured and defined as transverse asymmetry.
Volumetric asymmetry represents the difference in volume between the two sides
of the back. Hump severity derives from volumetric asymmetry and represents
the volume of the rib hump; its value is not presented on the scan but has to be
calculated from other parameters. In the sagittal plane, kyphosis and lordosis are
measured, either as distances from the vertical line or as angles. Finally,

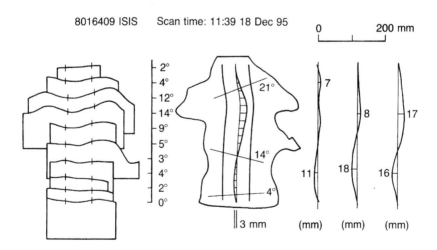

Figure 13.3 The ISIS scan

imbalance represents the distance of the mid-point of the sacrum from the vertical line passing from the spinous process of the seventh cervical vertebra.

The initial publications on ISIS were descriptive of the technique and its clinical application (Turner-Smith, 1988; Turner-Smith *et al.*, 1988). The reliability of the technique was found satisfactory by Harris *et al.* (1987). Further studies presented the use of ISIS in evaluation of scoliosis progression (Csongradi *et al.*, 1987; Tredwell and Bannon, 1988), bracing (Weisz *et al.*, 1989) and spinal fusion (Jefferson *et al.*, 1988).

The latest generation of optical scanners use video techniques. Pearson *et al.* (1992) presented their device which uses structured light to form a multi-stripe fringe pattern on the human back. A CCD video camera acquires an image which is transferred via a frame store to a microcomputer. The fringe pattern is analysed and the complete three-dimensional shape of the back reconstructed and displayed on the screen. The technique offers measurable parameters, is fast and economical. The authors claimed good accuracy and reliability.

Another video-based optical scanner was presented by Hill *et al.* (1992). Their technique includes three video cameras and a dot projection device, but is still undergoing development. The team are studying methods of improving the technique and eliminating error in measurements (Adams *et al.*, 1992).

Video-laser systems

Video-laser systems are high technology devices, with previous applications in the glass and plastic industry, animation and advertising. The medical application was first presented by Brunet (1990). A laser plane intercepts the object to digitise, producing a curved-light line along the relief of the object. A camera records an image of the trace and this is then digitised. Software converts the image into a corresponding co-ordinate system. The output is a picture which is very precise. Another video-laser system, the Auscan, was presented later (D'Amico *et al.*, 1992) with the same principle of function. In neither of the studies, however, was the reliability of the method tested.

Finite element models

Finite element (FE) analysis utilises structural engineering techniques to model the spine and the rib cage. Information from three-dimensional radiographs and surface data concerning the individual patient are combined with a defined spine and rib cage model contained in computer software (Andriacchi *et al.*, 1974; Stokes *et al.*, 1990). The three-dimensional geometry of the deformed spine and thorax can be displayed and studied. The software contains information on the mechanical properties of the skeleton and therefore surgery or bracing can be simulated and their effects can be studied before treatment is started (Aubin *et al.*, 1992; Matsumoto *et al.*, 1992; Stokes and Gardner-Morse, 1992).

Conclusions

A large number of methods of imaging the human back are available and for several of these reliability has been established. In most of the hospitals where these methods have been introduced, they are used in parallel with conventional radiography although they have probably reduced the number of X-rays required. Furthermore, these methods give information on body surface shape that radiography is unable to provide. Some also provide numerical data that may be compared from examination to examination.

Most of the methods outlined above provide a display of the human back where at least part of the cosmetic defect of the patient can be visualised and appreciated. Any deterioration of the condition will become apparent on back shape and any numerical data available will help monitor the deterioration. The question is which are the important cosmetic parameters to measure and monitor on back surface? This is discussed below.

Spinal deformity and cosmesis

Quantification of cosmesis

An attempt to quantify the cosmetic defect of spinal deformity has been made on patients with adolescent idiopathic scoliosis (Theologis, 1991; Theologis *et al.,* 1993a). Photographs of 100 adolescent idiopathic scoliosis patients were examined by ten non-medical judges. Each one of the judges gave a Cosmetic Spinal Score (CSS) for each patient, according to the cosmetic appearance of the patient's back. The CSS obtained for each patient was compared with an ISIS scan performed at the same time as the photograph. The CSS proved to be reliable. The correlation between CSS and Hump Severity Score, the ISIS parameter representing the size of the rib hump, was high. The rib hump, therefore, seemed to be the single major factor influencing cosmesis. Less significant correlations were found with Lateral Asymmetry and the Cobb angle. An equation based on a combination of two ISIS parameters (Hump Severity and Lateral Asymmetry) was developed, which could predict the CSS with sufficient reproducibility. The practical value of this equation is that the cosmetic appearance of a patient can be calculated from ISIS parameters with reasonable approximation. This provides the surgeon with a single figure that gives an impression of the severity of the cosmetic deformity.

Although the cosmetic importance of the rib hump and the patients' concern related to it seem to be common knowledge among orthopaedic surgeons, the literature in this field is rather poor and most authors simply state it as a fact. A study by Thulbourne and Gillespie (1976) showed that the rib hump is the feature of the scoliotic deformity most resented by the patient. They suggested a simple device to measure the size of the hump. Aaro and Dahlborn (1982) also considered the rib hump as the major cosmetic concern of their patients. The same observation has been made by several other authors (Pun *et al.,* 1987; Weatherley *et al.,* 1987; Edgar and Mehta, 1988).

The influence of treatment

In recent years, it has become clear that correction of the lateral deformity of the spine in scoliosis is insufficient to give a satisfactory cosmetic result (Weatherley *et al.,* 1987; Edgar and Mehta, 1988). It has been suggested that the three-dimensional deformity should be addressed and that derotation of the spine is needed to correct the sagittal plane deformity and the rib hump (Cotrel *et al.,* 1988; Cundy *et al.,* 1990). Some authors have also suggested that the problem of the rib hump should be addressed directly by costectomy or costoplasty (Owen *et al.,* 1986; Broome *et al.,* 1988). Although there has been some evidence of cosmetic improvement in the above studies, this has not been established with reliable statistical analysis. Furthermore, there has been evidence of late deterioration of the initial rib hump correction after spinal fusion (Edgar and Mehta, 1988; Webb, 1991).

In a study where the influence of treatment on back cosmesis was evaluated, it was found that bracing did not have a beneficial effect, while Harrington fusion offered an early cosmetic improvement (Theologis *et al.,* 1993a). The long-term outcome of cosmesis in those patients, however, was not evaluated.

Conclusions

Certainly 'beauty is in the eyes of the beholder' and human body aesthetics can vary enormously in different individuals and societies. Based, however, on the hypothesis that a number of persons can represent the general population and give their opinion on the cosmetic appearance of a scoliotic back, thus expressing the common feeling, quantification of cosmesis may be possible.

The single attempt to achieve this, outlined above, showed that cosmesis is quantifiable using one of the numerous methods of imaging back shape. Similar methods could be developed using other devices. Some of the most modern devices provide more detailed information and are not limited on the back shape only. They can measure and take into account deformity of the whole body, measure change with time and, it is hoped, provide a more precise cosmetic score. The use of high technology in this field could help more with evaluation of cosmesis. Three-dimensional images that can be rotated, translated and viewed and measured from all angles, perhaps in combination with finite element models, could help in better appreciating the cosmetic defect and planning and predicting the results of treatment. The problem at present is that many of these techniques have not yet acquired an ideal quantitative representation. They need to provide useful measures with clinical application and not only a picture showing the deformity. Since there is some evidence that these methods can detect progression of the deformity sooner than conventional radiography (Fabris *et al.,* 1992; Theologis *et al.,* 1993b), there is the probability that the need for repeated X-rays can be reduced or eliminated. Finally, the same methods can be applied to the study of spinal deformities other than scoliosis.

The cosmetic importance of the rib hump has been shown. Indeed, this part of the deformity which is the main concern of the patients, is also the single major factor influencing cosmesis in the eyes of the 'objective' observer. There is increasing emphasis amongst orthopaedic surgeons to correct the rib hump while performing surgery. Although the results of surgery are not at present entirely satisfactory in improving cosmesis in the long-term, the problem is well recognised and efforts continue.

Cosmesis is an important factor to be taken into account because of its psychological impact on the patient. More research is needed, however, on the psychological impact of the treatment of spinal deformity on the patient. It is not yet clear whether treatment has a beneficial effect on the psychological status of these patients. Nor it is shown whether it is the deformity itself or the treatment, involving long-term bracing or major surgery, which causes more psychological distress.

The representation of cosmesis as a numerical score has a clinical value. In controversial cases, where cosmesis is an important criterion of treatment, in cases with moderate curves, gross rotational deformity and/or rib prominence without severe spinal curvature, cosmesis can be measured. Furthermore, in cases in which the patient insists on asking for treatment when there is no significant deformity (or *vice-versa*), or in cases of patient and family disagreement, the surgeon can be guided by the cosmetic score and form his own opinion.

The old practice has been to document the three-dimensional spinal deformity by radiographs (two-dimensional), measure it using the Cobb angle and treat it with straight (linear) Harrington rods (Stokes, 1992). The new practice is to understand the three-dimensional nature of spinal deformity and its effect on body surface shape and to use implants which allow the correction of the deformity in three planes.

References

Aaro S, Dahlborn M (1982) The effect of Harrington instrumentation on the longitudinal axis rotation of the apical vertebra and on the spinal and rib cage deformity in idiopathic scoliosis studied by computer tomography. *Spine*; **7**: 456–462

Aaro S, Ohlund C (1984) Scoliosis and pulmonary function. *Spine*; **9**: 220–222

Adams W (1865) *Lectures on the Pathology and Treatment of Lateral and Other Forms of Curvature of the Spine*. London: John Churchill and Sons

Adams KD, Durdle NG, Raso VJ, Peterson AE (1992) Considerations for establishing the accuracy of a CCD video camera. In: Dansereau J (ed.) *International Symposium on 3-D Scoliotic Deformities*. Stuttgart: Gustav Fischer Verlag, pp. 364–369

Andriacchi TP (1974) A model for studies of mechanical interactions between the human spine and rib cage. *J. Biomech.*; **7**: 497–507

Aubin CE, Dansereau J, Labelle H (1992) Incorporation of costo-vertebral joints modelisation into a personalised finite element model of the scoliotic spine. In: Dansereau J (ed.) *International Symposium on 3-D Scoliotic Deformities*. Stuttgart: Gustav Fischer Verlag, pp. 400–407

Bengtsson G, Fallstrom K, Jansson B, Nachemson A (1974) A psychological and psychiatric investigation of the adjustment of female scoliosis patients. *Acta Psychiat. Scand.*; **50**: 50–59

Bernhardt M, Bridwell KH (1989) Segmental analysis of the sagittal plane alignment of the normal thoracic and lumbar spine and thoracolumbar junction. *Spine*; **14**: 717–721

Broome G, Simpson AHRW, Catalan J, Jefferson RJ, Houghton GR (1990) The modified Schollner costoplasty. *J. Bone Jt Surg.*; **72B**: 894–900

Brown R, Burstein A, Nash CL, Schock C (1976) Spinal analysis using a three-dimensional radiographic technique. *J. Biomech.*; **9**: 355–365

Brunet M (1990) The V3D 1/800/Medical videolaser system: a body digitizer. In: Neugebauer H, Windischbauer G (eds) *Surface Topography and Body Deformity*. Stuttgart: Gustav. Fischer Verlag, pp. 159–162

Burwell RG, Patterson JF, Webb JK, Wojcik AS (1990) School screening for scoliosis. In: Neugebauer H, Windischbauer G (eds) *Surface Topography and Body Deformity*. Stuttgart: Gustav Fischer Verlag, pp. 17–23

Carman DL, Browne RH, Birch JG (1990) Measurement of scoliosis and kyphosis radiographs. *J. Bone Jt Surg.*; **72A**: 328–333

Clayson D (1979) Psychological problems of scoliosis in early adolescence. In: Zorab PA, Siegler D (eds) *Scoliosis*. London: Academic Press, pp. 227–231

Cobb JR (1948) An outline for the study of scoliosis. *Am. Acad. Orthop. Surg. Instructional Course Lectures*; **5**: 261–275

Cochran T, Irstam L, Nachemson A (1983) Long-term anatomic and functional changes in patients with adolescent idiopathic scoliosis treated by Harrington rod fusion. *Spine*; **8**: 576–583

Cotrel Y, Dubousset J, Guillaumat M (1988) New universal instrumentation in spinal surgery. *Clin. Orthop.*; **227**: 10–23

Csongradi J, Jefferson RJ, Turner-Smith AR, Harris JD (1987) Predictive value of surface topography in the management of scoliosis. In: Stokes IAF, Pekelsky JR, Moreland MS (eds) *Surface Topography and Spinal Deformity*. Stuttgart: Gustav Fischer Verlag, pp. 21–28

Cundy PJ, Paterson DC, Hillier TM, Sutherland AD, Stephen JP, Foster BK (1990) Cotrel-Dubousset instrumentation and vertebral rotation in adolescent idiopathic scoliosis. *J. Bone Jt Surg.*; **72B**: 670–674

D'Amico M, Chiarelli G, Ferrigno G, Santambrogio GC (1992) Back surface reconstruction by the Auscan system. In: Dansereau J (ed.) *International Symposium on 3-D Scoliotic Deformities*. Stuttgart: Gustav Fischer Verlag, pp. 165–170

Drerup B (1992) 3-D acquisition, reconstruction and modeling techniques applied on scoliotic deformities. In: Dansereau J (ed.) *International Symposium on 3-D Scoliotic Deformities*. Stuttgart: Gustav Fischer Verlag, pp. 2–10

Dutkowsky JP, Shearer D, Schepps B, Orton C, Scola F (1990) Radiation exposure to patients receiving routine scoliosis radiography measured at depth in an anthropomorphic phantom. *J. Paediat. Orthop.*; **10**: 532–534

Edgar MA, Mehta MA (1988) Long-term follow-up of fused and unfused idiopathic scoliosis. *J. Bone Jt Surg.*; **70B**: 712–716

Fabris D, Taglialavoro G, Constantini S, Nena U, Gentilucci G (1992) The clinical features and the prognostic value of rib cage deformity in thoracic idiopathic scoliosis and its relationship with vertebral rotation and lateral somatic wedging. In: Dansereau J (ed.) *International Symposium on 3-D Scoliotic Deformities*. Stuttgart: Gustav Fischer Verlag, pp. 217–220

Ferguson AB (1930) The study and treatment of scoliosis. *South Med. J.*; **23**: 116

Frobin W, Hierzholzer E (1984) A metric rasterstereographic camera for simplified patient recording. In: Harris JD, Turner-Smith AR (eds) *Surface Topography and Spinal Deformity*. Stuttgart: Gustav Fischer Verlag, pp. 3–10

Frobin W, Hierzholzer E (1990) Video rasterstereography: a method for on-line surface measurement. In: Neugebauer H, Windischbauer G (eds) *Surface Topography and Body Deformity*. Stuttgart: Gustav Fischer Verlag, pp. 155–157

Groves D, Dangerfield PH, Pearson J (1990) Advanced computer analysis of moiré contour images of the human back. In: Neugebauer H, Windischbauer G (eds) *Surface Topography and Body Deformity*. Stuttgart: Gustav Fischer Verlag, pp. 107–114

Halioua M, Liu HC, Chin A, Bowins TS (1990) Automated topography of human forms by phase measuring profilometry and modal analysis. In: Neugebauer H, Windischbauer G (eds) *Surface Topography and Body Deformity*. Stuttgart: Gustav Fischer Verlag, pp. 91–100

Harris JD, Jefferson RJ, Turner-Smith AR, Thomas D (1987) Transverse asymmetry, a measure of the progression of scoliosis. In: Stokes IAF, Pekelsky JR, Moreland MS (eds) *Surface Topography and Spinal Deformity*. Stuttgart: Gustav Fischer Verlag, pp. 85–94

Hierzholzer E, Drerup B (1990) Three-dimensional reconstruction of the spinal midline from rasterstereographs. In: Neugebauer H, Windischbauer G (eds) *Surface Topography and Body Deformity*. Stuttgart: Gustav Fischer Verlag, pp. 53–55

Hierzholzer E, Drerup B (1992) Which requirements must be met in order to replace radiography by surface topography. In: Dansereau J (ed.) *International Symposium on 3-D Scoliotic Deformities*. Stuttgart: Gustav Fischer Verlag, pp. 131–138

Hill DL, Raso VJ, Durdle NG, Peterson AE (1992) Designing a video based technique for trunk measurement. In: Dansereau J (ed.) *International Symposium on 3-D Scoliotic Deformities*. Stuttgart: Gustav Fischer Verlag, pp. 157–161

Hoffman DA, Lonstein JE, Morin MM, Vischer W, Harris SH, Boice JD (1989) Breast cancer in women with scoliosis exposed to multiple diagnostic X-rays. *J. Natl. Cancer Inst.*; **81**: 1307–1312

Houghton GR (1984) Cosmetic surgery for scoliosis. In: Dickson RA and Bradford DS (eds) *Management of Spinal Deformities*. Oxford: Butterworths, pp. 237–251

Ions GK, Whittingham TA, Saunders PJ, Leonard MA, Stevens J (1984) Radiation free imaging of the scoliotic spine. In: Harris JD, Turner-smith AR (eds) *Surface Topography and Spinal Deformity*. Stuttgart: Gustav Fischer Verlag, pp. 71–75

Jefferson RJ, Weisz I, Turner-Smith AR, Harris JD, Houghton GR (1988) Scoliosis surgery and its effect on back shape. *J. Bone Jt Surg.*; **70B**: 261–266

Karras GE (1990) Calibration and accuracy of shadow moiré topography. In: Neugebauer H,

Windischbauer G (eds) *Surface Topography and Body Deformity.* Stuttgart: Gustav Fischer Verlag, pp. 143–145

Klein P, Rooze M (1990) Close range moiré topography: an error analysis. In: Neugebauer H, Windischbauer G (eds) *Surface Topography and Body Deformity.* Stuttgart: Gustav Fischer Verlag, pp. 147–149

Mauritzson L, Benoni G, Ilver J, Lindstrom K, Willner S (1984) Three linear array back scanning with airborne ultrasound. In: Harris JD, Turner-Smith AR (eds) *Surface Topography and Spinal Deformity.* Gustav Fischer Verlag, pp. 47–51

Matsumoto T, Kitahara H, Minami S *et al.* (1992) Computer simulation of corrective surgery for scoliosis. In: Dansereau J (ed.) *International Symposium on 3-D Scoliotic Deformities.* Gustav Fischer Verlag, pp. 96–101

Mehta M (1972) The rib-vertebra angle in the early diagnosis of resolving and progressive infantile scoliosis. *J. Bone Jt Surg.*; **54B**: 230–243

Merolli A, Tranquilli-Lealli P (1990) Preliminary clinical experience with a back surface topography automated recorder (STAR). In: Neugebauer H, Windischbauer G (eds) *Surface Topography and Body Deformity.* Gustav Fischer Verlag, pp. 101–105

Moe JH, Winter RB, Bradford DS, Lonstein JE (1978) Scoliosis and other spinal deformities. Philadelphia: Saunders WB

Morrissy RT, Goldsmith GS, Hall EC, Kehl D, Cowie GH (1990) Measurement of the Cobb angle on radiographs of patients who have scoliosis. *J. Bone Jt Surg.*; **72A**: 320–327

Mouchref K, Billat R, Quézel G, Ponzio P (1992) A real time spinal deformity measurement and visualization apparatus. In: Dansereau J (ed.) *International Symposium on 3-D Scoliotic Deformities.* Gustav Fischer Verlag, pp. 42–49

Nash C, Moe J (1969) A study of vertebral rotation. *J. Bone Jt Surg.*; **51A**: 223–228

Oates CP, Whittingham TA, Leonard MA (1990) The Newcastle ultrasonic spine imaging system. In: Neugebauer H, Windischbauer G (eds) *Surface Topography and Body Deformity.* Gustav Fischer Verlag, pp. 31–33

Owen R, Turner A, Bamforth JSG, Taylor JF, Jones RS (1986) Costectomy as the first stage of surgery for scoliosis. *J. Bone Jt Surg.*; **68B**: 91–95

Pearson JD, Dangerfield PH, Hobson CA, Li Y (1992) An automated visual system for the measurement of the three-dimensional deformity of scoliosis. In: Dansereau J (ed.) *International Symposium on 3-D Scoliotic Deformities.* Stuttgart: Gustav Fischer Verlag, pp. 50–56

Perdriolle R (1979) La scoliose: son etude tridimensionnelle. Paris: Maloine SA

Propst-Proctor SL, Bleck EE (1983) Radiographic determination of lordosis and kyphosis in normal and scoliotic children. *J. Pediatr. Orthop.*; **3**: 344–346

Pun WK, Luk KDK, Lee W, Leong JCY (1987) A simple method to estimate the rib hump in scoliosis. *Spine*; **12**: 342–345

Stagnara P (1974) Examen du scoliotic. In: Deviations laterales du rachis. Paris: Encyclopedie Medicochirurgicale

Stagnara P, DeMauroy J, Dran G, Gonon GP, Costanzo G, Dimnet J, Pasquet A (1982) Reciprocal angulation of vertebral bodies in the sagittal plane: approach to references for the evaluation of kyphosis and lordosis. *Spine*; **7**: 335–342

Steinnocher K, Jansa J, Kausel W (1990) Recognition of scoliosis by automated evaluation of digital Moiré images. In: Neugebauer H, Windischbauer G (eds) *Surface Topography and Spinal Deformity.* Stuttgart: Gustav Fischer Verlag, pp. 115–116

Stokes IAF, Bigalow LC, Moreland MS (1987) Three-dimensional curves in idiopathic scoliosis. *J. Orthop. Res.*; **5**: 102–113

Stokes IAF (1990) Three-dimensional osseo-ligamentous model of the thorax representing initiation of scoliosis by asymmetric growth. *J. Biomech.*; **23**: 589–595

Stokes IAF, Gardner-Morse M (1992) Three-dimensional simulations of the surgical correction of idiopathic scoliosis. In: Dansereau J (ed.) *International Symposium on 3-D Scoliotic Deformities.* Stuttgart: Gustav Fischer Verlag, pp. 89–95

Stokes IAF (1992) 3-D spinal deformity measurement methods and terminology. In: Dansereau J (ed.) *International Symposium on 3-D Scoliotic Deformities,* Stuttgart: Gustav Fischer Verlag, pp. 236–243

Suzuki N, Ono T, Tezuka M, Kamiishi S (1992) In: Dansereau J (ed.) *International Symposium on 3-D Scoliotic Deformities.* Stuttgart: Gustav Fischer Verlag, pp. 124–130

Takasaki H (1970) Moiré topography. *Applied Optics*; **9**: 1467–1472

Theologis TN (1991) Quantification of the cosmetic effects of adolescent idiopathic scoliosis using the ISIS scan. MSc Thesis, Oxford

Theologis TN, Jefferson RJ, Simpson AHRW, Turner-Smith AR, Fairbank JCT (1993a) Quantifying the cosmetic defect of adolescent idiopathic scoliosis. *Spine*; **18**: 909–912

Theologis TN, Turner-Smith AR, Fairbank JCT (1993b) Study of the progression of adolescent idiopathic scoliosis using the ISIS scan. 9th Phillip Zorab Scoliosis Symposium, Cambridge

Thulbourne T, Gillespie R (1976) The rib hump in idiopathic scoliosis. *J. Bone Jt Surg.*; **58B**: 64–71

Tredwell SJ, Bannon M (1988) The use of the ISIS optical scanner in the management of the braced adolescent idiopathic scoliosis patient. *Spine*; **13**: 1104–1105

Turner-Smith AR (1988) A television/computer three-dimensional surface shape measurement system. *J. Biomech.*; **21**: 515–529

Turner-Smith AR, Harris JD, Houghton GR, Jefferson RJ (1988) A method for analysis of back shape in scoliosis. *J. Biomech.*; **21**: 497–509

Weatherley CR, Draycott V, O'Brien JF, Benson DR, Gopalakrishnan KC, Evans JH, O'Brien JP (1987) The rib deformity in adolescent idiopathic scoliosis. A prospective study to evaluate changes after Harrington distraction and posterior fusion. *J. Bone Jt Surg.*; **69B**: 179–182

Webb JK (1991) A comparison of modern surgical techniques in scoliosis. Combined British and Nordic Scoliosis Societies Meeting, Newcastle

Weisz I, Jefferson RJ, Carr AJ, Turner-Smith AR, McInerney A, Houghton GR (1989) Back shape in brace treatment of idiopathic scoliosis. *Clin. Orthop.*; **240**: 157–163

Windischbauer G, Neugebauer H (1990) Reviewing proposals of evaluating the scoliotic spine curvature without exposition to ionizing radiation. In: Neugebauer H, Windischbauer G (eds) *Surface Topography and Body Deformity.* Stuttgart: Gustav Fischer Verlag, pp. 49–52

Wojcik AS, Burwell RG, Webb JK, Moulton A (1990) A new ultrasound method for measuring spinal torsion in scoliosis. In: Neugebauer H, Windischbauer G (eds) *Surface Topography and Body Deformity.* Stuttgart: Gustav Fischer Verlag, pp. 25–30

Chapter 14

Biomechanical measurements

JF Orr and IC Revie

Introduction

The topic of biomechanics acknowledges, through the title itself, that natural structures may be subjected to engineering analysis. The engineering sciences of dynamics, statics and strength of materials are often associated with biomechanics, also subjects such as fluid flow and thermodynamics contribute. This chapter will concentrate on topics primarily of application to the former three areas. Engineers seldom regard a structure in its complete form but prefer to consider parts which can be analysed and understood in order to build up knowledge of individual contributions to structural integrity or to study those parts involved in a particular mode of failure.

Such approaches are essential in natural structures which are very complex, although it can be difficult to identify unique functions for any particular feature. The concept of rationalisation includes: resolution of forces into orthogonal components; degrees of freedom to describe relative movements; free body diagrams to represent the interaction of structural segments with their environment.

Spatial considerations

Anatomical geometry and lines of action of resultant forces are oriented in three-dimensional space. It is often convenient, for analysis, to resolve the variable of

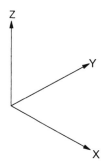

Figure 14.1 'Right handed' cartesian co-ordinate system

interest and to describe it in terms of components within a co-ordinate system (O'Conner, 1992). Force components are usually resolved as orthogonal, or mutually perpendicular forces, in x, y and z directions of Cartesian co-ordinates. In engineering convention a 'right handed' system is preferred (Figure 14.1) in which rotation of the x axis to the y axis would advance a 'right handed' screw along the z axis in the positive direction. However, consideration of body symmetry and the desire to keep positive directions in the same sense relative to right and left structures requires both left and right handed systems (Figure 14.2). The application of Cartesian co-ordinates to the hip joint is demonstrated by Brown *et al.* (1984). A co-ordinate system must be defined relative to a structure which is taken to be fixed as an origin. The ground surface is often appropriate, as in gait analysis; however, it may be convenient to position the origin of axes within a body structure, for instance at the centre of rotation of the hip joint. The choice is made for convenience in any particular study but must be defined at the outset. The directions of axes are usually chosen to be vertical and horizontal but care should be taken relating to the conventional anatomical reference planes since they may be used to describe structures which are approximate to, rather than truly lying in, the planes. It should be noted that Cartesian co-ordinates are not universally used. Mapping of body surface shape is an example when a polar system may be convenient (McCartney and Hinds, 1992). However, there are still three values to be quoted to define a point in three-dimensional space.

A point is uniquely defined in three-dimensional space by three co-ordinates. Three co-ordinates will not be sufficient to define the position and orientation of a structure. If a point in the structure is defined, then rotation may be considered to occur about axes parallel to each of the co-ordinate system axes, and hence three further values are required to establish position and orientation. Thus, there are six *degrees of freedom* of any object in three-dimensional space. Any movement of position of an object may be considered as a combination of three linear translations and three rotations about perpendicular axes. Such treatment is particularly appropriate for description of articulating joints where some degrees of freedom may be suppressed to support forces and maintain functional alignment of body segments, while others are free to permit movement and function. Suppression of all six degrees of freedom may be desired in the case of bone

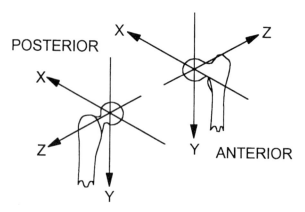

Figure 14.2 Co-ordinate systems at hip joints

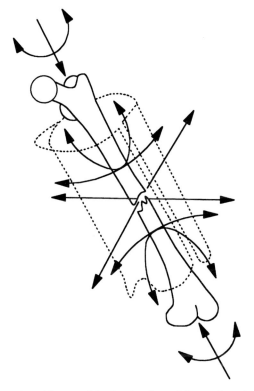

Figure 14.3 Suppression of degrees of freedom in a femoral fracture brace by containment of soft tissues

fracture immobilisation. Individual consideration of each is very helpful in understanding the design features of orthoses, such as a femoral fracture brace (Figure 14.3).

Further simplification can be made by consideration of only that part of a structure which is of direct interest. In the example of force analysis at an articulating joint the behaviour of adjacent bones as structures may be of secondary interest. In such cases it is usual to represent the parts of interest in *a free body diagram* (Figure 14.4). It is valid to perform such a simplification only if forces and moments which are transmitted outside the selected boundaries are represented by their reactions on the model.

Stress and strain

Engineers usually consider the strengths of materials in terms of stress, that is force per unit area. This is a derived quantity from knowledge of deformation expressed as strain (change in length divided by original measured length). The relationship between stress and strain is found by experiment. Stress, therefore, cannot be measured directly but must be derived from strain measurements. Stresses and strains are not purely linear but are considered in two-dimensional

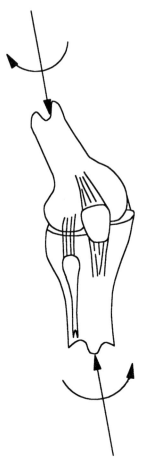

Figure 14.4 Free body diagram of the knee joint showing resultant forces and moments

or even three-dimensional fields. The analysis of such fields is complex. The complete description of stresses and strains in a particular direction requires knowledge of direct (tensile or compressive) and shear components. The two-dimensional case is a special case of the general situation and is often the subject of experimental measurement of strains. The stress or strain field at a point may be completely defined by orthogonal 'principal' values and their directions. Principal stresses or strains are direct in nature and occur along directions where shear components are zero (Benham and Crawford, 1990). In isotropic materials the principal stress and strain directions are coincident; however, this is not necessarily the case for non-isotropic materials. Bone is a notable example of a non-isotropic material.

The relationships between stress and strain need to be known for materials. The relationships are often described with reference to characteristic points of a graphical plot of stress versus strain. The data for such a graph are usually obtained from a tensile material test for which loads and deformations are measured. These are converted to stresses and strains by division by the cross-sectional area (for stress) and original length (for strain) before loading of the specimen. A typical graph for a ductile metal is shown in Figure 14.5. Normally initial strain is proportional to stress, obeying Hooke's Law, the gradient is often quoted as the *modulus of elasticity* or *stiffness*. As stress increases this initial relationship is lost at the *limit of proportionality*. The *elastic limit* marks the point beyond which complete recovery to pre-test dimensions will not occur when the load is removed. Even though plastic deformation is now occurring the stress may still increase to the *ultimate strength* of the material before localised gross yielding causes reductions in area and failure. The apparent reduction of stress at failure is an artefact of calculating stress with respect to original cross-sectional area, a procedure which is not strictly valid as the test proceeds. Brittle materials can generally be regarded as following the same initial stress/strain behaviour but reaching their failure or fracture stress before an elastic limit is attained or may even fail before the limit of proportionality. Polymers behave in a similar manner to ductile metals; in this case, even the initial relationship is not proportional, so there is no straight portion of the curve.

Strain measurement

There are many methods of measuring strain and each offers special character-istics which may render it most suitable for a specific application. Details of methods are available (Miles and Tanner, 1992) aimed at assisting researchers to make a suitable choice and to start practical applications, however a brief overview of popular techniques is described in this section.

In engineering most design and determination of stress and strain in structures is performed theoretically, using formulae derived from first principles or empirically and then complemented by a knowledge of material properties. On occasions it may be necessary to resort to experimental measurements when a structure geometry is complex or material properties and boundary conditions are not known. This often applies to biomechanical structures.

Brittle coatings

The method of covering a structure with a coating which cracks due to surface deformation dates back to early orthopaedic research. In the late 1800s, Meyer

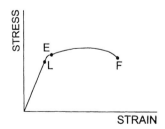

Figure 14.5 Stress/strain behaviour of a ductile metal showing limit of proportionality (L), elastic limit (E) and fracture (F)

and Wolff were studying bone structure and Roux was investigating bone deformation by applying paraffin wax to rubber models. Brittle coating has become an established engineering technique for strain measurement. Coatings can be applied to a substrate which cracks on tensile loading, or if pre-loaded, when the structure is allowed to relax. The techniques are quite difficult to use successfully with cracking being dependent on ambient temperature, humidity and coating material choice (Humphreys et al., 1990).

The relationship between cracking density and known strains can be determined from cantilever calibration specimens. In practice the technique is usually used to identify points of maximum strain and hence, stress. The orientation of the cracks give good indication of principal strain directions. They may not coincide with principal stress directions in non-homogeneous materials such as bone and composites. Further quantitative measurement is usually performed by other devices such as strain gauges. There are several studies on implants using brittle coating (Markolf and Amstutz, 1976; Brockhurst and Svensson, 1977; Humphreys et al., 1990) and some earlier applications to bone (Evans, 1948; Kalen, 1961). It is likely that there will be difficulties with the technique, especially if wet specimens are being studied.

Strain gauges

The most common method of measuring strain is using electrical resistance strain gauges. The term 'strain gauge' is often used synonymously with these devices. However, there are gauges which sense change of length by other principles such as capacitance, acoustic resonance and optical interference. Traditional mechanical extensometer devices may also be used. In practice there have been few reports of these other devices being used in biomechanical applications. The electrical resistance strain gauge relies on the fact that an electrical conductor changes its resistance when strained. Electrical resistance may be expressed as being proportional to the product of resistivity and length divided by the cross-sectional area. All three factors change to support either an increase in resistance due to tension or a decrease due to compression. The application of pre-printed foil gauges and the measurement of resistance changes appears deceptively easy. However, there are many factors which can substantially influence results and users are strongly advised to seek advice on gauge selection and application. Gauge manufactures can often give excellent technical guidance notes. Dabestani (1992) showed it is possible to bond strain gauges to wet bone surfaces. We have gained satisfactory results from a cadaveric pelvis and femur using gauges secured with cyanoacrylate adhesive.

An early and ambitious application of strain gauges to measurement of joint forces was reported by Rydell (1966) who measured forces in prosthetic femoral components in patients with hip joint replacements. The components themselves formed pre-calibrated dynamometers with strain gauges bonded within the hollow necks in appropriate positions to measure forces and moments. The experiments were curtailed by the requirement for transcutaneous connection leads for power and signals. It is interesting that this work was directed at understanding the forces in the intact hip joint rather than to the design and development of artificial components (Hirsh, 1965).

Optical methods

Optical measurement in biomechanics embraces numerous techniques and applications. These have the advantage of avoiding contact but the disadvantage of exposing the structural surfaces under study. The use of optical methods to record body segment motion during gait is a common application (see Chapter 8). Methods of strain and displacement measurement will be described here.

Photoelastic stress analysis relies on some materials, notably epoxy based polymers, exhibiting the characteristic of birefringence when strained. Polarised light can be regarded as travelling along the planes of principal stresses in a loaded, two-dimensional model, parallel to the axis of propagation. Interference of the light from the two transmission paths causes dark and light fringes to be formed (Orr, 1991) (Figure 14.6). Colourful photoelastic images are often seen in publicity material. The method allows quantitative measurement in models of principal stress directions and shear stress magnitudes. Individual principal stress magnitudes may be derived. Three-dimensional modelling is also possible but a method of analysis has to be used which allows fringes to be recorded in a series of planes within the model. The frozen stress method, where models are physically sliced after a thermal cycle under load, is most common (Dally and Riley, 1991). Some advanced methods of 'optical slicing' have been reported for biomechanical applications (Kihara *et al.,* 1985, 1987).

Photoelastic stress analysis has been used in orthopaedic applications since about 1940 (Milch, 1940) when suitable polymer materials became available (Orr *et al.,* 1990; Orr, 1992). Early studies tended to concentrate on modelling bone with reference to functional structure and prediction of response to operative intervention (Dylag *et al.,* 1964; Williams and Svensson, 1971; Steen Jensen, 1978a). Comprehensive use of photoelastic models was made by Pauwels to explain body structure and even cancellous bone remodelling. The papers describing the studies have been published in book form (Pauwels, 1980). Few authors have addressed problems regarding the representation of bone by homogeneous models (Holm, 1981). Implants, particularly joint replacements, do not present the same difficulties (Steen Jensen, 1978b; Fessler and Fricker, 1989).

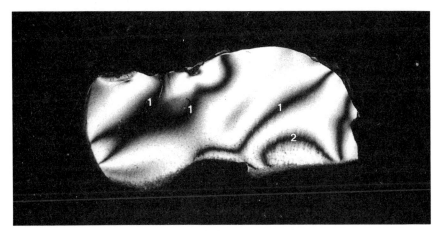

Figure 14.6 Isochromatic fringes in model of talus

An alternative to using polymer models is to bond a photoelastic sensitive coating to prototype structures with reflective adhesive and view fringes with polarised light (Zandman *et al.*, 1977). There are still problems relating to surface reinforcement but the technique is appropriate for comparative studies (Finlay, 1992).

Holography describes the recording of the three-dimensional shape of a structure using laser illumination. If the structure has such holograms recorded at two different loads by double exposure then relative deformation will result in interference fringes on the image. The technique is extremely sensitive and requires the elimination of movement of the structure during exposure, either from its load response or external vibration (Shelton, 1992). The conventional holographic technique described measures movements along the direction of the incident light; however, there are further laser interference methods, such as speckle interferometry, which have the potential to measure in-plane movements.

Modelling of joints

The study of forces and movements of human joints has been conducted from experimental and theoretical approaches. The difficulty of making measurements *in vivo* encourages theoretical studies which may be based on measurements external to the body. A well established example is ground reaction force data recorded during gait analysis and subsequently used to calculate joint forces and moments with consideration of muscle forces to maintain joint stability. The work of Paul (1967) is widely quoted in the development of such techniques and demonstrates how further knowledge of muscle force distributions is necessary to solve a large number of equations in such statically indeterminate problems.

If muscle forces and their lines of action are known relative to bone anatomy, theoretical models may be developed to allow parametric investigations of joint disorders and treatments. Such analysis requires the free body consideration described above in order to keep the study within practical and relevant limits. *In vitro* experimental modelling also tends to adopt a parametric approach, that is a comparison of trends rather than absolute values comparable to *in vivo* conditions. Both types of study have been reported for the hip joint. These have concentrated on the strain response of the femur to loading, joint and muscle loads.

Case study: experimental measurement of muscle loads and bone strains at the hip joint

The following example has been selected to introduce considerations of muscles acting about the hip joint, to demonstrate the free body concept in experimental modelling and present some experience of strain measurement in a biomechanical model.

The authors wanted to investigate the implications of movement of the hip joint centre of rotation, from its anatomical centre, for strains in the pelvis. The study was part of a design project for custom acetabular components. While it was not suggested that any position other than anatomical was appropriate, it was important to understand the effects of misplacing the centre through necessities of implant selection or anatomical abnormalities.

Model development

The muscles represented in the experimental model are listed in Table 14.1, together with those previously modelled by earlier researchers (Revie, 1995). The structures represented, or preserved in the case of ligaments, are comprehensive compared to some studies. Even these more complex models

Table 14.1 Muscles considered by researchers for theoretical and experimental models of the hip joint

	Muscle models & loads									
	Revie (1995)	Johnston et al. (1979)	Dalstra (1994)	Delp and Maloney (1993)	Finlay et al. (1986)	Goel et al. (1978)	Jacob et al. (1976)	McLeish and Charnley (1976)	Oonishi et al. (1983)	Petty et al. (1980)
Adductor	▨		▨	▨					▨	
External obliqus						▨				
Gemellus			▨							
Gluteus maximus	▨	▨	▨	▨	▨			▨	▨	▨
Gluteus medius	▨	▨	▨	▨	▨	▨	▨	▨	▨	▨
Gluteus minimus	▨	▨	▨	▨	▨	▨	▨	▨	▨	▨
Gracilis			▨							
Hamstring	▨	▨				▨			▨	
Internal obliqus	▨					▨				
ITB	▨		▨	▨	▨		▨			
Obturator externus/internus	▨		▨							
Pectineus	▨		▨							
Piriformis	▨		▨	▨	▨				▨	▨
Psoas major/iliacus		▨	▨	▨		▨				
Quadratus lumborum						▨				
Rectus abdominous						▨				
Rectus femoris	▨	▨	▨	▨		▨				
Sartorius	▨		▨	▨						
Tensor facia latae	▨	▨	▨	▨	▨			▨	▨	▨
Transverse abdominous						▨				
Iliofemoral ligament	▨					▨				
Iliolumbar ligament	▨					▨				
Pubic symphysis ligament	▨					▨				
Sacroiliac ligament	▨					▨				
Sacrospinous ligament	▨					▨				
Sacrotuberous ligament	▨					▨				

have usually been theoretical. The aim of representing as many muscles and ligaments as possible is justified by noting that pelvic strains were under study. Even so, the lack of abdominal muscles limits the interpretation of results. Most work at the hip has concentrated on the femur and femoral implants, for which simpler models may be justified (McLeish and Charnley, 1976; Delp and Maloney, 1993).

An articulated cadaveric pelvis and left femur was dissected and the insertions and lines of action of the muscle groups identified and measured with reference to a pair of stainless steel rods, fixed at approximately 90° through the distal femur before dissection. The hip joint was reconstructed using high stiffness cord (Spectra, SD3-Racing, Marlow Ropes Ltd, Hailsham, UK) and load dividing pulley systems to distribute muscle forces. Final attachment to bone was made using cyanoacrylate adhesive with rubber filler to enhance its toughness (Loctite Prism 480, Loctite, Welwyn Garden City, UK) (Figure 14.7). As noted above, there was no muscle representation proximal to the iliac crest. Muscles and the ilio-tibial band on the lateral side of the femur had their lines of action preserved and terminated in a stainless steel anchorage plate around the distal femur, where it was embedded in epoxy resin and attached to a universal ball clamp permitting rotational alignment about three axes.

Electrical resistance strain gauges were used in load transducers to measure muscle forces. The transducers were of two types; axial tensile rods, loaded through springs (range 0–1000 N) and miniature beam transducers for lower load ranges (0–300 N) (Figure 14.8). Both types of transducer were designed for the study, each used four strain gauges wired in full bridge configuration to give enhanced sensitivity and were individually calibrated on a tensile testing machine.

Rosettes, each comprising three gauges (WA-06-060WR-120, Measurements Group Inc., Basingstoke, UK) were bonded to the pelvis using cyano-acrylate

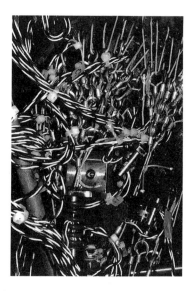

Figure 14.7 Attachment of muscle cords to bone using cyano-acrylate adhesive

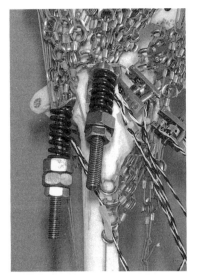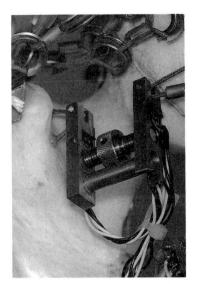

Figure 14.8 Axial and beam force transducers

adhesive. They permitted calculation of principal strains and also strains along axes defined by the bone structure. No attempt was made to calculate stresses since there was insufficient knowledge of the underlying bone properties. It was a parametric study to compare strains for the intact joint with strains resulting from a prosthetic joint with various centres of rotation.

The complete model (Figure 14.9) was loaded through the 5th lumber vertebra using dead weights up to 25% body weight. Higher loading was precluded by

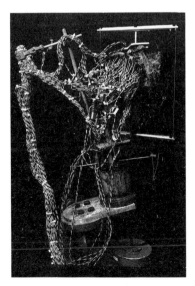

Figure 14.9 Cadaveric femur and pelvis with reconstructed muscles

bone deformation, principally the distal femur close to its point of embedding. However, this region was well outside the areas of measurement. Strains from the load transducers (nine channels) and from 18 strain gauge rosettes on the bones (54 channels) were recorded through a data logging interface (Datascan 7000, Measurement Systems, Newbury, UK) and software (Labtech Notebook, Labtech, Massachusetts, USA).

Results

Muscle forces were found to lie within the ranges calculated and measured from the reported theoretical and experimental studies (Figure 14.10). Bone strains were rather more complex to interpret. Trends were comparable with those predicted by previous workers and changes of strains around the acetabulum were determined as a consequence of joint replacement and movement of the centre of rotation.

The outcome of this study was valuable knowledge of the effects of total hip replacements on bone. The results of the muscle measurements complement trends reported in literature and hence give confidence for the further strain results. The experimental model was complex and the practical strain measurements bear some discussion. The bonding of the gauges was satisfactory, with only one rosette giving unreliable readings. The bone specimens did suffer creep deformation under load so a strict time plan was required for loading, with measurements taken during relaxation to compensate for this phenomenon.

Experiments of this type should be conducted over as short a time period as possible, due to dehydration of the bones. Bones can be kept moist at the earlier stages of preparation and sealed prior to bonding muscle cords and gauges. Inevitably, the preservation of moisture becomes more difficult as the complexity of the model and instrumentation increases.

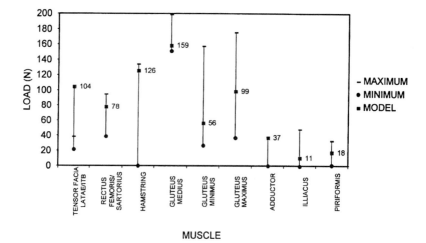

Figure 14.10 Comparison of experimental muscle forces with ranges reported in literature

Further developments

Much of the foregoing discussion has addressed the measurement of strains in bone. Soft tissue measurements are required and present their own problems (Shrive, 1991). New technology has also presented opportunities for further development of research measurements. Thermal emission from a cyclically stressed body was reported by Lord Kelvin in 1878 and the phenomenon now forms the principle of operation of SPATE (Stress Pattern Analysis by Thermal Emission). This instrument displays coloured fringes which are proportional to the cyclic change of the sum of the principal stresses at any point on a model or prototype structure. This data is complementary to photoelastic fringes which are proportional to shear stress or the principal stress difference. Bone has been found to produce measurable thermal emission (Duncan, 1992).

On the topic of model making, rapid prototyping methods and stereo-lithography (3D Systems, Valentia, CA), offer a new means of reproducing anatomical structures. Stereo-lithography involves building objects, layer by layer, by polymerisation of liquid resin on exposure to an ultra-violet laser controlled by computer. The models may be made from acrylic or epoxy polymers, the latter having good photoelastic properties. Models of isolated anatomical structures can be built from data from clinical digital images. So far, these models have been reported as being used for operative planning and implant design. There will undoubtedly be many further applications of this technology (Mahoney, 1995).

The emphasis on experimental research reflects the authors' experience and it is acknowledged that much work is performed theoretically. Experimental measurements and modelling can yield very valuable information and are amenable to the representation of practical operative procedures. The techniques available for strain measurement should be regarded as complementary, each having its own unique capabilities. Selection of an appropriate technique depends on the application and researchers need to be sufficiently familiar with the options to make an informed selection. Once this decision is taken, there is a great deal of information and experience available for guidance. Methods need not be expensive or unduly time-consuming before useful results are gained. This chapter can only address topics superficially but the references which follow represent leads into the techniques described.

References

Benham PP, Crawford RJ (1990) *Mechanics of Engineering Materials*. Essex: Longman Scientific and Technical

Brockhurst PJ, Svensson NL (1977) Design of total hip prosthesis. *Medical Progress Technology*; **5**: 73–102

Brown TRM, Nicol AC, Paul JP (1984) Comparison of loads transmitted by Charnley and CAD Muller total hip arthroplasties. *First International Conference on Engineering and Clinical Aspects of Endoprosthetic Fixation*, Inst Mech Engrs, C210/84, 63–68

Dabestani M (1992) *In vitro* strain measurement in bone. In: Miles AW, Tanner KE (eds) *Strain Measurement in Biomechanics*. London: Chapman & Hall, pp. 58–69

Dally JW, Riley WF (1991) *Experimental Stress Analysis*. New York: McGraw-Hill

Dalstra M (1994) Biomechanical aspects of the pelvic bone and design criteria for acetabular prostheses. PhD thesis, Biomechanics Section, Institute of Orthopaedics, University of Nijmegen, Netherlands

Delp SL, Maloney W (1993) Effects of hip centre location on the moment generating capacity of the muscles. *J. Biomech.*; **26**: 485–499

Duncan JL (1992) Strain measurement by thermoelastic emission. In: Miles AW, Tanner KE (eds) *Strain Measurement in Biomechanics.* London: Chapman & Hall, pp. 156–168

Dylag Z, Kreczko R, Orlos Z (1964) Photoelastic study of the effect of McMurray osteotomy on the mechanism of work of the hip joint. Bulletin de L'Academie Polonaise Des Sciences; **12**: 281–287

Evans FG, Lissner HR, Pederson HE (1948) Deformation studies of the femur under dynamic vertical loading. *Anat. Rec.*; **101**: 225–241

Fessler H, Fricker DC (1989) A study of stresses in alumina universal heads of femoral prostheses, Proc. Instn. Mech. Engrs. Part H: *J. Engineering in Medicine*; **203**: 1–14

Finlay JB (1992) Photoelastic coating techniques. In: Miles AW, Tanner KE (eds) *Strain Measurement in Biomechanics.* London: Chapman & Hall, pp. 126–138

Finlay JB, Bourne RB, Landsberg RP, Andreae P (1986) Pelvic stresses in vitro-II. A study of the efficacy of metal-backed acetabular prostheses. *J. Biomech.*; **19**: 715–725

Goel VK, Valliappan S, Svensson NL (1978) Stresses in the normal pelvis. *Comput. Biol. Med.*; **8**: 91–104

Hirsch C (1965) Forces in the hip joint – general considerations. In: Kenedi RM (ed.) *Biomechanics and Related Bio-engineering Topics.* Oxford: Pergamon Press, pp. 341–350

Holm NJ (1981) The development of a two dimensional stress-optical model of the Os Coxae. *Acta Orthop. Scand.*; **41**: 608–618

Humpreys PK, Orr JF, Bahrani AS (1990) Testing of total hip replacements: Endurance tests and stress measurements. Part 2: Stress measurements, Proc Instn Mech Engrs, Part H: *J. Engineering in Med.*; **204**: 35–42

Jacob HAC, Huggler AH, Dietschi C, Schreiber A (1976) Mechanical function of subchondral bone as experimentally determined on the acetabulum of the human pelvis. *J. Biomech.*; **9**: 625–627

Johnston RC, Brand RA, Crowninshield RD (1979) Reconstruction of the hip: a mathematical approach to determine optimum geometric relationships. *J. Bone Jt Surg.*; **61A**: 639–652

Kalen R (1961) Strains and stresses in the upper femur studied by the Stresscoat method. *Acta Orthop. Scand.*; **31**: 103–113

Kihara T, Unno M, Kitada C, Kubo H, Nagata, R (1985) Three dimensional stress distribution measurement in a model of the human ankle joint by scattered-light polarizer photoelasticity, Part 1. *Appl. Opt.*; **24**: 3363–3367

Kihara T, Unno M, Kitada C, Kubo H, Nagata R (1987) Three dimensional stress distribution measurement in a model of the human ankle joint by scattered-light polarizer photoelasticity, Part 2. *Appl. Opt.*; **26**: 643–649

Mahoney DP (1995) Rapid prototyping in medicine, Computer Graphics World (February), 42–48

Markolf KL, Amstutz HC (1976) A comparative experimental study of stresses in femoral total hip replacement components: the effects of prosthesis orientation and acrylic fixation. *J. Biomech.*; **9**: 73–79

McCartney J, Hinds BK (1992) Computer aided design of garments using digitized three-dimensional surfaces, Proc Instn Mech Engrs, Part B: *J. Engineering Manufacture*; **206**: 199–206

McLeish R D, Charnley J (1976) Abduction forces in the one-legged stance. *J. Biomech.*; **3**: 191–209

Milch H (1940) Photoelastic studies of bone forms. *J. Bone Jt Surg.*; **22**: 621–626

Miles AW, Tanner KE (1992) Strain Measurement in Biomechanics. London: Chapman & Hall

O'Conner JJ (1992) Load simulation problems in model testing. In: Miles AW, Tanner KE (eds) *Strain Measurement in Biomechanics.* London: Chapman & Hall, pp. 14–38

Oonishi H, Isha H, Hasegawa T (1983) Mechanical analysis of the human pelvis and its application to the artificial hip joint – by means of the three dimensional finite element method. *J. Biomech.*; **16**(6): 427–111

Orr JF (1991) Photoelastic Stress Analysis, Workshop for Strain Measurement in Biomechanics, Canadian Medical and Biological Engineering Society, Ontario, 13–30

Orr JF (1992) Two- and three-dimensional photoelastic techniques. In: Miles AW, Tanner KE (eds) *Strain Measurement in Biomechanics.* London: Chapman & Hall, pp. 109–125

Orr JF, Humphreys PK, James WV, Bahrani AS (1990) The application of photoelastic techniques in orthopaedic engineering. In: Hyde TH, Ollerton E (eds) *Applied Stress Analysis*. London: Elsevier Applied Science, pp. 111–120

Paul JP (1967) Forces at the human hip joint, PhD Thesis, University of Glasgow, UK.

Pauwels F (1980) *Biomechanics of the Locomotor Apparatus*. Berlin: Springer Verlag

Petty MD, Miller GJ, Piotrowski GP (1980) In vitro evaluation of the effect of acetabular prosthesis implantation on the human cadaver pelves. *Bull. Prosthet. Res.*; **17**(1): 80–92

Revie IC (1995) The Manufacture and Evaluation of Custom Acetabular Components or Total Hip Replacement, PhD Thesis, The Queen's University of Belfast, UK.

Rydell NW (1966) Forces acting on the femoral head prosthesis. *Acta Orthop. Scand.*, Supplement 88

Shelton JC (1992) Holographic interferometry. In: Miles AW, Tanner KE (eds) *Strain Measurement in Biomechanics*. London: Chapman & Hall, pp. 139–155

Shrive NG (1991) Measuring strain on soft tissues, The Workshop for Strain Measurement in Biomechanics, Canadian Medical and Biological Engineering Society, Ontario, 87–96

Steen Jensen J (1978a) A photoelastic study of a model of a proximal femur. *Acta Orthop. Scand.*, **49**: 54–59

Steen Jensen J (1978b) A photoelastic study of the hip nail-plate in unstable trochanteric fractures. *Acta Orthop. Scand.*; **49**: 60–64

Williams JF, Svensson NL (1971) An experimental stress analysis of the neck of the femur, *Med. Biol. Engng.*; **9**: 479–493

Zandman F, Redner S, Dally JW (1977) Photoelastic coatings: SESA Monograph No.3, ed. B.E. Rossi, Society for Experimental Stress Analysis, Westport, CT

Chapter 15

Neurophysiological investigations

JA Finnegan

Introduction

Clinical neurophysiology is now routinely used in the investigation of patients but not always to the best effect. This chapter aims to outline the basic principles and applications of particular orthopaedic interest. The investigation is essentially an extension of the clinical examination and is logical and deductive. It demonstrates normality or abnormality at different sites and levels of the nervous system, showing that the problem is confined to one or more individual nerves, or certain nerve roots.

Alternatively, evidence of a more widespread neuromuscular disorder may emerge. The best results are obtained when the clinician has a clear question in mind and has regular contact with the neurophysiologist, results must always be interpreted in the light of the clinical situation.

Basic physiology

Nerve and muscle cells have electrical properties, which are exploited by the neurophysiologist in the assessment and diagnosis of nerve injuries and neuromuscular disorders. The resting electrical potential, maintained by the distribution of ions across the cell membrane, is altered on stimulation and an action potential is generated which travels along the nerve by saltatory conduction. A surface recording electrode, overlying a peripheral nerve records the summated action potentials from all the underlying nerve fibres. Stimulation of a mixed peripheral nerve and recording over an appropriate muscle, allows selective assessment of motor function. Study of exclusively sensory nerves, such as the digital branches of median nerve in the hand or the sural nerve in the leg, provides information specific to sensory fibres.

The latency in milliseconds is the conduction time between the applied electrical stimulus and the recorded nerve or muscle action potential and directly reflects the conduction velocity; the fastest conducting fibres make the earliest contribution to the recorded potential, and the slowest fibres the last. The duration of the potential therefore reflects the range of different conduction velocities shown by nerve fibres of varying diameter. Normal myelination is essential for normal conduction along the fastest fibres.

The amplitude or vertical size of the potential, measured in microvolts or millivolts, is indicative of the number of normal functioning nerve fibres making a contribution to recorded response. Thus a peripheral nerve in which axonal loss has occurred will show potentials of low amplitude but a reasonably normal conduction velocity, while a nerve with significant demyelination with intact axons produces marked slowing of conduction but reasonably normal values for amplitude or area of the recorded potential. In practice, there is commonly a combination of these pathological processes in a particular clinical situation.

In the laboratory, excitation of a peripheral nerve generates an action potential simultaneously conducted with equal facility in both directions from the site of stimulus. The retrograde or antidromic response travels back along motor fibres, and depolarises some anterior horn cells, triggering a further series of motor potentials, recordable as a 'late' response in the relevant muscle. This is called the 'F wave', which occurs about 40–50 ms (in the small muscles of the foot) after motor nerve stimulation at the ankle (Figure 15.1). It usefully reflects both motor neurone function and conduction along the entire length of the nerve, including the proximal and radicular sections inaccessible to direct peripheral stimulation.

The 'H reflex' is another late response occurring after a similar time interval to the F wave but is fundamentally different. It travels along the afferent sensory fibres, entering the cord via the dorsal root and initiating a genuine reflex. It is recordable in normal adults in soleus and sometimes extensor carpi radialis but not usually in other muscles. Like the F wave it may provide information about proximal nerve conduction, particularly at the S1 root level.

Electrophysiological activity within muscle at rest and during voluntary contraction is recorded by a concentric needle electrode. Normal muscle fibres are electrically silent at rest, but generate abnormal spontaneous activity of

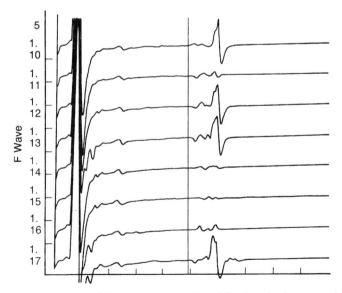

Figure 15.1 F Wave: normal F wave responses at 49 ms following stimulus to posterior tibial nerve at ankle. Note slight variability in timing and form

different kinds after denervation or in certain neuromuscular disorders. Voluntary contraction is initiated and maintained by recruitment of motor units, which is the fundamental electrophysiological event underlying muscle excitation and physical contraction (Figure 15.2). A motor unit is the summated electrical activity of all the individual muscle fibres supplied by a single anterior horn cell (recordable within a radius of about two millimetres around a concentric needle electrode). The system allows continuous grading of muscle contraction by progressively increasing the numbers of recruited motor units and their rate of firing to cope with different physical workloads. The study of motor units involves assessment of their size, morphology, numbers, recruitment pattern and firing rate, it provides useful clinical information.

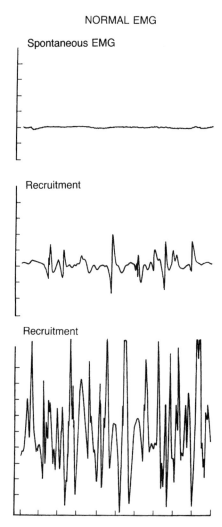

Figure 15.2 Top trace (10 ms/div and 100 μV/div): normal electrical silence at rest. Middle and lower traces (10 ms/div and 250 μV/div): moderate and full motor unit recruitment

Normal and abnormal EMG findings

At rest

Fasciculations are visible clinically, and although commonly benign, especially in fatigue states, may also indicate serious disorder in the peripheral motor system, especially at the level of the motor neurone. They represent abnormal spontaneous discharges of the entire motor unit.

Fibrillations are discharges of individual muscle fibres, not clinically detectable, but recordable only with a concentric needle electrode, and are always pathological (Figure 15.3). They imply a disruption of axonal continuity, and hence indicate denervation, and recovery that will at best be prolonged, and possibly incomplete. Positive sharp waves have the same significance. Spontaneous high frequency discharges of motor units in the resting state are always abnormal and occur in a variety of neuromuscular disorders, typically polymyositis, myotonic muscle disease and some neuropathies.

On voluntary contraction

In a normal muscle there is motor unit recruitment which is appropriate to the subject's effort. At maximum voluntary contraction all available units are recruited and firing at maximum rate, so individual potentials cannot be clearly discerned; the monitor screen is filled with continuous motor unit activity, sometimes referred to as the 'interference pattern' of full recruitment (Figure 15.2). When motor units have been lost, in anterior horn cell disorders, motor neuropathies, or following nerve injury, this full motor unit pattern is replaced, even at maximum effort, by one in which discrete individual units are prominent,

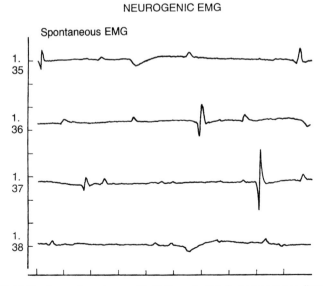

Figure 15.3 EMG: abnormal spontaneous fibrillation potentials in motor neurone disease (10 ms/div and 100 μV/div)

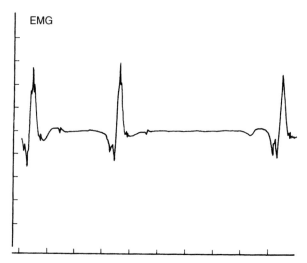

Figure 15.4 EMG: left deltoid. Severely neurogenic pattern. Discrete rapidly firing large motor units in patient with traumatic left brachial plexopathy (10 ms/div and 2mV/div)

and firing rapidly; at the extreme only one or two units will be observed, or even perhaps none at all. Neurogenic motor units are commonly 'polyphasic' containing four or more turns across the baseline, or 'phases'.

In primary muscle disorders, such as myositis or dystrophy, the muscle fibres are diseased or disordered but normally innervated. The motor unit pattern produced by voluntary muscle contraction shows normal numbers of motor units but of highly abnormal morphology; they are characteristically of low amplitude, brief duration and polyphasic (Figure 15.5). In fact, because of the poor physiological capacity of these fibres, motor unit recruitment often needs to be greatly increased to achieve even a weak physical effort, producing a surprisingly 'full' motor unit pattern in this situation.

Disuse atrophy shows entirely normal EMG findings, at rest and on voluntary contraction. Patients with non-organic or functional muscle weakness show normal motor unit morphology and recruitment, the latter fluctuating in keeping with the patient's uneven voluntary effort. In the presence of upper motor neurone pyramidal lesions, motor unit recruitment is reduced but with a low firing rate of individual units, in contrast to the rapidly firing neurogenic motor units with a lower motor neurone or peripheral nerve problem.

Evoked potentials

An evoked potential is an electrophysiologial potential, recorded in brain or spinal cord, following an external stimulus. Visual or auditory evoked potentials are of limited interest in orthopaedic practice but somatosensory evoked potentials, obtained by electrical stimulation of a peripheral nerve, are often of relevance. In all cases the evoked potential demonstrates the integrity of the connections between the external sensation and the highest levels of the neuraxis,

MYOPATHY

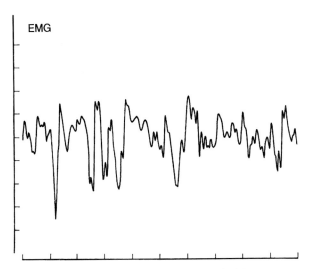

Figure 15.5 EMG: myositis: note abnormal small motor units of brief duration and highly polyphasic (10 ms/div and 500 μV/div)

such as the spinal cord, brain stem, or cerebral cortex, providing information about damage or dysfunction along peripheral or central afferent pathways. This includes neurological deficits at cervical or lumbosacral radicular level, obviously of orthopaedic interest. Somatosensory evoked potentials are continuously monitored during spinal deformity surgery and provide reassurance of continual normal function as the correction proceeds, or an early warning of impending danger to the cord.

Pathology and neurophysiology

Diverse traumatic and medical conditions result in similar pathological changes in peripheral nerves, those of axonal degeneration and demyelination. Although in some disorders one or other of these pathological processes predominates, in practice the two commonly coexist, and each may be secondary to the other, reflecting the interdependence between the Schwann cells, from which the myelin sheath is derived and underlying neurones and their axons.

Wallerian degeneration indicates disruption of axonal conduction, whether or not the nerve is transected or merely severely crushed or stretched. Medical disorders or toxic effects on the cell body or axon may initiate the same process by disruption of axonal transport mechanisms. In this latter situation, predictably it is the longest axons serving the extremities which fail first, underlying the 'dying back' or 'glove and stocking' neuropathy. Wallerian degeneration and fibre loss is signalled by low amplitude nerve action potentials and the characteristic electromyographic abnormalities of fibrillation potentials and motor unit loss in the affected muscles. Demyelination results in gross slowing of nerve conduction velocity.

Penetrating knife or gunshot wounds, which injure nerves, will inevitably lead to transection of the nerve bundle or at least some fascicles and hence Wallerian degeneration. This may also arise, however, from acute severe compression by adjacent fractures, dislocations or haematoma if the pressure is sufficiently intense or prolonged; with less severe injury the damage may well be restricted to a neuropraxia. In practice, such blunt trauma or pressure injury will result in damage of varying degrees of severity in the individual component fibres of the nerve bundle, some showing mild neuropraxia, others with complete axonal disruption, and the recovery of function will be appropriately graded and variable.

If nerve stimulation above the lesion results in any recordable compound muscle action potential (CMAP) in the relevant muscle, some axons are obviously conducting. Similarly if electromyography in that muscle shows any motor units at all under voluntary control, axons must be conducting. If there is no such neurophysiological evidence that some fibres at least are conducting, one cannot distinguish, initially, between a nerve bundle that is physically transected and one which remains in continuity but which is so badly damaged as to prevent any electrophysiological conduction or motor unit recruitment. Repeating the studies in a few weeks may be informative; if there has been no improvement the suspicion will increase that the nerve has been divided, assuming that this is clinically a reasonable possibility.

Chronic localised entrapment produces lesser degrees of the same pathological and neurophysiological abnormalities. Localised demyelination causes local difficulty in exciting the nerve and slowing of conduction velocity across the damaged segment. A local conduction block may also be revealed by a low amplitude compound muscle action potential on stimulation proximal to the lesion, and higher amplitude CMAP distal to the lesion.

Neurological disorders

Patients with muscle weakness and wasting, posture and walking difficulties, are often referred to orthopaedic clinics and ultimately are shown to have an underlying neurological disorder. They can usually be distinguished by clinical assessment and neurophysiological investigation.

Neuralgic amyotrophy or brachial neuritis has many other synonyms, and is usually easily recognised from the clinical picture of acute severe shoulder girdle pain, followed by wasting of shoulder and upper arm muscles. Less commonly, the pain and weakness is in the distribution of a single peripheral nerve in the upper limb, such as the anterior or posterior interosseous. Routine nerve conduction studies are often normal, except for some reduction in action potential amplitude; however, a more selective study of proximal nerve conduction in the upper limb may be more rewarding. There is EMG evidence of denervation in the appropriate muscles.

Painless wasting of shoulder or hip girdle muscles may indicate limb girdle muscular dystrophy. This term has now fallen out of favour in the light of genetic advances which have shown a variety of dystrophic syndromes of autosomal dominant or recessive or X-linked inheritance. There is weakness in scapulo-humeral, scapuloperoneal, or facioscapularhumeral distribution. There may well be a family history. Nerve conduction studies are normal and there will be typical myopathic EMG abnormalities.

Painful restriction of shoulder movements and upper arm pain are common problems, particularly in the elderly, and have various causes. Polymyalgia rheumatica usually has normal motor and sensory nerve conduction studies and EMG. Proximal muscle tenderness and weakness due to myositis has marked EMG abnormalities; at rest there may be abnormal spontaneous high frequency pseudomyotonic discharges, fibrillations and positive sharp waves, attributed to involvement of terminal nerve endings in the inflammatory process. On voluntary contraction the motor unit pattern is typical of primary muscle disease (see above). Cervical radiculopathy may be indicated by abnormalities of the tendon reflexes and appropriate sensory loss. The routine nerve conduction studies are usually normal, although this is often useful information, excluding a separate peripheral nerve entrapment with paraesthesiae in arm or hand. There are neurogenic EMG abnormalities in the appropriate muscles. Cervical spine evoked potentials may be abnormal, but are usually normal in patients with cervical radicular pain but no physical signs. All these conditions may be complicated by a painful restrictive pericapsulitis or 'frozen shoulder'.

Asymmetric weakness in the arm or leg is sometimes due to motor neurone disease. Important clinical features are intact sensation, some additional upper motor neurone findings, the onset of bulbar symptoms, and visible muscle fasciculations. Nerve conduction studies show evidence of motor fibre loss but essentially normal conduction velocity. The F waves are absent or infrequent, and highly stereotyped in appearance, reflecting the diminished spinal motor neurone pool. Sensory nerve conduction studies are of course normal. EMG shows spontaneous fibrillation potentials and fascicultations, and on contraction there are discrete, high amplitude 'neurogenic' motor units. Typically the onset of motor neurone disease is in middle or later life; there is a paediatric equivalent, spinal muscular atrophy, with similar neurophysiological findings, reflecting the degeneration of anterior horn cells. Old poliomyelitis infection is another cause of such neurophysiological findings but with a static rather than progressive clinical course. Wasting of the small hand muscles, with the classical dissociated sensory loss, strongly suggests syringomyelia and magnetic resonance imaging should reveal the typical changes within the cord. Nerve conduction studies will show evidence of motor and sensory fibre loss, but normal velocities, and no evidence of any peripheral nerve entrapment to explain the clinical appearance. EMG of the affected muscles confirms the central neurogenic atrophy and denervation.

The thoracic outlet syndrome is another cause of hand paraesthesiae and muscle wasting, more commonly in the thenar rather than hypothenar muscles. It may therefore be confused with the carpal tunnel syndrome, except that the sensory disturbance in thoracic outlet syndrome is commonly in the medial forearm and fifth finger, reflecting involvement of the medial cord of the plexus. Radiology may show bony abnormality such as a cervical rib. Neurophysiology is very helpful, showing normal median sensory nerve conduction studies, with median motor fibre loss and ulnar sensory action potential abnormalities. A histamine flare test, comparing the responses from each arm may also be useful.

Nerve entrapment

Symptoms referable to an individual peripheral nerve are commonly encountered in orthopaedic practice, often in the expectation that they arise from a localised irritation or mechanical entrapment. Indeed this is often the case; particularly so for some obvious and well-known peripheral nerves but also in some more obscure entrapments. However, it should be remembered that individual peripheral nerve syndromes sometimes have a non-mechanical cause, for example mononeuritis, rather than a simple localised compression, remediable by surgical treatment.

Nerve entrapments typically present with symptoms of pain and parasthesiae in the relevant distribution, often provoked or exacerbated by prolonged activity or repetitive movements of the appropriate part. There may be sensory loss and weakness and wasting of supplied muscles. The underlying pathology is localised demyelination followed by axonal loss distal to the compression. Nerve conduction studies by this stage are always abnormal. Definite symptoms are often present before any obvious clinical physical signs, or neurophysiological abnormality. Much depends on the underlying cause and pathology; for example symptoms aggravated by fluid retention or endocrine effects in women with carpal tunnel syndrome, or associated with certain postures or positions of limbs may be transient and fluctuating, and commonly neurophysiological studies in these situations are normal. They are likely to remain so until some underlying structural disruption of nerve fibres occurs leading to fibre loss and conduction delay.

Conversely, subclinical neurophysiological abnormalities may be present with few troublesome symptoms, especially in some less perceptive patients, or those who have engaged in heavy manual work, sustaining repeated hand trauma, and sometimes the elderly. Localised peripheral nerve damage, such as osteophyte formation or post-Colles fracture, is much more likely to occur adjacent to some anatomical derangement.

The essentials for diagnosis of a single peripheral nerve lesion are appropriate symptoms and physical signs and the demonstration by nerve conduction studies that the abnormalities are confined to a single peripheral nerve, hence excluding a more widespread systemic peripheral nerve disorder. For convincing demonstration of a localised physical entrapment, ideally one should further demonstrate that the neurophysiological abnormalities are confined to one precise section of nerve, for example the ulnar nerve at the elbow, with normal conduction and function proximal and distal to this site.

Median nerve

The carpal tunnel is the commonest site of entrapment and the syndrome of nocturnal acroparasthesiae should be confirmed by nerve conduction studies. These should demonstrate a prolonged distal motor latency in the median nerve on stimulation at the wrist, recording the common muscle action potential (CMAP) in abductor pollicis brevis relative to the normal ulnar distal motor latency between the wrist and abductor digiti minimi (Figure 15.6). Sensory action potentials will be of low amplitude and careful study will reveal specific slowing of sensory conduction velocity in the transcarpal segment of the median nerve, compared with the digit to mid-palm segment. Some patients with convincing symptoms will have normal nerve conduction studies, typically in those patients whose symptoms are transient and associated with reversible factors such as fluid retention. Compression of the exclusively motor anterior interosseous branch of the median nerve proximally in the forearm shows a striking clinical picture, with selective inability to flex the terminal phalanges of first and

CARPAL TUNNEL SYNDROME

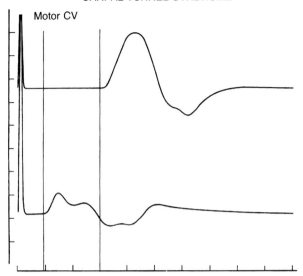

Figure 15.6 Carpal tunnel syndrome: top trace (2 ms/div and 2.5 mV/div): stimulation of median nerve at wrist recording from abductor pollicis brevis: prolonged motor latency at 6.0 ms. Carpal tunnel syndrome: lower trace (2 ms/div and 2.5 mV/div): ulnar stimulation in same hand as a control with normal distal motor latency of 2.0 ms

second digits. This is due to denervation in the flexor digitorum profundus, which can be confirmed electromyographically. Conduction in the main trunk of the median nerve is normal, however, and since this innervates abductor pollicis brevis electromyography in that muscle is normal, as are the sensory action potentials.

The median nerve is rarely trapped around the elbow, either by the heads of pronator terres or by the ligament of Struthers. With entrapment at this latter site, just above the elbow, EMG will show denervation in pronator terres. When the entrapment is between the two heads of this muscle, however, the innervation to the muscle itself, and its electromyographic findings, are usually normal. These more obscure median nerve entrapments, causing forearm pain and denervation, must be distinguished from neuralgic amyotrophy.

Ulnar nerve

The common site for ulnar nerve entrapments is the cubital tunnel. Nerve conduction studies are essential for confident distinction between peripheral entrapment and more proximal lesions at brachial plexus or C8–T1 radicular level. Typically neurophysiological studies will show localised slowing of motor conduction velocity in that segment of nerve crossing the elbow. A conduction block at this site will cause a significant reduction in amplitude of the compound muscle action potential in abductor digiti minimi on stimulation above the elbow, compared with better nerve function below the elbow. Absent or low amplitude sensory action potentials from the fifth finger to the wrist indicate distal degeneration. Stimulation of the ulnar nerve at the wrist evokes an absent or reduced mixed nerve action potential above the elbow.

This contrasts with ulnar nerve compression in the canal of Guyon at the wrist, when the ulnar mixed nerve action potential between the wrist and elbow is normal, as is electromyography in the ulnar supplied forearm muscles, since they receive their innervation proximal to the lesion, and hence are spared.

Trauma to the hand can cause a palsy of the exclusively motor deep palmar branch. Neurophysiological studies will show normal distal motor latency from wrist to abductor digiti minimi, which is not involved, but prolonged latency and abnormal compound muscle action potential in first dorsal interosseous muscle which is denervated. Sensory action potentials are normal.

Femoral nerve

This may be damaged by femoral fractures or haematoma, among other local causes, or may be involved in diabetic mononeuritis, formerly called diabetic amyotrophy. One sees the appropriate clinical weakness of hip flexion and knee extension and electromyographic evidence of denervation in quadriceps. Nerve conduction studies show especial difficulty in excitation of the femoral nerve at the inguinal ligament, with slowing of conduction and an abnormal and dispersed compound muscle action potential.

Radial nerve

With injury at the spiral groove of humerus the nerve is difficult to excite at this point and there may be EMG abnormalities in the wrist extensors, possibly a guide to prognosis. When the nerve is damaged at the level of the supinator tunnel, another distinctive syndrome is seen with a deficit confined to the exclusively motor posterior interosseous branch. Here there is normal function in triceps and brachioradialis. Weakness and EMG denervation is much more obvious in extensor carpi ulnaris than extensor carpi radialis. The preserved radial sensory action potentials are preserved.

Nerve injuries

The sciatic nerve is occasionally injured during hip or vascular surgery and the common peroneal component usually predominates in its clinical effects over damage to the posterior tibial portion. The patients often present with a foot drop and neurophysiological investigation is helpful in distinguishing between a palsy of the common peroneal nerve at the knee and a higher lesion at sciatic level. This is achieved by demonstrating electromyographic abnormalities above the knee in the hamstring muscles, as well as in more distal muscles which are not supplied by the common peroneal nerve, indicating a lesion above the division of the sciatic into common peroneal and posterior tibial branches. In this situation the common peroneal nerve shows normal excitability at the knee and normal motor conduction velocity across the knee, although fibre loss may cause a reduced amplitude compound muscle action potential without any conduction block across this site.

This contrasts with a lesion at the knee, in which abnormalities are confined to the common peroneal nerve, or one of its divisions, the anterior tibial or superficial peroneal branches. There is a reduction in motor conduction velocity in the section of the nerve crossing the knee, compared with the knee to ankle segment. The nerve is difficult or impossible to excite at the knee. A conduction block may be indicated by a lower amplitude compound muscle action potential on stimulation above the knee compared with stimulation below. Spontaneous fibrillation potentials and neurogenic discrete motor units are evident in the anterior tibial muscles. Much information may be obtained by stimulation at the knee and observing the resultant clinical twitch should one occur. If there is eversion of the foot, without dorsiflexion, the abnormality is likely to be chiefly in the anterior tibial branch, with relative preservation of the superficial peroneal. Less commonly the opposite situation is seen.

Brachial plexopathy and cervical root avulsion

Dislocations of the shoulder disrupt surrounding nerves to individual muscles such as the deltoid, or the brachial plexus trunks with consequences down the upper limb. Nerve conduction shows loss of motor and sensory fibres and there is electromyographic denervation in relevant muscles (Figure 15.7). Severe traction injuries or neck trauma may cause avulsion of intraspinal roots from the cord; they are fragile in this pre-ganglionic section in comparison to the post-ganglionic fibres and the damage is permanent and beyond treatment. In the rare event of this occurring without coexisting plexus damage, there is a curious paradox, of clinical sensory loss with intact sensory action potentials, which arises because the lesion is proximal to the dorsal root ganglion .

BRACHIAL PLEXUS EVOKED POTENTIALS

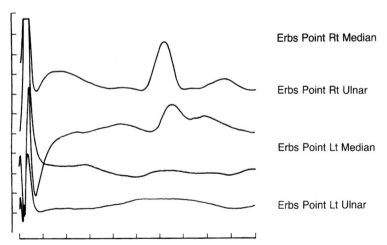

Erbs Point Rt Median

Erbs Point Rt Ulnar

Erbs Point Lt Median

Erbs Point Lt Ulnar

Figure 15.7 Brachial plexus evoked potentials: same patient as in Figure 15.4. Stimulation of right and left median and ulnar nerves at the wrist, recording from Erb's point. Absent responses on left (1 ms/div and 10 µV/div)

Peripheral neuropathies

The many causes of systemic generalised failure of cells in the peripheral nervous system result in the familiar pathological processes of axonal failure and demyelination. Although in many neuropathies one or other of these is prominent, the two commonly occur together. General disturbances such as metabolic disorders and the toxic effects of drugs or other chemicals or hypoxia may act either on the neuronal cell body or axon and lead to axonal degeneration. This is encountered in those neuropathies with a prominent vascular or vasculitic component or in the so-called critically ill polyneuropathy sometimes found in patients after several weeks on an intensive care unit. In contrast, acute demyelination is encountered in the acute post-infectious neuropathies (Guillain–Barré syndrome), while chronic demyelination is a feature of some hereditary motor and sensory neuropathies.

Peripheral neuropathy conditions have been greatly clarified by neurophysiological studies. The heterogeneous condition formerly known as peroneal muscular atrophy (Charcot–Marie–Tooth syndrome) has been classified into those in which the upper limb motor conduction velocity is severely reduced to below 30 metres per second and those of essentially normal conduction velocity. A further subclassification on the basis of underlying pathology and genetics can be made. Such patients commonly have pes cavus and may therefore present to orthopaedics clinics.

In all cases the diagnosis of peripheral neuropathy depends on the demonstration of widespread abnormalities, which may often be present when the clinical signs or symptoms are subtle or absent. Conduction velocities will indicate whether the neuropathy is one of significant demyelination or chiefly axonal degeneration, or whether the brunt of the pathological process is chiefly motor or sensory or mixed and whether its expression is predominantly distal or proximal.

There is a fall-off of peripheral nerve function with advancing age so that many patients in late life may have electrophysiological evidence of a peripheral neuropathy.

The distinction between lumbosacral radicular syndromes and peripheral neuropathy may be a little complicated, particularly in those neuropathies which are commonly expressed in an asymmetric distribution, such as those associated with collagen vascular or microangiopathic causes. There may be a mononeuritis multiplex overlying a background peripheral neuropathy. Neurophysiology may help in this distinction. Clearly, the presence of neurophysiological abnormalities in the upper limbs indicates a systemic peripheral nerve disorder rather than a localised lumbosacral radicular syndrome. Conversely, well preserved or normal amplitude sural sensory action potentials in the lower limbs is evidence against a significant peripheral nerve disorder, particularly in later life.

Lumbosacral radiculopathy

Somatosensory evoked potential studies may contribute to the assessment of patients with lumbosacral syndromes (Finnegan, 1986). Specifically, a stimulus applied over an area of skin subserved by a particular dermatome is followed by a cortical evoked potential which should be reasonably symmetrical in latency and amplitude between the right and left legs (Figure 15.8). The technique should be regarded as complementary to magnetic resonance imaging. These evoked potentials are better at reflecting loss of function than identifying a precise root level. They are sometimes useful, however, in demonstrating normal neurological function in a patient with a pain syndrome who may therefore be reassured or they may serve as a useful baseline for any deterioration as the patient is followed up.

Monitoring of spinal cord function during scoliosis surgery

Evoked potential techniques now play an important part in spinal deformity surgery in the hope that the surgeon may be provided with useful information about any deteriorating cord function during the correction phase of the surgery. This has become rather more important with the more ambitious and aggressive corrections which have become commonplace in recent years. In this way the small but tragic incidence of paraplegia or serious neurological disability following such surgery may be significantly reduced or abolished (MacEwan *et al.*, 1975; Jones *et al.*, 1982).

The best established technique involves stimulation of the posterior tibial nerves at knee or ankle throughout the surgical procedure, monitoring the evoked potential as it travels up the spinal cord, across the operation site, and hence up to the cortex. The most useful technique is recording the spinal potential via an electrode in the epidural space, inserted by the surgeon one or two segments above the levels of his fixation. This produces a stable potential which is not

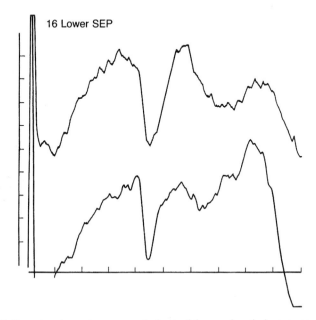

Figure 15.8 Dermatomal somatosensory evoked potential: normal cortical responses at 44 ms following stimulation of right and left lumbar L5 dermatomes (10 ms/div and 400 nV/div)

significantly affected by anaesthetic factors, unlike the cortical potential which can be greatly affected by anaesthetic agents and hypotension. The spinal epidural response typically contains at least three clearly definable peaks and these reflect conduction in afferent spinal tracts, conducting at different velocities (Figure 15.9). The first peak is attributed to activity in the spinocerebellar tract and the second to conduction in the dorsal columns. A sudden deterioration in the potential with loss of one or more peaks usually suggests some potential threat to the spinal cord and the surgeon can then be informed. Traditionally, a 50% fall in amplitude of the epidural response from the baseline potential obtained before any instrumentation or distraction is regarded as significant. There is now increasing evidence, however, that a drop in amplitude of 20–30% correlates with increasing incidence of neurological damage and in some centres these lower levels are taken as significant (Forbes *et al.*, 1991). It is essential to go on monitoring for at least 20–30 min after the completion of the correction because some cord damage will only become detectable after this period of time. Occasional 'false negatives' reported in the literature in which evoked potentials have failed to detect cord damage have possibly occurred because monitoring has stopped too early (Daube, 1989). Conversely, the term 'false positive' requires some clarification and will depend on the kind of neurological problem or impairment one regards as significant. The more closely one looks for neurological abnormalities following such surgery, the clearer it becomes that their incidence increases with even modest deterioration in the amplitude of the spinal epidural potential (Harrison, 1990). Often such deficits are minor and transient but they are nevertheless betrayed by the sensitive technique. If the outcome is judged merely in terms of crude motor and sensory function in the lower limbs then it is true that some patients have abnormal evoked responses during surgery but crudely 'normal' neurological function in the legs afterwards.

In all cases it is essential to obtain a series of baseline recordings before that part of the operation which may threaten cord function. These potentials then become the standard by which further recordings are judged (Figure 15.10).

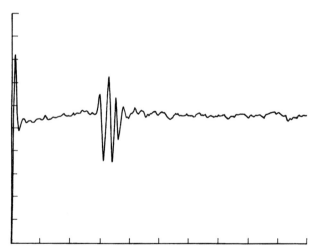

Figure 15.9 Normal spinal epidural evoked potential (5 ms/div and 0.3 μV/div)

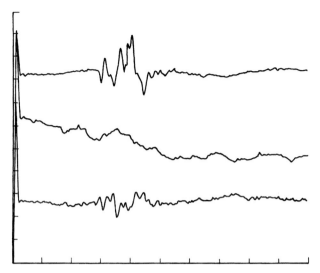

Figure 15.10 Spinal monitoring: top trace shows pre-correction baseline. Middle trace shows loss of potentials during distraction of spinal instrumentation. Lower trace shows return of modified waveform after slight alteration in instrumentation (5 ms/div and 0.62 μV/div)

Who should monitor and interpret the trace?

It is essential that an experienced neurophysiological technician, experienced in evoked potential work, is present to manage the formidable technical problems involved in recording in the electronically rather hostile atmosphere of the operating theatre. They should have sufficient confidence and seniority to be able to provide useful and reliable data to the surgeon. Ideally a clinical neuro-physiologist should be on hand to interpret the data either directly or indirectly, perhaps via a video or computer link. If no such person is present then clearly the orthopaedic surgeon must assume even more responsibility and should have some understanding of the neurophysiological data. In these circumstances it is essential to establish a detailed protocol between the surgeon and the neuro-physiology technician beforehand and the surgeon will need to feel confident that the data is accurate and the technique sensitive to impending cord damage.

Conclusion

Neurophysiology provides valuable data, sometimes quantitative, refining diagnosis and prognosis, or monitoring a changing situation. When the clinician has an awareness of its uses and limitations it becomes an essential component of orthopaedic assessment and research.

References

Daube JR (1989) Intraoperative monitoring by evoked potentials for spinal cord surgery: the pros. *J. Electrorencephalogr. Clin. Neurophysiol.*; **73**: 374–377

Finnegan JA (1986) In: Hukins DWL, Mulholland RC (eds) *Neurophysiological Assessment of Lumbo-Sacral Lesions in Back Pain*. Manchester: Manchester University Press, pp. 113–148

Forbes HJ, Allen PW, Waller CS, Jones SJ, Edgar MA, Webb PJ, Ransford AO (1991) Spinal cord monitoring in scoliosis surgery: experience with 1168 cases. *J. Bone Jt Surg.*; **73B**: 487–491

Harrison CA (1990) Monitoring of spinal cord function during scoliosis surgery. *J. Electrophysiol. Technol.*; **16**: 69–88

Jones SJ, Edgar MA, Ransford AO (1982) Sensory nerve conduction in the human spinal cord: epidural recordings made during scoliosis surgery. *J. Neurol. Neurosurg. Psychiatry*; **45[5]**: 446

MacEwan GD, Bunnell WP, Sriram K (1975) Acute neurological complications in the treatment of scoliosis: a report on the scoliosis research society. *J. Bone Jt Surg.*; **57A**: 404–408

Further reading

General

Aids to the Examination of the Peripheral Nervous System. Baillere, 1986

Kimura J (1989) *Electrodiagnosis in Diseases of Nerve and Muscle*. Philadelphia: F.A. Davies

Thomas PK, Dyck PJ (1993) *Peripheral Neuropathy*. London: W.B. Saunders

Spinal monitoring

Finnegan JA (1993) *Spinal Cord Monitoring During Scoliosis Surgery; Techniques and Applications*. Instructional video: Birmingham Neuroscience Centre, Queen Elizabeth Hospital, Birmingham, UK

Harrison CA (1990) Monitoring of spinal cord function during scoliosis surgery. *J. Electrophysiol. Technol.*; **16**: 69–88

Jones SJ *et al.* (1982) Sensory nerve conduction in the human spinal cord: epidural recording during scoliosis surgery. *J. Neurol. Neurosurg. Psychiatry*; **45**: 446

Somatosensory evoked potentials

Finnegan JA (1986) In: Hukins DWL, Mulholland RC (eds) *Neurophysiological Assessment of Lumbo-sacral Lesions in Back Pain*. Manchester: Manchester University Press, pp. 133–148

Nuwer M (1986) *Evoked Potential Monitoring in the Operating Room*. Philadelphia: Raven Press

Chapter 16

Bone density measurement

(*Methods and interpretation*)

R Smith

Introduction

The development of methods for the measurement of so-called bone density has been a useful advance in the clinical management of bone disease, especially since the amount of bone is the major determinant of its strength and, therefore, closely related to the likelihood of fracture. It is important to understand both the limitations and the advantages of bone densitometry methods. In order to do this we need to first consider briefly the composition, biology and structure of bone, second to review the changes which occur with age and lastly, to analyse the relationship between bone density and fracture. The main application of bone density measurement is related to the diagnosis, prevention and management of osteoporosis (Chatterton, 1993; Ross, 1993; Kanis *et al.,* 1994; Compston *et al.,* 1995; Hassager and Christiansen, 1995).

Bone biology

Bone tissue consists of a mineralised organic matrix in which hydroxyapatite is laid down on a regularly arranged fibrous structure composed of type I collagen. The strength of this structure and hence its resistance to fracture depends on the amount of both components and on the bone architecture. Poorly mineralised bone, as in osteomalacia, is weak, as is also bone with a defective matrix, as in osteogenesis imperfecta. However, an increase in the amount of mineralised bone does not necessarily increase its strength; a familiar example is fluoride-treated bone which is over-mineralised but weak. Bone tissue is constantly being removed and replaced by the activity of its bone cells, the osteoclasts and osteoblasts, respectively. This constant activity, which is more in the young skeleton than the old, repairs micro-architectural defects and provides a mechanism for laying down bone along lines of mechanical stress. It is the imbalance between osteoclast and osteoblast activity in favour of bone resorption which leads to bone loss with increasing years. Although age is the most frequent cause of bone loss, there are numerous situations such as corticosteroid excess, prolonged immobility and lack of sex hormone where bone loss is excessive in young adults. This is referred to as secondary rather than idiopathic or primary osteoporosis.

Bone structure

Structurally, bone is of two main types, trabecular or spongy and cortical. Trabecular bone occurs predominantly in the axial skeleton, the vertebral bodies and also in the femoral neck whereas the peripheral bones are largely cortical. Trabecular bone is metabolically more active than cortical and the changes in its amount and measured density occur more rapidly. This is seen particularly in the spine after the menopause and also in various secondary forms of osteoporosis particularly that associated with corticosteroid therapy.

Age-related changes in the skeleton

From infancy the size of the skeleton increases and so does the amount of calcium within it. Increase in size ceases after adolescence and amongst the last bones to stop growing are those of the vertebrae. Peak bone mass (as assessed by the amount of calcium in the skeleton) is achieved by the age of 30 and is less in women than in men. Subsequently bone is lost at a constant rate in both sexes but with a period of acceleration in the first 10 post-menopausal years. Late adult bone loss and increasing bone fragility is a constant process and contributes to the increasing tendency to fracture. The so-called fracture threshold (or range) defines a bone density below which fracture is likely. A diagram of these changes and their relevance to osteoporosis management (see below) is shown in Figure 16.1.

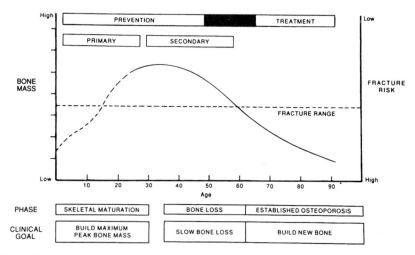

Figure 16.1 Changes in bone mass with age and their relevance to osteoporosis and fracture. Peak bone mass, attained by 30 years, is determined by genetic, nutritional and mechanical factors. The subsequent decrease in bone mass contributes to an increase in fracture rate. This figure emphasises the possibilities for prevention (primary and secondary) and for treatment of bone loss. In practice prevention and treatment can be regarded as continuous. The horizontal dotted line labelled fracture range indicates a value of bone mass below which fractures become more frequent. This is the same as the theoretical fracture threshold (Figure 16.3) (from Ross, 1993, with permission)

Bone density

The amount of bone is in practice measured by the amount of calcium it contains, since it is the mineral component of bone tissue which provides the image on the radiographs and is responsible for the absorption of photons, either from radio-isotope or X-ray sources. Ultrasound measurements can also give some idea of structure and quantitative computed tomography can measure a true volumetric bone density. Otherwise bone density is most often expressed as gcm^{-2} which is an area, not a volumetric, measurement.

Bone densitometry methods

For convenience, the methods used to measure the amount of bone may be divided into those which use a single or dual X-ray source (DXA) and those which do not. The reason for this division is that machines utilising X-ray absorptiometry (SXA) have overtaken previous techniques and work on osteo-porosis is now widely based on their use (Table 16.1). No method is yet ideal for measuring bone mineral density (BMD) but modern machines come close to it. The ideal BMD method should be accurate and reflect the true bone mass; be reproducible both in the short and long term (to allow serial measurements to be made); be acceptable to the patient and have safe levels of radiation.

Non-X-ray methods

These include conventional radiographs, radiogrammetry, quantitative absorptio-metric methods using radio-isotopes, neutron activation analysis and ultrasound. Severe osteoporosis was first recognised radiographically but it became widely accepted that bone loss could not be detected by this means until it had reached about 40%. Radiogrammetic measures included cortical thickness, which has been of considerable use in the past (Meema and Meema, 1972) and the Singh index which is related to the number and distribution of trabeculae in the femoral neck (Singh *et al.*, 1970). Radiographic photodensitometry attempts to compare radiographic density with controls such as aluminium step wedges (Chatterton, 1993).

Neutron activation analysis has also been used to give an idea of the amount of calcium within the body, but it is expensive and complex and exposes the patient to significant radiation. By contrast, ultrasound methods are relatively simple and give an estimate of the structure as well as the density of bone. When sound traverses the interfaces between bone and soft tissue it is scattered and attenuated. The more interfaces there are, the greater the loss of intensity, and in cancellous bone the amount of attenuation is an index of the amount of bone present. The velocity of sound is also much greater in bone than in soft tissues and this velocity also indicates the amount of bone present. Instruments have now been constructed to measure both the broad-band attenuation of ultrasound waves and the velocity of propagation. These are most applicable to peripheral bones and a reasonable correlation between the results obtained by ultrasound and by other non-invasive methods for BMD has been demonstrated (Baran *et al.*, 1991). It is likely that ultrasound will have a greater application in the future; one particular advantage is that it does not involve ionising radiation and another

Table 16.1 Advantages and disadvantages of methods of measuring bone mass

Method	Sites	Percentage of trabecular bone	Precision (%)	Accuracy (%)	Dosage	Comments
Radiogrammetry	Metacarpal and others	N/A	5-10	5-8	Low	Cortical bone only
Radiographic photodensitometry	Various sites	Various	2-5	5-10	Low	Many possible errors
Neutron activation analysis	Whole body	20	2-3	4-5	High	Requires facilities for simultaneous irradiation and detection
	Part body	Various	2-5	3-4	High	
Quantitative computed tomography	Axial	100	4-6	5-15	High	Can select entirely trabecular sites. Measures true volumetric bone density
	Appendicular		1	5-15		
Single photon absorptiometry (SPA)	Forearm (distal and mid radius)	5-60	1-3	5-8	Low	Limited by positioning errors. Replaceable isotope source
	Calcaneus	90	2-3	5-8	Low	
Single energy X-ray absorptiometry (SXA)	Forearm (distal and mid radius)	5-60	0.5-1	5-8	Low	
	Calcaneus	90	0.5-1	5-8	Low	
Dual photon absorptiometry (DPA)	Lumbar spine	70	1-3	4-8	Low	Influenced by soft tissue variation. Replaceable isotope sources
	Proximal femur	75	3-5	4-8	Low	
	Whole body	20	1-2	8-10	Low	
Dual energy X-ray (DEXA, DXA)	Lumbar spine (AP)		<1.0	4-8	Low	Dual X-ray, not isotope source
	Lumbar spine (lateral)		2-5	4-8	Low	
	Proximal femur		2-3	4-8	Low	
	Whole body		<1.0	8-10	Low	
Ultrasound	Calcaneus	90	2-6	Not Established	None	Can give information on structure

is the additional information about architecture and hence indirectly strength. However, broad band ultrasound (BUA) cannot be used to accurately predict axial BMD measured by DXA (Young *et al.*, 1993).

Quantitative absorptiometric methods

The following remarks apply whether the source is a radioactive isotope or X-rays. There is an absolute mathematical relationship between the attenuation of electromagnetic radiation and the quantity of material in its path. In earlier machines the source of the ionising radiation was generally a radio-isotope such as iodine 125, americium 240 or gadolinium 153. Radiation from these sources is confined to a narrow energy band, or two narrow bands in the case of gadolinium and it requires only a simple mathematical model to measure the amount of bone mineral present. Recently technological difficulties with the stability of electronics which supply power to X-ray tubes and the generation and detection of two energies of X-rays simultaneously, have been solved. The dominant technology now uses X-rays as the radiation source; other instruments include single photon absorptiometry, dual photon absorptiometry using isotope sources and a variety of computed tomographic techniques.

Single photon absorptiometry (SPA)
In SPA the procedure relies on rectilinear scanning with a finely collimated radioactive iodine source across a peripheral bone. Background soft tissue correction is made by surrounding the extremity in a soft tissue equivalent, such as a water bath. The calculation is only valid for a two-component model (of bone and water-equivalent soft tissue). A favoured site for SPA is the forearm, measuring either mid-forearm, distal forearm or ultra-distal forearm. There is progressively more cancellous bone in each of these sites. In careful hands the technique should have a reproducibility approaching 1% (Peel and Eastell, 1993).

Dual photon absorptiometry (DPA)
Initially radio-isotopes were used as the sources in dual photon instruments. Mathematically, it transpires that to resolve more tissue components than SPA *in vivo,* a knowledge of the attenuation of a greater number of photon images is needed. In addition, it is not practical to immerse or to surround non-peripheral parts of patients with tissue equivalents. To resolve the three components of soft tissue, fat and bone mineral, at least two photon energies are needed. For DPA the isotope source is gadolinium which has two different photon energies (44 and 100 KeV).

Quantitative computed tomography (QCT)
This X-ray based technique QCT can distinguish between cortical and trabecular bone. Since the sources and detector are rotated around the area of interest, it is possible to focus on a specific volume of bone and therefore to measure a true volumetric BMD. This has been particularly applied to the spine where there is a close correlation between QCT estimated density and vertebral fracture. However, sampling errors can lead to poor reproducibility.

X-ray absorptiometry
Single energy X-ray absorptiometry (SXA) is now available for peripheral (forearm) bone density measurements, compared with SPA, the source is constant and does not need replacing.

Dual energy X-ray absoptiometry (DEXA or DXA)
DXA has the advantage over DPA in not requiring a replaceable isotope source. The X-ray beam may be more highly collimated and the precision is better than DPA. The procedure is faster and the radiation dose less. Methods used for producing and detecting the radiation differ from one machine to another. Thus some machines produce two energies of X-rays whilst others use rare earth filters for selective absorption. The detector technology also differs, but in practice the final result is similar. However, the BMD measured by different instruments (for instance Hologic versus Lunar) may differ between 10 and 15% (Wahner and Fogelman, 1994). Modern systems now allow the estimation of bone density in almost any bone including the peripheral skeleton.

Despite the sophistication of modern DXA technology, it is worth emphasising that it still provides a two- rather than three-dimensional measurement which is a particular disadvantage in the case of serial measurements in growing children.

Indications for bone density measurements

The main purpose of bone density measurement is to predict the likelihood of fractures (Peel and Eastell, 1993; Eastell and Peel, 1994; Compston *et al.,* 1995). Recognised indications for bone densitometry include:

1. Oestrogen deficiency, especially where bone density measurement may affect the decision of a menopausal woman to take hormone replacement therapy.
2. Radiographic osteopenia or vertebral deformity where there is doubt about the bone density. Certain radiographic appearances (apart from fracture) may suggest that bone density is low (osteopenia); these include prominence of vertical trabeculae in the vertebral bodies. However, the radiographic diagnosis of osteopenia is often very misleading.
3. Clinical situations where there is recognised to be excessive bone loss, for instance long-term glucocorticoid therapy or primary hyperparathyroidism. In patients on corticosteroid therapy, a low BMD may give some guidance about treatment and reduction of steroid dosage (which is always essential). In primary hyperparathyroidism, some regard a low bone density as a relevant indication for surgery although not necessarily a strong one.
4. Research. These include monitoring therapy for osteoporosis, the identification of fast bone losers and the investigation of rare bone diseases.

In practice bone density measurement is probably most commonly used in patients with oestrogen deficiency. In addition to the assessment of BMD in post-menopausal women, this includes younger females with amenorrhoea, for instance due to anorexia nervosa or excessive exercise. Also, bone densitometry is quite widely used in assessing the effectiveness of treatment of osteoporosis. Since the annual changes in BMD are rarely more than 1 or 2% there is little point in repeating this measurement more frequently than once a year. A continuing frequent indication is the elucidation of radiologically reported osteopenia.

Interpretation of DXA results

One of the major difficulties in the use of DXA is the interpretation of the results and their relation to osteoporosis and fracture (Ross, 1993; Kanis *et al.,* 1994). Each commercial supplier of clinical instruments has solved the technical problems in a slightly different way and has also expressed the results of the analysis differently. The problems of expressing the bone mineral result in a readily understandable fashion are multiple. One general problem which is not yet overcome is in correcting the measured result for bone size. The derived unit of bone density is not in fact a true bone density, since it relates the absorption to the area which is being scanned and not to its actual volume. The results are therefore given in terms of gcm^{-2} (apart from bone density measured by QCT for which a true volumetric measurement can be made). Results for individuals are compared either with age-matched controls or with young adults using a reference range defined as the mean bone mineral bone density plus or minus two standard deviations, which is equivalent to the 95% confidence limits. Comparisons of the value observed can be made as a percentage of the mean or as the number of standard deviation units above or below the expected results. These are not necessarily comparable (Figure 16.2). The problem of how to describe BMD results and how to interpret them, requires thought. It may be that the absolute BMD (gcm^{-2}) is the most useful measurement in determining current fracture risk but, since it is difficult to explain the relevance of such figures to a patient, it is easier to understand the result in relation to a normal age and sex matched population. Again, since most patients will be used to the idea of percentages it is easier to use this as a basis for comparison with normal. The standard deviation of the BMD is approximately constant across life but alters according to the measurement site (Figure 16.2). This means that for an individual with a measurement at the lower end of the reference range at each site the BMD expressed as percentage of normal (per cent expected) varies with the site. However, because the mean BMD and reference range falls with age the decrease in the denominator with ageing results in a wider range of percentage values representing the normal range (examples are given by Peel and Eastell, 1993). Because of these difficulties in using percentage values, standard deviations have been widely adopted. They are expressed as a Z score when compared to age-matched mean and a T score when compared to peak adult mean. The normal age-matched range is therefore limited by $\pm$ 2 SD (Z score from −2 to +2) and is equivalent to the 95% confidence limits. The upper limit lies on the 97.5th percentile and the lower on the 2.5th percentile. Percentiles are familiar to those who use them, for instance, in studies of growth (see Chapter 11) but they are not included in the printout of current DXA instruments. In practice, the printout obtained (Figure 16.3) gives either percentages or Z scores, i.e. standard deviations above and below the mean for an age-matched normal group and T scores which are the standard deviations above and below the peak young adult mean. Since the main current use of DXA machines is to measure the bone density to give an indication of the likelihood of fracture the remainder of this account will be concerned with osteoporosis.

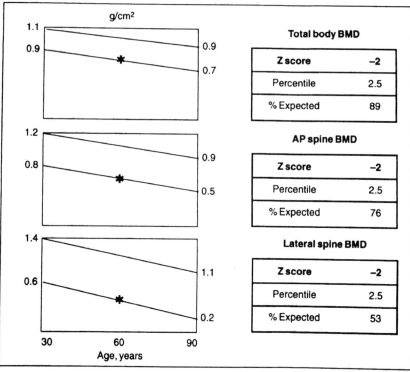

Figure 16.2 In this example, the standard deviation of BMD is constant throughout life but the width differs with the site measured, being narrowest for the total body (upper panel) and widest for the lateral lumbar spine (lower panel). The asterisk shows the result for a 60-year-old woman with a density at the lowest end of the reference range (i.e. −2.0 SD) at all three measurement sites. The age-matched Z score and the percentile are the same at all sites. The result expressed as percentage of the amount expected for age differs from one site to another (From Eastell and Peel, 1994 with permission)

Diagnosis of osteoporosis

Over the years many definitions of osteoporosis have been offered. A recent conference defined osteoporosis as a disease characterised by low bone mass and microarchitectural deterioration of bone tissue, leading to enhanced bone fragility and a consequent increase in fracture risk (Consensus Development Conference, 1991). For many this definition is too amorphous. The clinical significance of osteoporosis lies in its contribution to fractures. Many prospective studies now indicate that the risk of fragility fractures increases progressively and continuously as bone mineral density declines. Indeed fracture risk increases by about 1.5–3 fold or more for each standard deviation decrease in bone mineral density (Cummings and Black, 1995). Bone mineral mass can be utilised not only as a prognostic tool to predict fractures but also as a test for the presence of osteoporosis. The most recent definition of osteoporosis and osteopenia is as follows (Kanis *et al.,* 1994):

1. Normal. A value for bone mineral density or bone mineral content that is not more than 1 standard deviation below (or above) the young adult mean value.

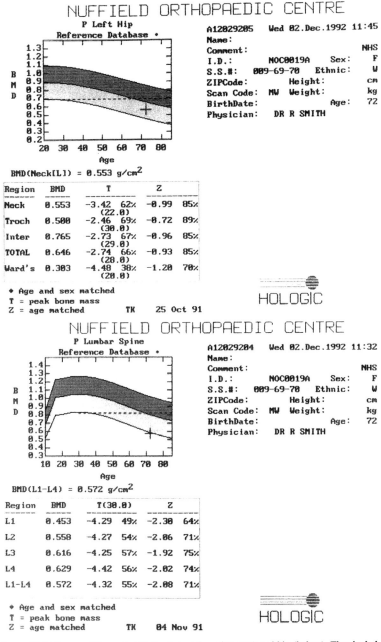

NUFFIELD ORTHOPAEDIC CENTRE

P Left Hip
Reference Database •

A12029205   Wed 02.Dec.1992 11:45
Name:
Comment: NHS
I.D.:   NOC0019A   Sex: F
S.S.#:   009-69-70   Ethnic: W
ZIPCode: Height: cm
Scan Code: MW Weight: kg
BirthDate: Age: 72
Physician: DR R SMITH

BMD(Neck[L]) = 0.553 g/cm²

Region	BMD	T		Z	
Neck	0.553	-3.42	62%	-0.99	85%
		(22.0)			
Troch	0.500	-2.46	69%	-0.72	89%
		(30.0)			
Inter	0.765	-2.73	67%	-0.96	85%
		(29.0)			
TOTAL	0.646	-2.74	66%	-0.93	85%
		(28.0)			
Ward's	0.303	-4.48	38%	-1.20	70%
		(20.0)			

♦ Age and sex matched
T = peak bone mass
Z = age matched   TK   25 Oct 91

HOLOGIC

NUFFIELD ORTHOPAEDIC CENTRE

P Lumbar Spine
Reference Database •

A12029204   Wed 02.Dec.1992 11:32
Name:
Comment: NHS
I.D.:   NOC0019A   Sex: F
S.S.#:   009-69-70   Ethnic: W
ZIPCode: Height: cm
Scan Code: MW Weight: kg
BirthDate: Age: 72
Physician: DR R SMITH

BMD(L1-L4) = 0.572 g/cm²

Region	BMD	T(30.0)		Z	
L1	0.453	-4.29	49%	-2.30	64%
L2	0.558	-4.27	54%	-2.06	71%
L3	0.616	-4.25	57%	-1.92	75%
L4	0.629	-4.42	56%	-2.02	74%
L1-L4	0.572	-4.32	55%	-2.08	71%

♦ Age and sex matched
T = peak bone mass
Z = age matched   TK   04 Nov 91

HOLOGIC

Figure 16.3 The usual form of a DXA printout for spine (top) and hip (below). The shaded area outlines the 95% confidence limit at different ages. BMD is given in absolute values, gcm⁻², and is related to the peak bone mass (T) and to the age-matched population (Z). The results are expressed as SD's below (or above) the relevant mean and as per cent of the mean. The dotted line is 2 SD below the peak mean and may be regarded as the theoretical fracture threshold (however see text). In this example from a 72-year-old woman the bone density (marked with a cross) is reduced particularly in the lumbar spine where it is 2.08 SD below the age-matched mean

2. Osteopenia (a low bone mass). A value for bone mineral density or bone mineral content, that lies between 1–2.5 standard deviations below the young adult mean value. Such individuals include those in whom prevention of bone loss would be most useful.
3. Osteoporosis. A value for bone mineral density or bone mineral content that is more than 2.5 standard deviations below the young adult mean.
4. Severe osteoporosis or established osteoporosis. A value for bone mineral density or bone mineral content more than 2.5 standard deviations below the young adult mean in the presence of one or more fragility fractures.

There are important limitations to the approach of using bone mineral density in osteoporosis irrespective of its variable contribution to fracture. The prevalence of osteoporosis with age is approximately exponential after the age of 50 (Figure 16.4) because the distribution of values for bone mineral density in the young healthy population is Gaussian. This exponential prevalence also occurs in many osteoporosis-related fractures. Since values for bone mineral density and fracture are continuously distributed in the population, there is no absolute

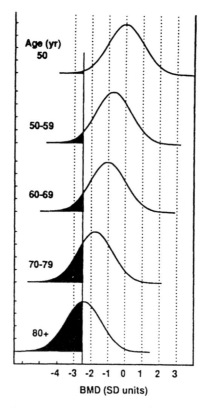

Figure 16.4 The relationship between BMD in women at different ages and the prevalence of osteoporosis. BMD is normally distributed at all ages but decreases progressively with age. The proportion of patients with osteoporosis defined as –2.5 SD or less than the young adult mean, increases exponentially with age. There is a corresponding exponential increase in the frequency of most fractures with age (from Kanis *et al.*, 1994 with permission)

Table 16.2 Examples of the distinction between risk factors and clinical outcome in different diseases

Risk factor	Associated disease	Clinical outcome
High cholesterol	Atheroma	Myocardial infarction
High blood pressure	Hypertension	Stroke
Low BMD	Osteoporosis	Fracture
High uric acid	Gout	Arthritis

criterion in the absence of fracture that can delineate an individual with disease from one without. In this sense several other diseases provide appropriate analogies, for instance hypertension or stroke (Table 16.2). The criteria for the definition of osteoporosis and osteopenia should be applied to men and to young individuals before skeletal maturity but there are insufficient data to establish them. Standards for women could be applied to men but the risk of fracture in men is substantially lower for bone mineral measurements within their own reference range. A criterion of –3–4 SD may therefore be more appropriate for the diagnosis of osteoporosis in men.

A number of factors impair the diagnostic accuracy of absorptiometric methods, particularly in the spine. Amongst these are the increasing frequency of extra-skeletal calcification – especially in the aorta – in the elderly, acquired and inherited deformity of the spine, additional new bone formation such as osteophytes around degenerative intervertebral discs, zygapophyseal joint arthritis and factors which affect mineralisation of bone itself such as osteomalacia. Other factors (apart from falls) which confuse the relationship between bone mineral density and fracture risk include the use of a two-dimensional density (discussed previously) and the inability to measure all the determinants of skeletal fragility. Most studies now suggest that there is significant correlation between bone mineral measurements made at one site compared with another (Melton *et al.,* 1993) and that the diagnostic criteria for osteoporosis are likely to change as experience increases, in much the same way as the cut-off value for hypertension has changed over the past 25 years. Nevertheless, it is important to have diagnostic guidelines to act as a frame for further investigation towards greater accuracy than hitherto possible in describing the extent and characteristics of the disease.

Osteoporosis and fracture

Not all patients with osteoporosis have fractures. The possession of a skeleton with a normal bone density does not make it immune from structural failure. It is obvious that under any circumstances a fracture will result when the forces through a bone are greater than its strength; also many fractures, especially in elderly people, are related more to falls than to reduced bone density. Nevertheless, it has turned out that bone density measured at any site is a good indicator of individual likelihood of future fracture and is certainly the best available predictor of such an event (Melton *et al.,* 1993; Cummings and Black, 1995). Certainly the analysis of so-called life-style factors, such as smoking, immobility, alcohol intake to predict osteopenia has turned out to have low

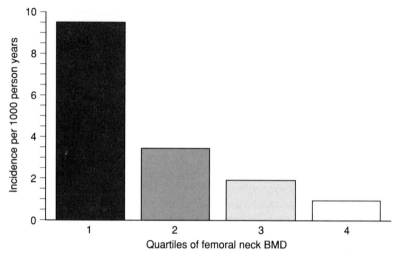

Figure 16.5 One example of the relationship between hip fracture and BMD. The incidence of hip fracture per 1000 person years doubles for each quartile decrease in bone density. Quartile 1 represents < 25th percentile (Z score, age-matched < −0.65) and quartile 4 represents > 75th percentile (Z score, age-matched > 0.65). The fracture rate in quartile 1 was 8 times higher than that in quartile 4 (from Eastell and Peel, 1994 with permission)

sensitivity. Several tables and formulae have been devised on the basis of current bone mass data to predict future fracture, and these are discussed in more detail by Ross (1993). Figure 16.5 shows that for fracture of the hip there is an almost exponential inverse relationship between bone density and fracture risk so that those in the lowest quartile have a risk eight times that of those in the highest quartile for bone density. One important implication of this finding is that for a person with a normal BMD, small changes will have little effect on fracture risk, whereas in the osteopenic individual a small change in BMD results in a large change in fracture risk. Another implication is that although most drugs currently available can cause or prevent relatively small changes in bone mass, it is nevertheless important to be able to measure them.

Optimum site for BMD measurement

Despite the dominance of DXA and consequent emphasis on the hip and spine for bone density measurement there are reasons such as expense, accessibility and reproducibility which mean that other sites (and methods) still require consideration. Since osteoporotic fractures typically occur in bones that are composed of a high proportion of trabecular bone such as the vertebral body, proximal femur and distal radius, these are the sites commonly chosen for measurement of BMD. Although BMD measurements are site specific in the sense that, for instance, BMD of the femoral neck predicts the risk of hip fracture better than BMD of the spine (Cummings *et al.*, 1993), in the majority of situations measurement of one site gives a reasonable indication of overall fracture risk (Melton *et al.*, 1993). The usefulness of spinal BMD in the elderly population is limited by inaccuracies arising from artefacts such as osteophyte formation, previously referred to. The recent introduction of lateral scans should remove most of these artefacts, but the precision of lateral measurements has yet to be established.

Recent technological advances

Current DXA gives an accurate measurement of bone present with no information on its structure. However, DXA technology continues to develop and new scanning modes have been introduced that supplement the standard spine and femur measurements. New applications include body composition measurement and the measurement of bone density in paediatrics. Fan beam scanning makes it possible to obtain an adequate spinal measurement very rapidly and the coupling of AP and lateral scans with a rotating scanning arm is a useful step towards estimation of true volumetric bone density. In addition, the further development of DXA will help to evaluate vertebral morphometry. All these aspects are discussed by Wahner and Fogelman (1994).

Current problems

The current problems which remain are the accurate measurement of volumetric density and the prediction of fracture. The likelihood of fractures may be approximately predicted by a DXA measurement at one specific time and more information on the rate of loss can be obtained by serial measurements. The rate of bone loss may be indicated by serial biochemical measurements, particularly those related to the excretion of cross-linked collagen-derived peptides, an indicator of bone resorption (Peel and Eastell, 1993). An increasing incidence of falls in elderly people means that fractures in the elderly are increasingly related to trauma rather than to osteoporosis. This increase is related to declining muscle strength (particularly quadriceps) and reduced sensory input (Evans, 1988).

References

Baran DT, McCarthy CK, Leahy D, Lew R (1941) Broadband ultrasound attenuation of the calcaneus predicts lumbar and femoral neck density in Caucasian women: a preliminary study. *Osteoporosis International*; **1**: 110–113

Chatterton BE (1993) Bone densitometry. In: Nordin BEC, Need AG, Morris HA (eds) Metabolic Bone and Stone Disease, 3rd edition. Edinburgh: Churchill Livingstone, pp. 360–364

Compston JE, Cooper C, Kanis JA (1995) Bone densitometry in clinical practice. *B.M.J.*; **310**: 1507–1510

Consensus Development Conference (1991) Prophylaxis and treatment of osteoporosis. *Am. J. Med.*; **90**: 107–110

Cummings SR, Black D (1995) Bone mass measurements and risk of fracture in Caucasian women: a review of findings from prospective studies. *Am. J. Med.*; **98** (supplement 2A): 245–285

Eastell R, Peel NFA (1994) Interpretation of bone density results. *Osteoporosis Review*; **2**: 1–3

Evans JG (1988) Falls and fractures. *Age Ageing*; **17**: 361–364

Hassager C, Christiansen C (1995) Measurement of bone mineral density. *Calcified Tissue International*; **57**: 1–5

Kanis JA, Melton LJ, Christiansen C, Johnston CC, Khaltaev N (1994) The diagnosis of osteoporosis. *J. Bone Min. Res.*; **9**: 1137–1141

Meema HE, Meema S (1972) Comparison of the micro-radiographic and morphometric findings in the hand bones with densitometric findings in the proximal radius in thyrotoxicosis and in renal osteodystrophy. *Invest. Radiol.*; **7**: 88–96

Melton LT, Atkinson EJ, O'Fallon WM, Wahner HW, Riggs BL (1993). Long term fracture prediction by bone mineral assessed at different skeletal sites. *J. Bone Min. Res.*; **8**: 1227–1233

Peel N, Eastell R (1993) Measurement of bone mass and turnover. *Bailliere's Clin. Rheumatol.*; **7**: 479–498

Ross PD (1993) Interpretation of densitometry. In: Nordin BEC, Need AG, Morris HA (eds) *Metabolic Bone and Stone Disease*, 3rd edition. Edinburgh: Churchill Livingstone, pp. 364–372

Singh M, Nagrath AR, Maini PS (1970) Changes in trabecular pattern of the upper end of the femur as an index of osteoporosis. *J. Bone Jt Surg.*; **52A**: 457–467

Wahner HW, Fogelman I (1994) *The Evaluation of Osteoporosis: Dual Energy X-Ray Absorptiometry in Clinical Practice*, 1st edition. London: Martin Dunitz

Young H, Howey S, Purdie DW (1993) Broadband ultrasound attenuation compared with dual energy X-ray absorptiometry in screening for post-menopausal low bone density. *Osteoporosis International*; **3**: 160–164

Index